SASS

A Novel

William Stuart Gould, M.D.

WMG LTD.

New York

WMG

WMG Ltd. Publishers
288 Lexington Avenue
Suite 6-F
New York, New York

Wmg.ltd.publishing@gmail.com

This book is a work of fiction. Names, characters, places, and incidents are either products of the author's imagination or are used fictitiously. Any resemblance to actual events, locales, or persons, living or dead, is entirely coincidental

ISBN: 978-0-9979804-6-2 (pbk)
ISBN: 978-0-9979804-7-9 (e-book)

ALSO BY BILL GOULD

At Yonah Mountain

Captain Iron Mustache

In Black Granite

C.O.L.A.

A Heart Wind from the Desert

Raphael's Blanket

Lincoln Friday

Sabrina's Suit

Marlene

Again and Forever

SASS

Reuben and Miriam Sassovitch emigrate from Romania to the promised land of the Bronx in the late 1970s. Crafting a new name and hearts brimming with hope, they enroll their only child, Elliott, in public school. Though a virtuoso in chemistry lab, his gifts do not extend to the classrooms, hallways, or streets.

His neuroses only deepen with time, nearly costing him his life in New York's drug underworld. Worse, though, it poisons his bond with a blemished, but magical woman he pursues across the world.

For Elliott, life is one sharp-toothed puncture wound after another, until a flicker of light transforms him. It is a coming-of-age tale, but one that crawls at a snail's pace. It is also the saga of a love not destined to be that succeeds.

PART ONE

CHAPTER ONE

Dean of Men/Vice-Principal Arthur Julian's office was decorated in a fashion that reflected both his temperament and sense of humor—the walls, once institutional green, were long faded to dusty grey, and they were bare. His workplace hadn't started out that way; bachelor's and master's degrees once hung beside pictures of Julian in goalie pads from the championship years back at Columbia. But over the decades the Dean of Men at Bronx's Isadore Goldstein High School of Science and Math had had his diplomas stolen, and every manner of Magic Marker desecration engraved on the evidence of his athletic career.

Much of the harmony in his life had been snuffed since pupils no longer needed grades and an invitation to join the student body. With the doors thrown open to the masses, there was little math or science taking place, unless one considered the subject of anatomy: boys groping girls, girls groping boys, and stairwells littered with the stripped bones of The Big Ugly Bear's Famous Fried Chicken.

In his first years, it had been the eighty-twenty rule in terms of discipline; four out of five kids were okay, and though all teens are mouthy, these were bright youngsters, and the majority greeted him in the halls with a wave, not an extended middle finger. Failing a test was rare, and a call to parents begot the wrath of God.

Now, quantitatively, it was still eighty-twenty, but, qualitatively, all had been turned on its head, less than twenty percent testing into pre-college courses. It had become a vicious cycle. Much of the faculty had fled, replaced by para-educators and teachers who pinched their noses in order to survive the two or three years left before their earliest retirement date.

The new eighty percent had felled Arthur. And this Monday morning presaged yet another awful winter week. Sitting across from him, yet again, was Elliott Sass. What surprised Julian was that Frequent Flier Sass had been one of the rare kids *recruited* to Isadore Goldstein from Jerome Junior High in the upper Bronx. The boy was famous for having flown through his math and chemistry courses in middle school, his final standardized test grades amongst the highest in the State of New York. He was, though, also infamous for mixing chemical substances behind his teachers' backs, rendering scented composites that reflected his mood. If a teacher or bully had glanced at him a trace sideways, Elliott's chem lab creation that afternoon was redolent of the public toilets on East 196th Street. If, rarely, his day was going well, that is, without a beating from the teen gangs that roamed the halls, mists suggestive of the Perfumatic on the cosmetics counter at Sachs Fifth Avenue drifted through the building. Sadly, as Elliott progressed through Jerome Junior, the former became the preponderance of his chemical offerings.

While his junior high teachers had touted his extraordinary skills on the Goldstein admission application, they had also quietly alerted the high school that Master Sass saw the world in hues somewhat darker than those of his contemporaries. And they peddled his ability to confabulate as simply another of the bequests endowed by the Creator. One teacher conned, "As with all gifted students, it requires a truly professional educator to guide these special children through the travails of our broken educational system."

Actually, all of his recommendations were driven by a single craving: Jerome Junior High shared a campus with Jerome Senior High, as well as many of the same facilities. The entire K-12 teaching staff found themselves interchangeable when subs were needed. Eventually, every teacher had had the opportunity to nurse Elliott in class. The consensus was that affording the boy a fresh start at a far-flung high school was a solid educational objective.

In mid-junior year at Isadore Goldstein High School of Science and Math, Elliott had found himself, once again a focus of attention, this time for peddling marijuana in the hallway before school. By itself, the few grains of pot that would have barely provided enough for two puffs of a joint were not grounds for a call to the local police precinct, or even a trip to Dean of Men Julian's office. Had even an ounce or two of dope been the standard for arrest at Isadore Goldstein, the doors would have been shuttered a decade before.

But Elliott's offenses were never isolated to a single infraction. There was always an extra bit of icing on his behavioral cake. This time, he stepped over the line by offering some of his better stash, the stuff from the left jeans pocket, to buy the silence of the teacher who'd caught him. That might have worked had the young businessman not made the frantic offer within earshot of the student to whom he'd just sold fibers of ground up stems. He had charged the kid a premium, explaining conspiratorially that he kept the good stuff in his right jeans pocket. Since this delinquent wasn't one of the gifted scientists promoted by the faculty of a top-notch junior high, he had believed Elliott's drivel about his purchase being a new strain from Panama, rough cut to satisfy real men.

The kid didn't even wait until the teacher walked away. He sprang back and belted Elliott in the side of the head. The teacher had little choice and brought the two to the Dean of Men's office. They sat outside trading spit and profane threats until Mr. Julian popped through the door and physically thrust them into the hallway. Crowds of milling students broke into gales of laughter as if patrons at a bar witnessing a pair of drunks being bounced into the cold street.

This was the fifth visit Elliott had made to administration during the fall quarter. On the fourth, a week earlier, Dean Julian called the boy's home. He learned from Elliott's earsplitting father that Elliott was a child of the Holocaust and had been through hell in Eastern Europe, beaten in the streets by Nazis and anti-Semitic communist teachers.

Papa Sass warned in fractured English that if there was to be trouble from the weak, stupid American teachers, he'd be down there with an AK-47 to straighten them out. At least that was what Dean of Men Arthur Julian thought he had heard through the foaming, Russian-sounding accent. When he asked Mr. Sass to repeat himself, the latter screamed, "I blow up school. You, too!" The next sound was a crash as loud as a pistol firing, but it was only Sass slamming the phone down.

Julian dug deeper. He called the cousin listed on Elliott's registration card as the backup emergency contact. In fact, Elliott had, indeed, been born in Romania, though it was his parents who were children of refugees of the Second World War. Actually, he had been raised by both parents in a middle-class flat in Bucharest, their expenses covered by Elliott's maternal grandfather, a doctor. Elliott's mother, Miriam, was a painfully shy, submissive woman, and his father, according to the unhappy cousin, was, "…a momzer, zat vun. You know vhat is a momzer? A no-good bastard, zhat's vhat."

Before Dean Julian could take a breath, the cousin went on. What the dean could gather was that Elliott's father had come to him in Bucharest and told him he had a dream about going to America. Apparently, the cousin's uncle had migrated to Philadelphia and long before sent back a booklet that described how to transition to American life. Elliott's father asked to see it, and while the cousin was making tea, Mr. Sass slipped the pamphlet into his crotch. At home, he read the suggestion that immigrants shorten their Eastern European names before reaching that sacred square of paradise, Ellis Island. It was the only way to circumvent the well-meaning clerks at the immigration center on the Island who were known to shorten Jewish surnames into foolish-sounding, impossible-to-pronounce, Gentile last names like Smith and Johnson.

Reuben Sassowitch tried various combinations. Sas, his first, was only three letters, far too short to elicit respect in any culture. But Sass, that had the ring of an authentic American name. Even better, according to his cousin's English-Romanian dictionary, one that had also slipped into Reuben's shorts, sass was defined as lively, bold, full of spirit, even cheeky. He looked these words up and was impressed to find that cheeky meant forward in an endearing way. Forward, he mused. "Yes, I will push forward." Of course, this was an abridged edition, and while there was a brief mention of impertinence and impudence, those words were far too difficult to look up.

CHAPTER TWO

Three months later, Papa Sass was shocked to find that Ellis Island was no longer a reception station for European refugees. He wondered if the suggestion to shorten his name had also been superceded, but there was no time to reconsider, for his family was being herded, practically at the double time, through a set of beaten offices in lower Manhattan. In less than two hours, it was all done.

They settled into a rent-controlled Bronx apartment on the corner of Jerome and Morris Avenues. Reuben took a job as a janitor at P.S. 86. A swarthy man, many people back home in Eastern Europe believed him to be Romany. At the school, the staff tried to decide if he was Puerto Rican or Mexican. On the other hand, his English *and* Spanish were so poor, and his mien so very sour, he was left to his own devices, treated more a leper than fellow traveler. It was a status, though, with which he was quite content, for it allowed even more time alone to pilfer the school supply room.

At first, it was just school paper, pencils, and vinegar for cleaning windows, all of which he was able to carry home in his lunch pail. But society was changing at warp speed, and more and more undocumented students were being jammed into classrooms. By the end of the school year, the census jumped from one thousand staff and pupils to two thousand. With the upsurge in bodies came an explosion in the largess over which he was master. Now there were ballpoint pens, typewriter ribbons, three-ring binders, toilet paper, paper towels, bags of detergent, and expensive florescent lightbulbs.

He offered the spirited goods at great discount, but only to neighbors a few doors to the left and right of the Sass apartment. With gained confidence, though, he expanded to the whole floor. As word spread, demand exploded. He added a floor a month. The day Elliott turned ten, Papa Sass began to advertise on the bulletin board next to the mailboxes by the main entrance, soon offering a door-to-door delivery service option for a small fee. Elliott was to be the instrument of distribution, promised fifty percent of the tips he could wrangle.

As the acorn seldom lands far from the tree, Elliott failed to report his full tip income, and with the extra few percent squirreled away, he bit his lip and let the corpus grow untouched over several years. With the fifty bucks he'd hidden under a loose floorboard in his bedroom, he invested in Transformers—foldable toy robots, good ones—which he leased to fellow students by the night or weekend. The most popular was Optimus Prime, brave leader of the Autobots. When the soldiers began to show signs of wear, for which the renters were held responsible—scratches a dime, chips a quarter—he used his mother's nail polish for touchups, then sold them as gently used. The purchasers of recycled stock, though, had to sign a no-competition clause which Elliott enforced with hired 9th grade muscle.

In 10th grade, he plunked his profits into selling pirated rock and roll cassettes, even some of the teachers patronizing his venture. By junior year, he moved on to pot sales, and in the summer between junior and senior years, he discovered Ecstasy. That endeavor, however, elevated him into circles that dealt far more vicious retribution than a single whack in the head from a weed sale gone awry. He retired from that venture after six days.

By the end of September, Elliott's mother was beside herself with the number of calls she was getting from Dean Julian, to say nothing of the black eyes and fat lips her son tried to hide as he ran to his room after school. She finally made him join Chemistry Club, and though he fought like a caged rat over being forced to spend one extra minute in school, he soon came up with a plan. He would behave for a few weeks, brewing only what the Chem Club's teacher assigned, then slowly move his experiments toward the rear corner, closer to the exhaust fan, where he would set up a still, boil down cheap wine, and sell the distillate to the alcoholic kids. With a month of good conduct under his belt, he approached the lab teacher submissively and proposed a deal allowing him to work on his own, *if* he promised, and signed a written contract, not to stink the place up with various iterations of his favorite, obscene, sulfur-laced mercaptans.

With his signature barely dry on the contract, chemicals and beakers flew from the shelves, Bunsen burners ignited, and in fifteen minutes, vapors of one of his teacher's favorite aromatic organic compounds filled that wing of the high school. In another beaker, he shifted his fortified wine production into high gear, impossible to detect the odor of ethanol under the cloying sweet scent of his fruity ester. On the mornings after Chem Club, the whole building was so agreeably scented, Dean Julian sought him out for a hesitant pat on the shoulder.

And that's all he did for the first few weeks, enhance the general atmosphere of the entire structure, collecting kudos from teachers and smiles from the girls, especially Buzzy Hawkins, a carrot-top, about whom he'd spent many an hour in bed fantasizing. There was even an up-curling of the lip from the one-eyed custodian, Mr. Sabotucci. With each week, he added another carbon molecule to his brew, graduating from simple, banana-scented, 2-carbon blends to graduate-level, 7-carbon creations. These chemical doings were far beyond the ken of the teacher, a permanent sub with a BS in phys ed. As the processes became more complex, the man spent less and less time poking his nose over Elliott's shoulder. In fact, the teacher soon devoted the bulk of Chemistry Club to activities in the private office/storeroom at the back of the lab. Eventually, Elliott would not see him all period.

In January that year, Elliott left the lab after dark, a full bottle of 180 proof spirits tucked into his backpack. At the entrance to the subway, a man approached him aggressively and seized his arm. Elliott tried to pull away, but the grip tightened. "Look, muther fukah, do as you're told or I'll fuckin' break your fuckin' nose. You hear what I'm sayin'?"

Elliott nodded shakily. "Okay, okay, whata you want?"

"Need a little help with a science project, brain boy. Lookin' for a dude, kinda guy who can keep a secret, if you know what I mean. Mix up some chemicals for me. My people at your school be sayin' you be da man for da job." Elliott's tremor deepened, which served to tighten the man's grip. "Look, asshole, you gonna do dis shit 'causin Reuben's health be dependin' on it. Dat make any sense to you?"

"What's my father got to do with this?"

"No questions. Dey tell me you smart. Use your mutha fuckin' imagination." The man gave him a small push. "This how it gonna play out. I gonna get you stuff to cook. Give you da recipe and how to get da finished product back to my associate. If you don't fuck up, you get, shall we say, a consideration."

Elliott whimpered, "I don't know what you mean."

"You don't need to know a gotdamn thing, 'ceptin' how to brew my shit. And no questions. That be da first rule, mutha fuckah. I told you what you gonna do, and we start next week. We be in touch." With that, the man squeezed Elliott's arm until it hurt and gave him an even harsher shove, almost sending him tripping down the subway entrance.

At home, Elliott wanted to tell his mother, to ask her for help, but as he walked into the bare apartment, she was, as always, in her tattered recliner next to the living room window staring down into the courtyard. To Elliott, it seemed she was indignantly appraising the piles of stinking garbage tossed uncaringly from kitchen windows by her uncouth, immigrant neighbors. Elliott was far too young to grasp that what Miriam saw was only wasted years of dreadful loneliness, the pointlessness of her sojourn so far away from home. It was the third time that week she was so mired in gloom, she did not turn to greet her son. He stood silently for a moment, finally calling to her, "Mama, is Tata okay?"

She turned to him slowly. "I don't know," then turned away again.

He went to his room and sat on the bed, shaking, too scared to cry. He thought about his father. Reuben Sass no longer lived at home. He had recently left to take up residence in a men's dorm at Sing Sing to do a nickel for dozens and dozens of counts of felony theft of New York State Department of Public Education property.

In the past, though Reuben had knocked the boy around the apartment a few times, when Elliott ran into trouble on the outside, his old man had always been right there to watch over him with a thick arm and a clenched fist, all the while spitting a creole of Romanian/English profanity. But other than his father, there had not been a single soul who had ever risen to shelter him, even, especially, his mother, her warmth so completely suffocated by the sad narrative of her yesterdays.

He sat quietly for a while, smoked a joint, took two shots of cheap rye, and spent the night tossing, weighing fantastic, violent schemes to escape his new business associate.

CHAPTER THREE

The next Wednesday, as Elliott got off the subway for school, a rail-thin man with long, stringy, greying hair bumped into him—hard. Elliott turned around, fists clenched and raised, but the man jammed a plastic Safeway bag in his face. "Do not look at me. Turn around and get your fuckin' ass to school."

At lunch, Elliott opened the bag. On a crumpled sheet of dirty paper were xeroxed instructions describing the production of a compound he was to fashion from the ingredients in the bag. He looked left and right cautiously then pulled free a box—pseudoephedrine pills. That ended the mystery of what he would now be spending Chemistry Club cooking.

The afternoon passed with Elliott hiding, contemplating the chemical smoke screen he'd need to cloak the cat-urine stink of what he was being forced to concoct. A decision was made minutes before Chemistry Club. He would brew his tour de force, a potent, wintergreen-scented ester. With the lab in a minty haze, he'd shuttle to a worktable even further into the depths of the lab to cook his felonious broth.

With the teacher occupied in the storeroom, disguising his product did not become an issue. When it dried to crystals, he snorted one granule. Though pleasant for a moment, the sensation scared him, and he scraped the residue into the bottle his handlers had placed at the bottom of the shopping bag.

After Chemistry Club, he left school in the dark, making his way, per instructions on another note in the bag, to the Foursquare Subway shop on 3rd Avenue. He was to order an Italian sub without peppers. Before Elliott could ask that the sandwich to be toasted, the teenage hoodlum behind the counter thrust the key to the bathroom in his face, sneered, and jerked his head toward the restroom. Elliott placed the package in the toilet tank as directed. When he came back out, he handed the cashier a five and got two twenties in change. Though he stood waiting, no sandwich was proffered, and the punk snapped, "Get the fuck outta here."

The procedure went without change for weeks, until there were no more boxes of pseudoephedrine in the Safeway bag. Instead, there was a directive to start buying pseudoephedrine on his own, spreading his purchases over several drugstores in the vicinity of his high school. He was not to speak a word to any of the clerks. Tuesdays after school turned into shopping sprees, and it all became fairly rote, even boring. When he turned his product over at the Subway, the sullen clerk suddenly began handing him an Italian sub, without peppers, and slipped him his five back as well as three twenties.

In late April, Elliott set out to reup his supply of pseudoephedrine, stopping first, as was his routine, at the Rite Aid on East 138th. He wasn't sure, but he thought a scruffy man, perhaps homeless, had followed him for a while after he left the drugstore. A few blocks later, as he was about to enter the CVS, he spotted the man again. Elliott dawdled in the pharmacy, pretending to be comparing bottles of mouthwash. When he left, it appeared the man was gone. Nonetheless, Elliott ducked into a doorway on East 147th, waited less than two minutes, and peeked out. There was the man, half a block behind, standing in the middle of the sidewalk talking on a cell phone. Seconds later, a featureless Chevy sedan pulled up and the mendicant bent forward to speak to the front seat passenger. Elliott jammed the bag of pills into his backpack, placed it in front of his chest, turned his coat inside out, took off his hat, and slipped into a gaggle of pedestrians. That afternoon, he skipped the Feel Good and Third Avenue Pharmacies.

Making do with but half the usual pseudoephedrine, he left a note in the bag at the Subway shop warning that he was being followed. At school the next morning, two New York City Police black and whites were double-parked, blocking the front doors. Elliott stopped abruptly across the street, hid behind a panel truck, and watched as the cops stood with Dean Julian scrutinizing each of the arriving male students. Slowly, he extracted himself and walked back toward his subway station. Cops were there as well, so he made his way west to the Grand Concourse, then north back home, walking the six miles.

He did not go to school the next morning, spending the hours watching TV with one eye and the building entrance three floors below with the other. The next morning, he was out of the house at dawn on the Bee Line Transit bus to Ossining, then on foot the half-block to Sing Sing. He walked in a daze past the unshaven correctional officer guarding the main gate until the man yelled at him. "Where *you* goin'?"

Elliott stopped but did not answer, standing motionless, gawking until the guard crooked his finger. Elliott took a few steps toward the cinder-block security bunker and stood rigidly.

The man barked, "State your business." The bit of color left in Elliott's face drained, and he turned, taking a step to walk back out the main gate. The man, though, softened his tone and called, "You here to see someone?"

"Yeah. I want to see my father."

"You can't just go walkin' in and out of the facility. You gotta make up your mind. You walk past that white line," he motioned toward a brightly painted, foot-wide stripe where the cement apron of the prison met the macadam of the City of Ossining, "and the rules change. What's it gonna be?"

"I want to see my father."

"Okay, now that we have that straightened out, you walk directly to that building." He pointed at a concrete structure over which a sign read, "Visitation Center."

As he turned back toward the mammoth complex, his head drooped. A step closer, his shoulders sagged even lower. At the entrance, he turned back toward the guard. The man was standing essentially at parade rest, hand on his baton, staring coldly at Elliott. He took a step into the administration building, nearly gagging on the institutional pong. It culled memories of his father dragging him along to Bellevue Hospital in Manhattan where his mother had been incarcerated after her second nervous breakdown.

That was the episode when she tried to throw herself from the window of their Bronx apartment.

Pine Sol, feces, and body odor, in that order, were the scents that drew him back to the hospital. But what sealed the deal was that, even where he stood, at the periphery of the complex, in this isolated building, his head already hurt from the howl of maddened residents, the banging metal, buzzers, and alarm bells; all of it, the stench, the cacophony, confirming that he had descended into Hades.

Following the scuffed floor arrows to the Inmate Visitation Desk, he came to a very, very portly woman in a skin-tight khaki uniform who played several more cards of computer solitaire before looking up to glare at him.

When Elliott stared back, she growled, "State yo business."

"I want to see my father."

"You got a appointment?"

"I don't think so."

"Well, you do or you doesn't."

"I just gotta talk to him for a minute."

"Don't matter, minute or hour. Ain't got no appointment, you gotta wait-n-see if we got time. What his name?"

The woman closed the solitaire screen and searched. She wrote a number on a slip of paper. "Take this. You gonna need it. And I need to see yo ID."

Elliott's eyes widened. "I'm not eighteen yet. I don't need an ID."

The woman pursed her lips and drew her head back irritably. "What you bangin' yo gums about? No ID, you don't get to see nobody in here. We got people younger'n you doin' time right over there." She pointed to a blockhouse a hundred feet away. "No ID? You jus' get yo butt outta my visitation center."

As the woman's pique rose, several people filed in behind Elliott and obediently formed a queue. As Elliott turned to leave the desk, an older man in priest's garb walked slowly to the counter. He asked the woman respectfully if he might speak to her supervisor. She looked up at him and spat, "State yo business."

"Officer, I'm Father Regan. You know me. I bring groups of visitors up from Bed-Sty. Today, we are privileged to have the neighborhood council. We are supposed to see Sergeant Winston. He's the supervisor, I believe."

"The woman picked up a filthy phone receiver and grumbled into it for less than three seconds. Half-a-minute later, a large man with three stripes on his sleeve appeared through a sally port. He greeted the priest and his entourage warmly. The reception officer pursed her lips again and shook her head indignantly as she went back to her computer.

The priest called the sergeant aside and spoke in a whisper. He nodded at Elliott, who had turned to shuffle toward the exit, his face as white as the prelate's collar. The officer called out, "Hang on there a minute, young man."

The officer walked to the back of the counter, typed into a different computer, and called the group forward. After the first three visitors were processed, he crooked his finger at Elliott and asked several questions, looked at his school ID, handed him a card on a lanyard, and told him to put it around his neck. He spoke gently to Elliott, asking him to wait with the others.

They were eventually escorted by yet another super-sized, khaki-clad, corrections officer into a room that looked more like a low-budget middle school cafeteria than the visiting chambers for the creme de la crème of New York State's twenty-thousand-plus incarcerated felons. Elliott placed himself at the rear of the group as if a first-year medical student trailing the procession of God's chosen on hospital rounds. The racket from the nearby cell blocks was so earsplitting, he did not hear the CO order the group to halt. He accordioned into several of the visiting women, a chorus of grumbling invectives accompanying his shoves backward.

He was told to take a seat at a warped, linoleum-topped card table. An hour passed until Elliott's father, in an orange jumpsuit and chains around his waist lashed to handcuffs, emerged with a guard walking behind him, right hand clasped to the waist chain. Reuben smiled broadly as his shackled wrists and hands parted to the heavens, thanking God for the miracle. The guard plopped him down and grunted, "Youse guys don't touch the other one. Got it?" Before they could answer, the man spat, "Fifteen minutes. Next time, make an appointment."

Reuben waited until the CO backed off toward the door. He gushed, "My boy, why is God so good to me? He lets me see my son, finally." He looked left and right. "You in trouble?"

"No, Tata."

"How's your Mama, and what are you doing here?"

"She's okay, I guess, but Tata, some guys who know your name made me cook drugs for them. They told me if I didn't do it, they were going to hurt you."

For an instant, Reuben's face hardened, though his eyes rolled in contempt. "Oh, them?" He puffed air through his lips scornfully. "They're babkas, nothing. Gangsters, yeah, but so stupid…" He flicked his middle finger in the air. "Forget about 'em."

"You sure Tata?"

"Of course I'm sure. See, there's all kinds of, may I say, clubs, here in the joint. Some got a little more influence than others. You know, we people from Eastern Europe, we take care of business. Not so loud, maybe, but we don't have to howl like animals to be heard. Now that I know, we gonna teach your friends a little manners. You don't worry. I'll take care of the momzers. And no drugs. I don't tolerate that shit. You wanna end up here?"

And just like that, time was up. It could not have been four minutes. "Sass, on your feet. Say good-bye." He did. Elliott wasn't sure if his old man's eyes reddened as he turned away, but he knew his had.

When he returned to school, Mr. Julian pulled up behind Elliott at his hall locker. He tapped him on the shoulder. "Mr. Sass, missed you last couple of days. Like to have a quick word with you after school."

Elliott froze, his lips trembling. He barely formed the word, "Okay."

As the day wore on, he left school several times, intending to run home, stuff his backpack with clothes and food, and board a Greyhound for California. He had saved more than five hundred dollars and planned to leave two hundred on the table for his mom. When he thought of what he'd write on the farewell note, he laughed dolefully that she would likely not realize he was gone.

Elliott again considered running when the final bell rang, but he also wanted it to be over, and he knocked feebly on the Dean of Men's door. "Glad to see you, Elliott. Proud of you for showing up. Some of your pals might not have had the balls. Have a seat. I want to talk to you about something that's happened. We're going to take a different tack dealing with this one. You're a senior now. Grown man, and I'm going to treat you that way."

Elliott flushed so deeply, Julian's eyes widened, and he leaned forward in his chair. "You okay, son?"

Elliott squeaked, "I know what this is about. They made me do it. Said they were going to hurt my father if I didn't. They can't hurt him, it turns out. But I didn't know that. What did you want me to do? I don't care what you do to me, what *they* do to me. It's not my fault!"

Now it was Julian's turn to go red. His mouth was open, but no words came. Finally, his color normalized, and a bare smile curled his lips. "Son, you didn't kill anybody, did you?"

"No!"

"Plant a chemical bomb?"

"No! What do you think I am?"

"Hurt anyone?"

"No!"

"You steal a lot of money?"

"No! No way!"

"Then whatever the heck you're talking about, I don't wanna know the details, not a single one." He paused for a moment and heaved a breath. "When you know you did something you shouldn't have, and every one of us does at one time or the other, and no one gets hurt, just keep your mouth sealed. Most of the time, a guy gets verbal diarrhea, and it gets him hanged. Remember that."

"Yeah, I guess so. I thought you knew…"

"Stop!"

"I'm sorry. It's just that…"

"Oh, my God. I just told you I don't want to know." Julian's eyes rolled toward the ceiling as he drew a breath. "Whatever it is, *just don't do it again.* Take it as a life lesson. Okay, now down to business. You missed senior English, Biology, and New York State History between fourteen and eighteen times this year. That's enough to keep you from graduating."

"But I turned in all my assignments."

"You did and got good grades on them. I'm sure you're proud of yourself. Problem is, paying the smart kids to do your homework doesn't count.

"So, if you want to graduate in seven weeks, you have a lot of homework and a bunch of minor papers to get done. Why am I offering this opportunity?" When Elliott stared back at him, the Dean shook his head. "Look, this is the first time I have ever had you in here for an infraction short of a felony. On the other hand, I'd like to think of myself as more than a policeman. Son, you have a talent in life, several actually, and you know what, my most important job at this school is to find kids like Elliott Sass and come up with a plan to help them become winners in life. I know you hate me, but, ready for this, I happen to like you. You remind me of me thirty years ago, but you're a lot more talented, smarter, and more of an individual. That's good."

Elliott sat a bit straighter. "Mr. Julian, how can you say that? I know I'm a crappy student. Were you as bad as me?"

"Let's put it this way. I failed senior English and had to take it during the summer to graduate. That sucked, let me tell you. Supposed to go to college in the fall, but that fell through, so I had to go into the army. Sent me straight to Vietnam. Heard of the place?"

"Yeah. Bet that sucked almost as much as school."

"Well, I'm glad you've enjoyed your time here, and yes, it was a nightmare. You don't know how good a life you have. And you are in a position to make it a lot better. Now, what I'm telling you is that finals are around the corner. You got a lot to make up for, but you're one of the smartest kids in this school. Start tonight. You got all the books, yes?"

"Yep."

"Tell you what we're gonna do. Make up your tests. I already got it arranged with your teachers. Get a B or better in English, history, and biology, take the State Regents Exams, and we'll base your final grades on the results. Now, you might graduate, but you aren't goin' to college next year. On the other hand, there's a new program at City College. If we recommend you, you can go to junior college right in your neighborhood. Department of Education pays your tuition and a stipend for living expenses. You get your AA after two years. You also need to get a job while you're in school, see what it's like in the real world. *Then* you can go on to a four-year college. You'll have it half-done and paid for. I'll get you in *if* you take it seriously *and* get Bs or above. Whata you think?"

Elliott sat, jaw hanging.

He forced his way through *The Scarlet Letter*, *Moby Dick*, *The Red Badge of Courage*, and *Beowulf* in ten days. In June, he aced his finals, except chemistry, but got an "A" anyway, the teacher terrified Elliott would go to the principal and squeal that he had walked in on the man fondling his student assistant, Gabby, in the chemical storage locker after class.

It was the first breast Elliott had ever seen for real, and it was an image he couldn't get out of his head, the aureole as red as her hair. And it was all reinforced by Gabby Hawkins' blush each time they passed in the halls of Isadore Goldstein High School. Elliott finally followed her after school onto the subway, trembling when she turned and crooked an index finger at him. She took him home, and it wasn't ninety seconds before her panties were pushed to the side, she pulled the Kotex free, his pants got as far as his thighs, and the whole thing was over.

They spoke nary a word in the fifteen-second afterglow, nor in the following thirty seconds when his pants came up, her skirt down, and he flew through the door to run home. He never did get to see her breasts during the brief dalliance, and it would remain a regret for the rest of his life.

They passed, ships in the night, for the next several weeks in the halls of Goldstein, until she pinched him in the arm after school and dragged him into an empty classroom. She cried and cried, managing to sob a few words that sounded like she had missed her period and had scheduled an abortion at Planned Parenthood, but it was a hundred and fifty dollars. She wept even harder when she showed him the seven dollars she had to her name. That night, Elliott dug into his kitty under the floorboards. He slipped her the cash wordlessly during chemistry club the next afternoon.

On the way home, he began to think about the whole thing. He remembered she had been on her period that day. How could she have gotten pregnant? He thought it was not possible, but maybe exceptions to the conception rule had been one of the biology lectures he had cut.

Though they never spoke again, he nervously asked one of her friends how she was doing. "Oh, she's great. She took all of us out for her eighteenth birthday on Saturday night. Bet it cost a hundred and fifty bucks."

It was a lesson he would not learn well.

CHAPTER FOUR

On June 16th, Elliott Sass walked with his class for graduation at Madison Square Garden. He stood when the designated Regents Scholars were announced. It was an honor bestowed by the State of New York, not the high school, and with it came scholarship funds that could be applied to college tuition, room and board, and books at any accredited university in the state he could get himself into.

The day after graduation, he went to see Dean Julian to beg for a letter of recommendation. Elliott had read in the paper that New York University sponsored a special admissions program for kids from disadvantaged homes who also held full Regence Scholarships. The dean demurred, citing his lack of time, a few words run together about the airport, catching a plane, and a vacation that began at noon, less than forty-five minutes later. Then he added succinctly, "I told you, you need to go get the AA, yeah, but you also need to get a job for a year, see how tough it is out in the real world. You need to become a man."

"But Mr. Julian, I have to use the scholarship in the fall of the year it's granted. And it's for four years, not two like the junior college thing you told me about."

"Yeah, the junior college *thing*. Elliott, like I said two months ago, you need to go out and prove yourself. Then come to me."

"I already proved myself here. You told me to do my homework, and I did."

Elliott relaxed as Julian stared at him for a moment then opened his desk drawer and reached around inside. Instead, however, of pulling free a sheet of letterhead, he poured the contents into a carboard box. "If you'll excuse me, I have packing to do."

Elliott marched from the room head hanging. He started toward the main exit but took a quick look back, ducked into a hallway, and jogged a full circle to the men's room just two doors from the Dean of Men's office. Behind a crack in the door, he waited until Dean Julian bristled from his office lugging a stuffed briefcase and an overflowing cardboard box.

As Julian had left the door slightly ajar to allow Mr. Sabotucci access for the yearly dusting and vacuuming of the ancient rug, Elliott slithered easily into the office. He hooked several sheets of school letterhead, envelopes, and a couple of Bic pens. He could not find the roll of stamps usually sitting on the desk and cursed aloud that Julian had probably stolen them.

The next morning, he showed up at the main office and asked the head secretary if he could sit in the corner and use the Selectric typewriter to fill out college admissions forms. She stared at him askance. "What's wrong with the typewriters in the library? And, *you're* applying to college?"

He knew better than to argue, for the only time he'd been in the office was to be punished with suspensions and to report back when his sentence had been served. He left with a little bow and a thank you, went out to the Valencia Bakery, asked in Spanish for a dozen of their most frilly donuts, then dropped his head servilely. The baker smiled, complemented his accent, and added two more.

He waited until half an hour before lunch break and marched back into the school office with the box held two feet in front of him as if a religious offering, the submissive bow of the head even lower than at the bakery. Drool formed at the corners of the ladies' mouths when he plopped the box onto the front desk. The head secretary giggled as she charged out of her chair to lift off the top. "You really are one for the books, aren't you, young man?" She bent over the box so far, the tip of her nose nearly touched the Puerto Rican Pineapple Rum Cake squares. She shifted her head a few inches to study each of the eleven pastries that had survived the walk back to school. She pulled free a sticky apple fritter the size of a rowboat and turned to Elliott. "What's such a big deal about the Selectric?"

At first, Elliott didn't hear the woman over the gallops of the staff toward the donuts. "What?"

"I said, why the big fuss over the electric typewriter?"

"Oh, the Selectric. Mrs. Connors, the portables in the library don't do a professional job. I really want to get into a good school and use my *Regents* Scholarship. I lose it if I don't start in the fall."

"That's right, you're the one who got the full ride, didn't you?"

"Yes, Ma'am."

"Okay, but don't tell anybody. Next thing you know, we'll have an admissions office going on in here."

"Oh, no Ma'am."

She stared over his shoulder several times for the first fifteen minutes, warning he was to use the typewriter *only* for admission applications, but she left to inhale a third donut and didn't come back. The instant the bell rang proclaiming high noon, her staff disappeared before Elliott could look up. The head secretary called back over her shoulder, "I'm locking the door so no one can get in. And," she wagged her finger, "don't you use the phones."

"Yes, ma'am."

When they were out of sight, he went to the box of donuts. It was essentially as empty as when the baker had pulled it off the shelf hours before, but grubbing around under the waxed tissue, he found a pinch of sugar dust and three sprinkles.

Then he pulled a sheet of school letterhead from his bookbag and started typing, one character at a time, lost in intense concentration, his work error-free. He wrote in Julian's voice, barraging the NYU admissions committee with the saga of a disenfranchised Romanian student, yet another victim of Hitler's madness, who came to America with nothing. Never mind the challenges, he had fashioned himself into a master chemist, creating compounds that he, Dean of Men, Arthur Julian, imagined had only ever been formulated in Harvard's Graduate School of Chemistry and Physics.

Elliott spoke of Elliott as an only child raised by a mother who had come to the U.S. already ill from the deprivations of post-war Europe, and who had spent so much time in the hospital since arriving in America, Elliott had essentially reared himself. "She came to me, this fragile woman, begging our school not to allow her son's *Regents* Scholarship to expire." Before leaving the room, Elliott snatched several postage stamps from the head secretary's desk and used them all. He wrote across the envelope "Airmail" in red Magic Marker.

Four days later, he received a call from NYU inviting him downtown for an interview. He pressed his father's tatty slacks and sports jacket, but not too well; washed his sneakers, unearthing the worn sole; and shaved, purposely nicking himself oh so lightly and innocently.

He was to meet the interviewer in a courtyard between research buildings at New York University's Langone Medical Center. He spotted her and started to walk across the thickly arboreal quadrangle where she sat on a wooden bench. A second later, though, he stopped short, startled by the bizarre twist of her features and the swollen warp of her lip, nose, and left eye. At first, he thought she was wearing orthodontic head gear, then he guessed it was merely the strong shadows of the New York summer playing through the trees. As he neared, he grasped the dark young woman suffered a surgically uncorrected cleft lip and palate. He had never seen an adult with that lesion, and his body seized. It had surely shown on his face as well. Her large, blue eyes averted by reflex, and this further unraveled Elliott's composure to the point he did not let his gaze drop to her breasts, as was his habit upon meeting a woman, any woman, of any age. He lifted his eyes from her lips to the deformed, swollen nose that was drawn to the left side of her face as if she had spent a career as a pathetic boxer. The woman turned back and saw his continuing disquiet, but was so used to the thoughtless rejection, she recovered quickly and offered a weak, misshapen smile.

She welcomed him in a strongly nasal Eastern European accent. Elliott brightened. Perhaps she was Romanian, and he quickly imagined the place at NYU that would certainly be carved for him. Then, she spoke her name. Despite the muted distortion, he clearly heard "Irena Ledderova," and knew immediately she was Russian. While taught from infancy, as were all Romanians, to despise Russia as a country and a culture, and to loathe profoundly every single Russian being, he made a quick exception and whispered, "So, we are brother and sister."

They spoke for an hour, the conversation warming until her face relaxed and her voice became gentle, almost feminine. She even told Elliott of her past, born on the Russian Steppes into a superstitious peasant commune where the disfigurement was the clear sign of a profane soul, a punishment thrust upon the otherwise godly community. There had been cries among the peasants during her first months, she'd learned later in life, that she be allowed to die. Not only was the monstrous face an augury of early death, more crucially, it was a harbinger of woe for the village. The extra food needed for her mother, Nita, to generate milk was, therefore, deemed a waste.

When Nita's postpartum bleeding did not stop, the baby was taken straightaway to the hut of a gnarled old woman, a sorceress, who set alight twigs from stunted aspens, scrutinized the curls of smoke, and extracted a final, phantasmal judgment. Shockingly, the vapors suggested this was a special child, and when the mother died hours later, the witch counseled the baby be afforded a wet nurse. However, the death of so beautiful a woman confirmed that not only was the infant's form obscene, its soul was tarnished well beyond redemption. The witch's advice was dismissed by the commune council, and she was ordered to place the neonate in a woven basket covered by shreds of straw and leave it on the banks of the river. She was not to check on the baby for twenty-four hours. It would live or die as the spirits chose.

Elliott was aghast at the chronicle of this woman's birth. His face lost so much color, Irena placed a hand on his shoulder. Her touch shocked him; it was soft, as delicate as any he'd ever experienced. Something flowed through her fingers into his heart, and his blood pressure climbed back through normal to rise until his face reddened. She smiled and explained, "Please forgive accent, grammar. I teach myself English when a student in Moscow. Many bad habits."

Elliott smiled and waved his hand. "No, it's fine. Completely clear," he lied. "What I don't understand is, why couldn't you learn English in your village, in school?"

"My village, oh my God, not Manhattan. Russian Steppes are so primitive, like Fourth World. I am not proud to say this. People in village never hear of English. No idea other people speak other languages, no idea there is world outside Steppes. They cannot imagine Moscow."

He was silent for a moment, absorbing what she was saying. "Okay, primitive, but they were going to let you die?"

"You see, not enough food to waste on organism will breathe for few hours. I am female. Killing girl babies not only in China. Council think in very pragmatic way. Even if I, one demon, survive to childhood, I never become strong enough to furnish labor for collective, never produce enough food to balance scale of food invested in Irena's childhood.

"Anyway, my father was not of that community blood. He is banished out there, sent from Moscow to dirt-poor commune. Punishment is for high crime against Supreme Soviet. He is petroleum engineer, just throw him away. But another story for another time. My father disobeyed local council. Kept me inside cabin, fed me his share goat's milk. Even when I thrive, but still council refuse me full ration, medical care, formal education.

"You do not want to hear this. Not important. You need to hear about NYU chemistry program."

"No, no. You can't stop now. Please."

Irena shrugged and spoke softly, "Okay, but if you die with boredom, you never enter program because deceased, you must promise not to blame Irena Ledderova."

"I swear to God."

She went on, Elliott perched at the edge of the park bench. On her fifth birthday, still on diminished rations, the council decreed she be sent to the fields to work on a horse-drawn combine, the fat old men assuming that would do the trick. She would die within a month by accident or weariness. But she didn't die, becoming stronger than any of the other children, her hard labor on the dray finally buying her entry to school at age eight. Having been home-schooled by her engineer father, she was ahead of her contemporaries by the end of the first semester. That bought her an excuse from the fields and appointment as a teacher's assistant. The staff hid Irena away and tutored her privately, conferring a shield from the bullies, both fellow students and the hamlet's dirty old men who felt no compunction about grabbing her breasts and giving them a twist or two.

At eighteen, she became the only child from her commune ever sent to Moscow for college, working furiously to graduate at the top of her chemistry class. She also slogged away the evenings as a waitress at an American restaurant in Moscow, but the food was so bad, few speakers of English ever patronized the place. She learned little English though saved her kopeks to escape Russia, which she did barely a millisecond after the diploma touched her palm.

When the story was over, she sighed and leaned back, her eyes red, soon glistening. After a hushed minute, she whispered quaveringly, "I am lucky, I guess. I do not know, maybe not lucky." There was another pause. "To live like this not bearable. No chance for normal life." She stopped and stared into the sky. "I believed America will be very different. Educated citizens. I am wrong. I am cursed."

"No!" Elliott blurted, "you're really exotic. I mean, and I know I shouldn't talk like this anymore, but I think you're really sexy. Oops, I'm sorry. I said it. Are you mad at me?"

She suddenly bent her head forward, a poor attempt to hide the tears rolling down her cheeks. Elliott awkwardly reached for her hand. She hesitated but took it and let him help her off the bench. He tried to guide her to the door of the chemistry faculty, whispering, "Let's go get dinner."

She shook her head. "No. I must not. Do not worry. I support Elliott Sass application to NYU. Good luck here."

When Elliott refused to turn and leave, she relented, but first went to a hallway locker to pull out a gargantuan hoodie and long-brimmed baseball cap. Elliott maneuvered her through the streets, all the time telling puerile jokes, finally stopping at a hole-in-the-wall pizzeria. When they finished a large pepperoni pie and several glasses of beer, she led him to her campus apartment.

While her imperfection was seemingly profound, Elliott was stunned to discover her body was thin, muscular, in fact, flawless. In all the porn mags he'd snuck into his room and hidden under the floorboards, he did not remember a body so perfect. As things progressed, she undid the bandana and let her chestnut hair down. It flowed to her thighs, and Elliott wrapped himself in a cocoon of her silk, overwhelmed with the scent of expensive European shampoo. Though she'd whispered over and over that she did not have a lot of experience, that she was sorry to be such a disappointment, Elliott kissed her neck and told her she was the sexiest woman he had ever been with. He meant it and did not leave her until after one A.M.

The next morning, a Saturday, he bought roses at the Safeway and left them by her door. Three days later, another letter arrived from the NYU Department of Chemistry. Not only had he been admitted to the fall freshman class, the school agreed to supplement his Regents funds. They even offered on-campus living quarters, available immediately. Elliott took it the next day then subleased it to a kid he'd known in high school. The renter signed a contract not to further sublease, and Elliott agreed to charge far less than the place was worth.

Irena did not have Elliott's telephone number, so she snuck into the faculty office, looked in his file, and called the number. His mother answered but hung up when she recognized the accent as Russian. Despite the summer heat, Irena obscured her face once again in the hoodie and long brimmed baseball cap, took the subway to the upper Bronx at the corner of Morris and Jerome, and knocked on Apartment 2-H. She could see an eyeball at the peephole, though it was gone in a trice. She tried again on Sunday with the same result. On Monday, she sent Elliott a letter, but after a week without an answer, she boarded the IRT Woodlawn Line and camped out across Jerome Avenue, hiding behind a steel pillar supporting the elevated. When Elliott appeared at noon, hungover, weaving as he made his way to the local grocery store for beer and cigarettes, she waited a couple of minutes and slid into the tiny store. As she approached him coming up an aisle, her nose flared at the reek of alcohol, tobacco, pot, and BO, as if he had not washed since the night they had shared.

"Elliott! I am so surprised. Do you live nearby?"

He stuttered a few words and half-pointed toward his building. "How come you're here?"

"My friend lives at apartment house up block." She pointed in a direction where there sat only structures belonging to Hunter College. She drew a deep breath. "I really enjoyed day together." She fumbled with her purse then blurted, "You would, you like get together again?" He faltered, but she reached out clumsily and touched his hand. "I promise I am better next time. I guess I am little scared, no, very scared. But it is extremely nice to be close." She took a step toward him and whispered, "Very nice."

The warmth of her breath on his neck caused the slightest shiver. It was unexpected, but pleasant, and he reflexively inhaled through his nose. As the hair on his arms lifted, she brought her mouth just centimeters from his ear and whispered again, "I promise I am better."

With Elliott's mother at work, they went to his place and showered together. When the sun set over Hunter College, Irena sat up and whispered she should be going but left a long pause and made no move to get out of bed. Elliott, however, jumped up and slipped into a robe. A minute later, she dressed and left quietly. He sighed in relief, standing by the window as he watched her climb the stairs to the elevated station, then waited until she boarded the train. He got a drink and tried to pay attention to the TV, but he found himself thinking about her and forced himself to ignore the feelings. When the phone rang an hour later, he ignored it.

CHAPTER FIVE

Classes at N.Y.U. began the third week of September. Elliott had been issued new textbooks, which he sold at a discount to less affluent freshmen, then bought years- old, beaten copies for himself. He cleared a desk at home and snatched a few cinder blocks from the maintenance room in the basement, then a couple of planks from a police barricade after a murder on Morris Avenue. He created a library over which his mother smiled, as much of a gush of pride as she'd ever displayed.

He took his classes seriously, but it was all review, and he became bored after eight or nine weeks. He began sleeping in, attending class every other day, and two weeks later, every third. He spent the hours in his living room, occasionally glancing at his books, but mostly, he became increasingly engrossed in the soaps.

He also began spending time with an older, though handsome, widow from upstairs in 5-H. He'd met Gladys in the laundry room. Her apartment was rent controlled, and with her husband's pension and savings, she was able to lavish gifts and cash on Elliott for certain chores at which he became, under her tutelage, quite proficient. As the weeks wore on, she seemed to act younger and younger, even trying pot and ecstasy.

Sometimes, she'd knock on Elliott's door after his mother left for work and entice him upstairs. Sometimes, they stayed at his place. One morning, after an hour at Elliott's, she dressed and walked toward the front door to leave. He followed, naked, snickering as Gladys turned the door handle, pulling with a jolt as Elliott pinched her butt. Taking a step to leave, she looked back over her shoulder to give a wily smile. With the door fully open, Elliott's eyes flashed in panic, and he reached forward to arrest

Gladys' momentum. It was too little, too late. Her body bounced against a woman standing at the threshold, hand raised to knock. The two ladies fell together, and after the initial stages of bilateral apologies, Gladys' eyes locked on the visitor's twisted deformity, her face warping in dread that the apparition's disease was communicable. Gladys was, though, not as startled as Elliott, who covered his post coital shrinkage with trembling hands.

His first reaction was to slam the door, but Gladys' behind was in the way as she disentangled from Irena's arms. Finally, he left the door and fled to his bedroom. It gave him time to come up with a plan, the first of which was to lock himself in his room and let the two of them duke it out. Then it crossed his mind that if the confrontation became too heated, the neighbors would flood the hallway, and that would be the end of his gravy train with Madame Gladys. He threw on a pair of sweats and walked back to find the women staring at each other.

"Irena, I would like you to meet Gladys. She's a masseuse. You know, what with my back and the pain. She's fully licensed, no different than a doctor, for real."

Taking a full two seconds longer than it should have, Gladys turned to him and spoke hoarsely, "Okay, Mr. Sass, we'll see you next week, same time, right?"

"Yes, ma'am."

Gladys' sickly smile lasted until the elevator doors closed. Elliott did not know if Irena saw which button Gladys had pushed, but he dragged her inside before she could watch the arrow on the elevator point north.

He invited her to sit in his mother's recliner and asked if she wanted a cup of coffee. She shook her head barely perceptibly, so Elliott retreated into the kitchenette and started to boil water for himself. While a watched pot never boils in real life, this one was roiling in microseconds, curtailing Elliott's stall for time to think. When he returned to the living room, he took a seat on the couch, as far from her as he could.

Irena looked at him for a moment, as if gathering steam to start the journey. "I can smell sex on her, you know."

"No, you're wrong. You smelled it on me. Okay, I'm going to level with you. When she gives me a massage, I get a little horny. I begin thinking about you. So, like halfway through, I excuse myself and go to the bathroom and pretend I'm feeling your silken hair around me, and, I'll be honest, I come right away. That's what happened. Really. I'm sorry." He paused, "No, I'm not. There, I said it. I think about you a lot."

"Really?"

"Really, all the frickin' time, if you must know. I spend half the day relieving the pressure."

She stared in his eyes. "Elliott Sass, I am to believe you?"

Elliott shook his head as if a little irritated. "You think I'd touch that old bag—I mean, after you?" He feigned deepening anger, "I'm not a perv, you know. She gives good massages. Period."

"Maybe I should go. I only have come only to tell you Dean gave me telephone call. He asked me to talk to you about attendance. I mean deficiency of attendance."

"Oh, that. I know. Told you I spend my time letting go of the tension." He laughed. She blushed. "Also had a cold last week. Was worse than the flu. Made my back so bad. That's why I had to call Gladys. She gives my mother massages. I don't know, maybe it was the flu. Hardly get out of bed. You may not want to get too close to me."

"Well, you are now well and going back to class?"

"Yep, plan to on Monday. Look, you sure you don't want coffee or tea?"

"Yes, I am sure."

They sat for a bit, and it did not take long before the tingling began to creep into his nether parts, and his eyes slowly drifted down from her sad face to lock on her breasts. When he saw through the thin blouse that her nipples had begun to perk, so did he, and just that fast he was unveiling one of the new skills he'd mastered at Gladys' tutelage. It was a success, and it was several hours before she left.

CHAPTER SIX

And then he did not hear from her for many weeks. That was okay, for he was busy with Gladys and a seventeen-year-old who bussed dishes at the student hub. Occasionally, though, there was a crumb of disquiet in Elliott's groin when he thought of how long it had been since he had been swathed in Irena's silken hair. The anxiousness grew until thinking of her became so throbbing, he couldn't sleep. He warned himself not to get drawn in, for it was easy to get involved with a woman, but so irksome to extricate oneself. Yet his chest remained heavy. It was almost as if he missed her for her.

He took a sheet of three-ring binder paper and reviewed his circumstances. On the left of the line drawn down the center were the positives, on the right, the liabilities. Irena fell into both categories, but most important at the moment, he realized, was the number of lecture absences he was racking up at school. He decided returning to class was a must do, and the next morning, before sunrise, he worked his way south from the Woodlawn Line to the West Fourth Street-Washington Square Station and NYU.

His first class on Mondays was Chemistry 153 lecture, basic inorganic chem for chem majors. The lecture began at eight, and Elliott fought to keep his eyes open, but in minutes, he was scrunched in his seat, lids drooped, a sweater behind his head. As he began to drift off, he thought he heard the professor smirk, "Okay, it's finally here. Time to separate the men from the boys," then go on to introduce another lecturer, one who would begin the course's section on physical chemistry.

Though Elliott had heard of p-chem, he had been forewarned by his high school science instructors that this was torture of unconstitutional proportions, cruel and unusual. The rumors were that even if you sweat night after night over the p-chem text, letting your other classes lapse, you flunked the weekly quiz, and the one after that, and, along with most of the rest of the class, the mid-term and final exams. By the end of the course, a good sixty percent of the would-be professional chemists morphed overnight into sec-ed, econ, and music majors.

He was still clearing his head when the new lecturer appeared from the wings, torso canted toward the whiteboard. Elliott wasn't sure if this was a man or a woman, but it mattered not, for in one fluid moment, without a word of introduction, or greeting, the professor started throwing up Greek-lettered equations and words like motion, energy, force, time, thermodynamics, quantum chemistry, statistical mechanics, analytical dynamics, chemical equilibrium, and worst of all, triple integrals.

It was happening so fast, the first Magic Marker soon ran dry, a second quickly shifted from the half dozen clutched in the professor's right fist. All he gleaned from the equations was that the script was decidedly European. It made him think of Irena, a flash of her perfect body, of her delicate touch, of her gentleness. He thought it was time to give her a call, positive she would drop everything to see him, forever available as his whims came and went.

He let his eyes sag and his head extend back into the folded sweater, preparing to resume his nap, but a second later, he reopened his eyes, castigating himself for not having checked out the teacher's butt. He looked down. The instructor was definitely female, one with a most sensational ass outlined in tight black slacks.

"What I would do for thirty minutes with that one…pay whatever she wanted, anything!" he fantasized aloud. The guy next to him winked. When the woman turned slowly toward the audience, there was an audible gasp as the silhouette of her breasts preceded her. *That* was what captured the attention of her teen students, not the brilliance of her teachings. A tingling expectation rose in the air as she faced forward, but that was muted by a groan as the boys' eyes eventually rose to her face.

Irena Ledderova began her discourse, standing regally, clearly in command of her material. It was the most complex discussion he'd ever encountered in a classroom, or anywhere else. While he did not grasp the concepts, he saw she was moving from point to point, deriving thermodynamic principles that followed each other logically, or so she said. He looked around at his colleagues, the bulk of whom had stopped taking notes and were gazing about the lecture hall, mostly staring furtively at the clock. After a few minutes, though, she'd wrestled back her audience, the notetaking so robust, the stuffy air was filled with the chirr of pens flying across paper.

It was the first time he'd seen her face from a distance without the hoodie or hat. He could not tell if he was attracted or repulsed. He did not know what to think and soon it did not matter, for he had begun to get hard, his mind drifting, not hearing her interspersed admonishments that genuine chemists did more than just admix powders and liquids, heat the brew, and make a lot of money.

In her Stalinesque, Russian-accented English, she peered out into the mass of pubescent faces and warned, "No, you have, first, to learn how much energy needed, heat required to make creation. You must know every calorie to make chemical join, maybe come apart. In real world, in industry, every degree to raise temperature, boss ask how much money you cost me in electricity, gas? You want employer to pay high energy bill because you get C in p-chem? No. You must know every penny to spend to make company product. This p-chem. Not as easy as mix vinegar bicarb make foam, stink up house. Maybe your company make product, not *use* energy, but *give off* energy, heat, exoth..." She stumbled over exothermic and gave up. "Maybe give off so much heat you burn factory to ground. CEO never to take NYU chemist again. That is why NYU does not award chemistry degree when you fail p-chem. So better pay attention."

Elliott was quite moved, not so much by the compelling ball of fire that lived within so exquisite a body, but because he had *been* with this woman, a spirit upon whom all eyes were now locked, a dignified soul, one who had already proven she was an exceptional member of her generation. It was tough to fathom why she had accepted him, cared for him, let him touch her. Why had she touched him with a gentleness he'd never before imagined? Elliott Sass shook his head in disbelief, closed his notebook, leaned back, shut his eyes, and smiled.

After lecture, he sat in his chair for a few seconds and wrote her a note, "Who knows? This evening could be a repeat performance. Got a *lot* saved up!" He walked two steps toward the floor of the lecture hall before a lab tech came from the staff entrance and presented Irena with what appeared to be a folded sheet of paper. He watched as she opened the note, her eyes growing as round as chemistry beakers. Because of the damaged facial musculature, he was not sure if she was smiling or grimacing. He tried to move down the stairs toward her but was blocked by a frontal wave of students flowing in the opposite direction. By the time he reached the lectern, Irena had rushed off through the staff exit. His chest gripped to think the note was from a new lover, and her silence had been contrived to annul so critical a lapse in judgement.

Confused, but also uncomfortable in his groin, he left the lecture hall to check his student mailbox. Perhaps she'd sent a message. It was the first time he'd visited the cubbyhole, and it was so stuffed with fliers to join clubs, fliers for cheap tickets to basketball games, fliers for cheap textbooks, and coupon books for local eateries, he almost missed the white business envelope with the dean's office as the return address. He placed it irritably back in the pile and continued sifting through the ream of paper until he accepted there was nothing from Irena. He found the official envelope once again, rolled his eyes and smirked, but he also felt a shot of adrenalin in the center of his chest. It was a feeling little different than when Dean Julian had requested his presence over the years.

He made his way to the Starbucks next door, dropping down at a table before ordering coffee. He tore nervously at the envelope, unfolding a single sheet of letterhead bearing the austere greeting, "Mr. Sass." He was to present himself to the office of the Dean of the Department of Chemistry at eight the next morning. The correspondence, though, was dated two weeks before.

The man was towering and grey-haired, his three-piece suit sharply pressed, shoes shined to a fare-thee-well. He met Elliott in the outer office, placed himself directly in front of his hostage and peered down, an eagle sizing prey. He did not offer Elliott a seat. "Mr. Sass, I want you to know that the program in which you are enrolled is both selective and coveted. We expect exceptional effort on your part, one that matches the resources we are investing in your future. At the very least, that demands perfect attendance. Am I understood? And this is not the first time you've been so advised."

Before Elliott could draw a breath to deliver the litany of absolutions for his lecture absences and tardiness in reporting as directed, the man heeled around and disappeared into his corner suite. The secretary eyed him and added, "I imagine we won't be seeing you up here again, will we?" Her head dropped back to her typewriter.

Elliott went to the rest of his classes that day, introducing himself to the lecturers, explaining that he had been ill but was now ready to invest himself without reservation in the course work. But as the sun faded toward the end of the last class, he lost the train of the lecturer's words and began fantasizing about Irena, watching her reach orgasm then melting into her.

He was gone in a shot as the lecturer droned his final words, walking then trotting to Irena's. When there was no answer to his increasingly insistent knocking, he banged with his fist. A neighbor, a tall, handsome man, opened a door across the hall and asked guardedly, "What can I do for you?"

Elliott stuttered, "Just seeing if my friend's at home."

"Irena?"

"Yeah."

"Well, the university prefers visits be prearranged. We don't want strangers prowling the halls. And how did you get in here?"

"Door was open."

The neighbor did not change expression but stood silently until Elliott turned toward the stairs. When Elliott heard the door shut, he ran down the steps into the dark street and across campus to Irena's lab. A petite Asian graduate student smiled plastically at Elliott's increasingly pressured questions, finally answering in a quavering, heavily-accented voice, "I am sorry. He not here."

Elliott's head cocked and responded impatiently, "He? No, Irena. She is a she, like you."

"Oh, I am sorry, yes, yes; she not here."

A large man with a scruffy beard walked warily from a corner office over which hung the sign: Laboratory Director. He stood behind the woman, his belly touching her shoulder as he undertoned menacingly, "Yeah, we're quite busy, as you can see. Thank you. And how did you get through the security door?"

Elliott was about to tell him that Irena had been assigned to tutor him, that it was all part of the special program he was in, and that he was supposed to meet her there that evening for the first session. It was such an obvious lie, even Elliott accepted he couldn't sell it. His head clouded with an image of the angry dean, and he could conjure the special session of principals from the chemistry faculty convening that evening to create the expulsion documents they'd hand deliver to his apartment before sunrise.

In fact, Elliott had accompanied Irena to the lab once before, and watched carefully as she'd typed in her PIN. He feared revealing that would speed his expulsion to before midnight.

CHAPTER SEVEN

Irena Ledderova had just read a note from the Dean's office informing her that her father had been hospitalized with end-stage liver failure. She left for Russia that afternoon.

Anatoli Ledderov was sixty-nine. He had been exiled to the commune in the Russian Steppes in his mid-thirties, an enemy of the people, a capitalist roader, a mad dog transmogrified from potent government official to peasant in a matter of hours. His trial, in which he had not taken part, lasted eight minutes. He had not even been informed that day was to be the one his case was finally brought before a magistrate in Moscow. He had spent the time standing at attention in his cell, much as he had for the seventeen months since he had been arrested for sedition.

Irena's father had not begun his adult life a likely felon. He had graduated from the Gubkin Russian State University of Gas and Oil, "Kerosene U.", scholastically on the level with MIT, and socially advanced for taking Jewish students when the other Soviet universities had shuttered their doors to God's Chosen People. Assigned to the USSR's Petroleum Bureau in Moscow after graduation, he rose in the hierarchy by honing his skills as the maven of oil exports, waking the Kremlin to the wealth sitting under their tundra. As with all Russian bureaucrats, even the medium-sized potatoes like Anatoli, there were constant visits from foreign investors, unctuous men offering lavish dinners, limousine service, women, and piles of rubles in paper grocery bags. Anatoli's ship came in, literally, when Turkish smugglers in Armani suits showed up at his office offering dramatically reduced shipping costs for Russian oil on its way to the West. With a wink and a nod, they opened binders with pictures of Chinese steamers, names painted over with Cyrillic letters. Some of the boats were long-retired passenger vessels, entire floors gutted, the walls covered in polyethylene—shake and bake oceanic oil tankers. They sailed from Vladivostok on the Russian East Coast, their names painted over mid-ocean to make them appear of Venezuelan registry. The oil was then mixed on the high seas with Turkish petroleum and sold at a fantastically marked-up rate to U.S. refineries, where the government was thankful for any non-Arab or Russian oil.

Anatoli squeezed a lot of fat out of the deal, smearing it across swarms of apparatchiks as one would spread thick pats of butter on hot toast. His Turkish friends invested his share in American oil company futures, the market in which Anatoli's pencil soon became the decisive factor. At first, it was only the diversion of a few tens of thousands of gallons of crude per week, peanuts, untraceable, all of it loaded in a flash aboard the prehistoric steamers. Aside from the mile-wide oil slick trailing the vessels, who could have known these ships were refiguring the world economy?

But the right people in Moscow instantly became the wrong people as gusts of political wind begat yet another Soviet purge. As accusations flew about the halls of the Kremlin, entire bureaus were decimated overnight, though Anatoli felt safe, for he had greased palms on both sides of the political spectrum. Further, he had plowed his profits into overseas corporations, the documents held in Turkey. Essentially, there existed not a shred of evidence to implicate him in high crimes and misdemeanors, at least not in the USSR.

He kept fresh in his mind that as a Jew, his star would sooner or later tarnish, and like most before him, he would eventually have to run for his life. He devoted his days to creating a future that would play itself out in Europe or the U.S. He held enough back from each payoff to buy fake passports, several sets, for himself, his wife, and his son; and falsified papers, registering the family as having not a drop of Jewish blood for at least three generations. He also beefed up their cache of rubles with each transfer, secretly engaging a travel arranger to purchase train tickets from various cities between Moscow and the Black Sea in case there were emergency route changes. Each stash contained a Bible-thick folder of identical papers and cash. He knew well that when he got the call from some co-conspirator that the KGB was on the way, there would be little time to retrieve more than one set.

But when it actually came time, it was not the way he'd imagined. In Russia, it seldom was. He was forced to implement Plan D: pack his wife and their son into a beaten East German Trabant sedan he kept hidden under rags and debris in a shed two blocks from their apartment. They would drive the thousand miles to Sochi on the Black Sea and from there contact his pals in Istanbul. The stacks of ESSO stock certificates held in the smugglers' safe deposit boxes were to be used as collateral for a boat the Turks would dispatch to rescue the family.

In the end, as with most things in Mother Russia, meticulous preparation made no difference. In fact, planning most often generated failure. This was an upside-down world in which there was a hazard point with every element of a plan that involved another human being. Any relationship in the USSR was simply a node at which the secret police could gain entry and ruin lives. The hard work for the KGB investigators was to isolate that single juncture between two suspicious lives, arrest one, then beat a confession out of the other—a two-fer. Then the street cops were dispatched to arrest families, pilfer homes, round up distant relatives, pilfer *their* belongings, and banish the lot to the gulags.

Nothing in the Soviet Union was predictable except, perhaps, the imminent demise of Anatoli's East German Trabant, to this day still considered the worst car ever produced. The man from whom he had purchased it took the cash, handed over the keys, and disappeared around a corner. No more than a day later, the seller was arrested in a liquor store, buying the place out, splashing cash around like water. The manager called the KGB, who beat him until he admitted he'd sold his Trabant on the black market. The cops sent a bulletin out to the authorities in a hundred-mile radius to be on the lookout for the jalopy.

Soon after, when the day came to leave Moscow, the Ledderovs got only eighty miles before both the engine and transmission caught fire simultaneously, flames eventually licking inside the car. Their belongings burned, including the title for the vehicle. Without proof of ownership, the local authorities arrested them for grand theft auto.

What angered the police was that the wad of cash they found jammed between the gas tank and the chassis had also been charred. They demanded the Ledderovs come up with an amount of cash equal to—because they were fair men—only half of what had burned. On the other hand, the family was not afforded a telephone to call friends for money. And, anyway, all their contacts were already rotting in Siberian labor camps.

It was after a month in jail that the urgent all-points bulletin from Moscow about the fleeing Ledderovs finally reached the local cops. Another few days passed before they realized a prize beyond their wildest dreams had been seized. Anatoli Ledderov, a fugitive of the highest rank, was worth untold sums in extradition negotiations with the KGB. The family was separated, thrown into fetid mud huts, and barely fed while the local cops entertained bids from the central police.

In a final gasp, Anatoli told the local authorities he had access to an American oil company's stock certificates worth millions. He would surrender them, free and clear, *if* he and his family were released. His only condition was to spend the night with his wife,

"The police chief snorted, "So you can take it out of her thing? Don't bother, I got it the first night."

Anatoli warned that the documents were worthless unless accompanied by a fresh signature and fingerprints, both of which would have to be authenticated at ESSO headquarters in Houston. He warned that any stock certificates over a million dollars were subject to new technology that could detect if a signature or fingerprints had been obtained under duress, He grinned, "Just the newest kind of lie detector machine." The cops stared at each other blankly.

Several days of negotiations followed, during which neither Anatoli nor his wife and son were given more than a crust of dry bread twice a day. Finally, the man who had been sent to Moscow to do research on the stock certificates returned, and the authorities agreed to allow the family to emigrate to Turkey. Anatoli signed the documents, which were simply non-negotiable copies of the originals, and was allowed to hold his wife's hand as his fingerprints were taken. A moment later, he was wrenched away, handcuffed, and thrown into a truck for transport to Butyrka prison in Moscow.

As his wife shrieked at the guards to honor their promise, they spit on the ground. It enraged her, and she attacked the chief, scratching at his eyes and biting his ear, the fray going on until Anatoli prevailed upon her to quieten. When she calmed, the police chief lifted his chin, sending Anatoli's paddy wagon on its way.

That night, his wife was raped again, though the next morning, she and her son were purportedly tossed onto a bus and taken to a fishing boat bound for Turkey. Or that was what Anatoli was told years later, the account coming from a new prisoner, one who claimed to have been a black-market travel arranger in Sochi. He swore he remembered the comely woman and young boy, and his dates were within the realm of possibility.

CHAPTER EIGHT

Anatoly's future was adjudicated in that eight-minute trial. While he had not been invited, the full complement of judicial officers, i.e., a prosecutor and a judge, were present. They lounged in chambers, enjoying bowls of borsht. The judge reviewed Anatoli's dossier and commented on the note that the prisoner had been sent by his Petroleum Bureau to the tundra a dozen times to inspect oil rigs. The fact that he actually made the journey so many times was the mark of a madman, *or* one involved in sedition. Especially damning was a letter the judge found in the file written in Anatoli's hand requesting permission to be allowed to remain in the tundra for an extra three weeks on his last trip. "Probably had a mistress out there," the prosecutor laughed. "Mighty expensive one!"

The judge grinned, "If it wasn't a woman, it was clearly incitement to rebellion. There isn't anything else, is there?" Without waiting for an answer, he mumbled. "Not much here to support the death penalty. We'll give him the benefit of the doubt. The man loves Siberia so much, good, I sentence him to sixty years there on a communal farm. And if he doesn't like my style of justice, I'd be thrilled to send him six kilometers up the road from the commune to the gulag. Why, I'll even take twenty years off the sentence if he prefers the prison camp."

The two dozen other men on trial that day faced charges for crimes ranging from stealing a telephone book to burn for heat to pilfering hay for his family's beds. The judge blotted a drop of soup from his jacket and shook his head. "Petit crimes?" the man asked rhetorically. "No. Not even close. These are blatant anti-communist actions denigrating the most just distribution of wealth on Earth. Soviet citizens in good standing get from the government what they need to live comfortably. The act of stealing basic human needs reveals criminal avarice, gluttony, and worse, antisocial tendencies."

Months later, Anatoli was placed on the floor of a 1932 Zis-5 army truck with those other men who had run afoul of the established order. Riding through the primitive wilderness for days on end, they finally came to Lake Baikal. The officer in the front stopped the vehicle and commanded the men to turn out and stand at attention, eyes closed, the burlap sacks of the impedimenta they'd lugged from prison to prison lined up dress right dress on the ground in front of them. He ordered the convicts to open their eyes. "Behold the lake. It is the largest and deepest body of fresh water in the world, holding more volume than the American, so-called, *Great* Lakes. Very few law-abiding Russians are given this opportunity. Why in Lenin's name you are being afforded a single moment of decency is beyond me. But here we are, and I hope you will remember what you are seeing. It is to be for the last time."

A few miles farther on, they began stopping at a string of communes, one prisoner dropped at each. The bags they had so closely guarded for years were left behind. "They will be delivered when you have successfully passed your probation." Finally, Anatoli was kicked off the truck, his belongings also tossed onto the growing pile. He never saw them again.

Anatoli stood on the frozen road and eyed his new home: Forty huts, some fashioned of mud and straw, some stone, and a few wood structures spread over several acres. Miles of yellowed fields swept into the flat horizon in all directions. He walked to a shanty over which read a placard: Communist Party Headquarters. Inside sat a toothless old woman who pointed him to a plywood shack in which thirty of the commune's undesirables lodged foot to head. He cleared an area in a corner, put his toothbrush on the ground, and so claimed his living space. Never once was he told what to do, nor did he ask. Anatoli simply followed the others to menial jobs in the fields and muddled through on the thin soup and bread, "Leftovers from the gulag," his compatriots groused sourly day after day.

He was so withdrawn, it took months before the authorities discovered he was literate, and it did not take long to rise from hand tilling vegetable fields to the camp logistical staff. While he was eventually responsible for much of the farm's material goods, and soon for creating lies on government reports about the level of commune production, he knew he would never go an inch higher. He had come there an enemy of the revolution, was reminded of it daily, and so it would remain for all of time. The council particularly disliked that he wore glasses and despised that he had, one day, up and marched out of the communal barracks, walked to the edge of the village, and manufactured a small house out of leftover scraps of wood, mud, and straw. When nothing happened after several days, he realized they were scared to stop him, probably fearing anyone with such chutzpah must be a KGB plant. So, he bought an oil drum from a travelling merchant, placed it on his roof, and captured rainwater for a primitive indoor plumbing system, even a toilet with a septic field. It was the first his comrades had ever seen or heard of.

Always reminding himself that he was lucky to have received a life sentence on a Siberian farm, not in the gulag, he rationalized that he was better off there than drowning in the blood sport bureaucracy back in Moscow that had been his life for so long.

Eventually, he married Katarina Anosov, a comely teacher, the most highly educated woman in the commune—she had gone through eighth grade. The daughter of a man who had also been labeled an enemy of the people, she and Anatoli led a lonely life as pariahs. Katarina buried her misery in books, Anatoli in vodka.

Two years later, Irena was born. There were complications, and Katrina died from blood loss shortly after the birth, a result of the ministrations of a poorly trained, toothless midwife. The woman massaged Katrina's uterus so violently after the birth to quash what was actually quite normal post-partum bleeding, she precipitated a rupture. Katrina nursed her baby but once.

Anatoli was quietly furious that, because of his political status, the commune was only willing to pay for an incompetent old lady to deliver his daughter. He went before the commune council and stated his outrage, though in hushed tones, as always. He petitioned the men to pay reparations and transport Irena to Moscow for facial surgery. The council actually let him finish his sentence before breaking out in peals of laughter and derision, declaring the pregnancy had been cursed long before the midwife came on donkey-back to attend. "Why, just look at your daughter. Deformed. It is her fault her mother died, and your fault that she became pregnant with such a monster. You are an evil influence on everything you touch. And, anyway, the demon will die in no time. Just look at it."

It had come time to make a river change, if not in his life, then in Irena's. He set about bribing officials on inspection tours, paying them to sneak cryptic letters into the hands of his first wife's closest friends in Moscow. He hoped against hope that they were in secret contact with her. He asked her to arrange an escape. It was the least she could do after the fortune he'd left for her in Istanbul. After four years, a dozen tries, and thousands of rubles pilfered from the commune with his creative accounting skills, there was not a word from the outside. He hadn't even an inkling if she and his son were alive. For all he knew, they never made it out of the USSR. Perhaps her friends had understood the code and stolen the stash in their apartment, using the largess to buy passage out of the Soviet Union to live in the south of France, the Ledderov name long forgotten.

As even more years passed, and with no opportunity to escape on his own, especially if he tried to take Irena with him, he slowly drank himself into a cage where he was soon physically so ill, he was dismissed from his accounting duties and assigned to shovel waste from the cesspools at the edge of town onto the vegetable gardens.

Irena had not been permitted to go to school, her face considered a distraction for the unmarked students. At five, though, Irena asked her father to teach her to read and write and cipher numbers. He agreed heartily but became so drunk each night after work, he failed at that as well.

Instead, Irena befriended two kids, helping them with their extra duties in exchange for rudimentary tutoring. On her eighth birthday, she marched into the school and wrote a composition about the importance of literacy for the future of Mother Russia. The teachers, all of them wives of the commune councilmen, demanded she be matriculated. They won, easily, as they always did, and while they held her back a year to learn arithmetic, in two years, she skipped a grade and became a teacher's aide.

By twenty, she was working at the school as a barely compensated teacher. It was that year the commune educational board received an order to send a single student to Moscow for university training. The teachers met, agreeing unanimously that Irena would go, no matter what their husbands might say. In concession to the council members, the women agreed to submit three names for final consideration, as long as Irena was the one chosen to go to Moscow.

The teachers said nothing to anyone besides their husbands about the plan until the Wednesday afternoon of the commune council's monthly meeting. Afterwards, to keep him away overnight, the men sent Anatoli out to the far reaches of the commune in his honey wagon to spread his load of excrement on the most distant fields. Then they sat the three candidates on a wooden bench outside party headquarters to await the final decision. The women disappeared into the Ledderovas' hut to gather her things and purloin what they could of coins lying around the shanty.

While cruel, they had no choice but to put Irena on a bus that afternoon before her father got involved and, more importantly, before the rest of the commune got word of the politically unsavory selection. There would surely to be recriminations, but if Irena was gone before the sun set, the matter would be forgotten in four days, like most things in life.

One of the grubby old men asked Irena to leave the other two girls and wait by herself in the supply room. He left the door open a crack, allowing Irena to hear them discuss the candidates and the pronouncement that she was the winner. She began shaking with excitement, but that lasted only seconds as the men noisily calculated the bribes Anatoli would pay to complete the deal. With each ruble, her heart sank. Anatoli had drunk away all the nefarious proceeds from the commune's books, and when the women showed up with just kopeks, the council grumbled it was less than a hundredth of what had been bandied about. Irena heard the entire conversation and sat solemnly, waiting to be given the sad news. Even the women discussed withdrawing their nomination.

Angry talk went on for some time until Commune Council Communist Party Chief Smokalov left the meeting room and stood above Irena. As he explained the process, she stuttered a few gloomy lines of acknowledgment, but she perked when the man suddenly bent forward and whispered that there was a way to surmount the difficulties. If she allowed a couple of the men to touch her, "very gently, nothing more," the bribes might be obviated.

She began to shake, mild tremors at first, then as if suffering a grand mal seizure as he pulled her off the bench and had her bend over. He lifted her skirt and entered her so quickly, she began to lose consciousness. He sneered that, as everyone expected, she was not a virgin, never considering she had been riding horses bareback her whole life. And even if he had known, he felt not a seed of guilt as he finished and called aloud for the next councilman. The instant the first man let go of her, though, she collapsed in a heap onto the concrete floor, weeping in howls. The rest of the men were so scared, they locked her in the council outhouse until the women loaded her aboard the bus.

Anatoli did not know she was gone until he returned the next night. He had wanted to share with her the location of loot the family had amassed and hidden in Moscow. While he knew he could never write a word of it in a letter, he had to satisfy himself with the thought of revealing the secret when she returned on the vacation she was never granted.

CHAPTER NINE

In the four years Irena attended the Lomonosov Moscow State University, she had not been permitted beyond the city limits, and all mail to and from the commune had been censored. She did not know if the letter telling her father she had graduated at the top of her class ever made it to the tundra. When the acceptance for graduate studies at NYU came a month later, she tried again, but the letter came back weeks later as undeliverable. Perhaps, the village cadres were scared that she was now closer to power than were they, or maybe her father had died. She knew well the government would not allow passage to her father's commune in Siberia, especially now that she was going overseas. Even if she paid to be smuggled out there, the odds of making the round trip without being spotted and turned in by someone, no matter how low on the social totem, were slim to none. All Russians knew that anyone could be a human trafficker, and once beyond the Moscow environs, market their cargo to the highest bidder, usually the local police, who then sold the payload to the KGB. She would be risking her future, and maybe her life, on the chance he was still alive. She would simply have to be a good Russian and, like her countrymen, bury her heart and forget hoping for anything that would make life a bit more tolerable.
She left Russia for New York the next day.

She assumed she would never see her father again, probably not even visit his grave, and she'd have been correct if it had not been for Glasnost. In the mid-1980s, censorship in Russia eased slightly and primitive mail service opened to the West. At the commune, Anatoli's neighbor was given permission to send Irena a letter about her father's illness, but it was several weeks old when she read it that day at the end of her lecture. She knew the prognosis was so hopeless, she imagined he had already passed, a trip home for naught. And even if she was able to get a visa, there was the impossibility of travel papers to the commune once she got to Moscow. Still, she went to the Russian embassy in New York and asked. After a breathtaking bribe, an emergency visa to allow her entry to Mother Russia was proffered. Another prodigious payoff garnered preapproved domestic travel papers.

Not twenty-four hours after boarding the plane at JFK, she found herself in the very same truck-converted bus that had taken her from the commune to Moscow so many years before. Bouncing along scarcely paved roads into her old provincial capital, the local police commanded her to wait in an unheated I for permission to enter the hospital. An orderly finally poked his head into the shop, snapped his fingers, then gasped and sharply averted his eyes when she looked up. He grunted over his shoulder for her to follow then left her at the front door of the hospital with a snarled, "Top of stairs."

The unpainted concrete bunker of a sanitarium rose a hundred feet into the frozen tundra, the tallest, most exquisite structure north of Irkutsk. It was serviced by two inoperative elevators, the lift doors on all floors jammed partially open, greasy pits exposed into which a good deal of the daily detritus was tossed by staff unwilling to venture outside to the garbage cans, especially during the Siberian winter.

Anatoli was on the fourth floor, his rusting gurney in a corridor, head facing an alcove by the stairs. He had been there for over three weeks, in that exact spot, not having conversed with anyone other than the food service man who brought him, twice a day, a bowl of soggy noodle soup laced with lumps of fat. Sandy sediment, actually debris from the hospital well, formed a layer on the bottom of the bowl. Anatoli had been told it was pepper, and he made great efforts to stir it into the slough water of the offering, savoring each grain of the faux spice.

Late in the afternoon of Irena's arrival, Anatoli's head was cocked uncomfortably to gaze at the open stairwell, which he did around the clock, that is other than when he was mired in increasingly frequent hepatotoxic stupors. His liver had all but ceased processing his body's wastes, the huge organ poisoned by the tanker cars of vodka he'd guzzled to numb the years on the commune. By this stage in the disease, the hepatic lobes had shrunk into golf balls of rock-hard scar tissue.

A normal liver produces bile, a syrupy, yellow-green fluid, from dead red blood cells and other wastes, then squeezes it into the gall bladder where it is stored until undigested fats pass by in the small intestine. With that the signal, the bile is injected into the intestine and mixed with lipids, allowing them to be absorbed into the body. Extra bile flows into the stool giving it its brown color. In Anatoli's case, the scar tissue blocked the flow of bile from what was left of the liver. With no route of escape, it was forced back into the circulation. The stool turned grey, and when the blood became saturated, the bile leached out into the skin, the eyes, urine, and even the hair, which would have shown an ugly yellow tint, were anyone to live long enough with that intensity of cirrhosis to grow out his hair. Worst of all, though, it infiltrated the brain and distorted one's thoughts.

Anatoli's stairwell was his soap opera, great adventures unfolding before him, outlandish visions more and more convincing as the bile and other unfiltered toxins permeated his brain. It thwarted some memories, warped others, and created new ones from whole cloth. He spent most of his final hours drifting deeper and deeper into mad dreams, hallucinations of dining in fine European hotels—mostly in Paris—savoring Stroganov and the finest Żubrówka Vodka. Once, he was a cosmonaut landing on Saturn, and one freezing evening, he even had the visage of Irena's face appearing at the top of the stairs. Gathering the few remaining neural fibers in his brain with the potential to fire, he assured himself it was just another of his delusions.

Then Irena passed his soiled gurney. While she was unaware it was her father, he was suddenly sure it was her, and he gathered every filament of spirit to extend a tremulous arm.

"Irochka," he whimpered, his voice fading as his arm slumped. She startled, turned back, focused on the sallow near-corpse, and involuntarily took a step away in disbelief. Anatoli's consciousness ebbed with the tapping of his last ounce of strength. Irena sighed, defeated, and as stoically as she tried not to let a fellow Communist see her weakness, she failed in even this most rudimentary rule of Russian behavior. Tears trundled along her cheeks. Of all the worst possible nightmares, her presence had become the very instrument of her father's demise. Palms rose to cover her wet eyes, as if so banal a maneuver might hide her frailty from the phalanx of peasants gathering in the hall. Woozy for only a few seconds, her chest slackened as she accepted this was but one of the unceasing, miserable dreams she'd woven through during the days of mad travel. She was getting used to them and quickly sensed a dash of relief as she recognized this as simply another sad fantasy. When she began to let her hands drop from her face, a harsh snore brought her back to the wretched hospital. The rumble was so loud, it shocked the gawkers, and even roused her father.

Her hand extended to touch his face, though the instant her fingers met his cheek, her arm withdrew as forcefully as if Anatoli's body was a bare electric wire. The sandpaper bite of his skin was shocking, as unpleasant a tactile sensation as she had ever encountered. Reflexively, she eyed her fingertips, confused by the glaze of what looked to be finely ground salt. She wiped her hand on her slacks before turning back. Focusing away from his face, she saw both arms covered with patches of jagged raw flesh from constant itching; deeper black and blue areas at the base of the barbs had coalesced into one grand tattoo. And there was more of the fine coating of salt. Fresh blood also oozed along the entirety of both extremities, and she again looked away, her eyes locking on the glaring spectators, now some twenty peasants strong. By their facial expressions and body language, she could see they were more offended by her behavior than her deformity.

She steeled herself and focused back on her father's face. It was worse than his arms. Semi-dried red crystals glistened over spurs of crusted blood in his nostrils, the itching there more intense than anywhere else. A slow stream of watery plasma dripped from his nose, over his lips, and into his mouth.

Irena took a corner of the dirty sheet, dipped it in the glass of murky water stored out of the patient's reach at the far end of the gurney, and patted away blood from his nose. No sooner was it gone than the bleeding started again. She left to get a tissue but had to settle for a roll of raspy toilet paper that did more trauma than healing. At the time, she did not realize that her father's blood was barely able to clot, the cirrhosis long ago having killed the liver's ability to generate coagulation factors.

As she patted the oozing, Anatoli looked up and tried to speak but began to cry. She kissed his cheek though pulled away, her face distorting as the taste of stale urine sullied her mouth. While she assumed it was poor hygiene generated by the staff's neglect, it was, in fact, uremic frost, a fine coat of crystallized uric acid that appears on the skin when the kidneys fail and can't rid the body of urine. It was part of the hepato-renal syndrome, the dying liver spreading its poison to destroy the kidneys.

She pulled a chair from one of the wards and sat there holding his hand. An orderly brought a bowl of what looked like soup which he handed roughly to Irena, spilling half as he shot back wordlessly to the kitchen. Basically vegetable peel water with two lumps of lukewarm lard, the best she could do was wet his lips with the spoon. After a few minutes, his mouth opened, and she was able to drip in broth, milliliter by milliliter, until the calories generated enough energy for Anatoli to keep his eyes open for more than a couple of seconds. Eventually, he rolled his head toward her and whispered, "Irochka, you are not here, I know. It is too much to ask, but my heart can see you. It is a gift, a gift."

"No, Papa, I *am* here. To care for you. It is not a dream. I will not leave you alone ever, ever again."

With that declaration, he seemed to gather strength, and she walked to the kitchen with a five ruble note flapping in her hand to buy another cup of soup. "Put some noodles in this time. Just noodles and broth. You're killing him with the fat."

There was a discussion amongst the help; one turned haughtily, though everted his eyes from her face. "And who the hell are you?"

She tightened and with pursed lips cautioned, "I am from the Russian Embassy in New York. *America*! That is my father. Any more questions?" She dropped the money on the chopping table, the worn bill soaking up a pool of grease, Lenin's face soon translucent.

There was silence until an old woman squatting by a bucket of dirty water sneered, "And I'm Catherine the Great."

Irena walked back to Anatoli's gurney, dug through her purse, and pulled free the NYU ID and her green card. She returned to the kitchen at a march to shove the documents under the woman's nose. The old lady rotated the cards several times before the cook snatched them away, grimaced at Irena's picture, and then harder at her face. He flipped the certificates back to Irena with one hand and pocketed the five ruble note with the other. He lobbed a handful of noodles into a bowl then pressed it into Irena's face.

Anatoli chewed slowly, the calories amongst the few he had consumed in a week. His liver lacked the potency to process much other than carbohydrates and light proteins like egg whites or a scrap of salmon, as if an ounce of fish had ever found its way into that infirmary. In half-an-hour, Anatoli's eyes drooped for a moment, but they suddenly shot open, and he grabbed Irena's arm. He pulled her close and whispered, "You are here! Wait until these bastards go away for the night. You'll stay until then, yes?"

"Yes, Papa, I have come to be with you."

They sat together for hours; Anatoli mostly slept. At sunset, she went down four flights into the street, shivering, entering the first restaurant she came to. It was a dark hole in the wall, dilapidated, filthy, though perhaps not as unsanitary as her father's hospital. She ordered a platter of potatoes and cabbage with a wedge of half-cooked pork belly. She could scarcely stomach looking at the meat and turned away from it as had the staff from her face. She held her breath rigidly and spooned the slab of lard onto a sheet of newspaper, which she folded. She thought to bring it back to a patient she'd encountered on the second floor, a skeleton also forced to face the stairs. This soul was so cachectic, his bed had appeared empty. Yet as she had passed him, a broomstick of an arm holding a bowl had materialized from under the sheet. A faint voice had begged, "Meat, meat."

She sliced the rest of the potatoes and mashed the cabbage, scooping the pulp into a zipper baggie. Climbing to the second floor, she stopped at the dying man's gurney. The arm was still extended, and grabbing a corner of the newspaper, she jiggled it until the slice of pork fat plopped into his bowl. As he had not moved a muscle since she'd first seen him, Irena thought he'd probably already departed for his eternal home, rigor mortis keeping the bowl from falling. As she turned away, though, a commotion erupted behind her; the squat, elderly woman from the gurney directly across the hall had slid from her bed to limp across and seize the bacon. That, however, woke the cadaverous man, who snatched it back, launching a pork pulling skirmish, one Irena studiously ignored as she climbed the stairs back to her father.

When she crested the stairs by Anatoli's gurney, a patient four beds down screeched that one of Russia's new crop of ill-mannered youngsters had stolen Irena's chair. She walked the hall, peeking into rooms until she saw the seat with the short leg occupied by a teenaged boy sitting by the door of his grandfather's room. The rest of the family was busy at the bedside helping the old man onto a bed pan. As he moved, the sheet slid up and Irena could see the mattress was nothing more than a sheet of warped, feces-stained, quarter-inch plywood.

A second ward farther down the hall was chairless, so she descended a flight and came to a pile of furniture. She shook her head at the enmity on the employees' faces as she pulled free a chair. As the attendants rose, now growling, to take back their property, she drew a few kopeks from her jeans pocket and tossed them on a table. With the angry attendants pawing at the money, she backed off the floor and descended one more flight to check on the man to whom she'd given the pork fat. Toothless, the man was chewing with difficulty but seemed happy. The woman across the hall, though, was on the ground, surrounded by staff who were wrapping the body in a sheet. Irena did not stay to watch.

The next bowl of soup had come for Anatoli. Irena lifted out the lumps of fat and added the sliced potatoes and mashed cabbage. She slipped the orderly a few kopeks and he returned with noodles in broth. Anatoli ate the vegetarian stew with increasing vigor, and as the calories fortified him, he perked even more, again begging her to stay until the staff went home. She kissed his forehead, the bitter taste of bile and uric acid causing her mouth to pucker, but she told him again that she would not leave his side.

CHAPTER TEN

Elliott had spent the weekend of Irena's disappearance at home, high, but cemented to the chair at his desk, catching up on the physical chemistry with which the smart-looking students seemed at ease. As it started to come to him, he found himself looking forward to Monday, the day Irena was next scheduled to lecture.

But she was not there, and a new lecturer introduced himself as a long-term substitute. Still there had been no answer at her door early Monday morning or late that evening. An empty feeling bore into his chest. He was not sure if it was jealousy or anger at her obstinance. He asked himself rhetorically, "Who would want her, anyway?" Then he answered himself, grumbling that some men were attracted to bizarre women. What if she had gone to bed with another guy, and it had been better than with him? He would now be no more than excess baggage in her life. The thought sparked an even deeper resentment.

Weeks passed—still no Irena. He began spending evenings at a bar near NYU getting drunk and trying to meet co-eds, his advances garnering only snubs, the same response he marshalled at the Chem Department offices when he tried to make inquiries into Irena's whereabouts. With the approaching Christmas break, most of the local watering holes stopped serving at nine to clear the place for the annual staff party. Forced to leave after just a few drinks, he trudged home early, afraid his mother might still be awake and forced to watch her son stumble, disheveled, to his room. At the apartment, though, she had already gone to bed. She'd left an airmail letter for him on the kitchen table. At first, he ignored it, but it looked quite foreign, and a longer glance revealed it was covered in Cyrillic letters. The glued edges had been cut open and resealed sloppily with Scotch Tape on which were smeared grimy fingerprints, far too large to be Irena's. He worked the tape from the envelope, preserving as much of the inner handwriting as he could. In fact, the letter had been written in the center of the paper, as if the writer knew it would be hacked open by censors.

Дорогой Elliott,

*I am wondering, you are still interested in coming to Moscow for International Chemistry meeting in December, Christmas break? Your paper on new plastics very well received. Professors so excited for chance to meet you. Especially your kind offer to teach chemical process. You remember Professor **Nikolay Demjanov**, discover of Demjanov rearrangement in organic chemistry. His son is head of department, very dear friend. He wants to meet you, hear of work in the new plastics. He is happy you agree to share discovery. It is exciting time between our two countries.*

He is to make arrangement for two-week stay. You must apply for emergency educational visa. Naturally, expenses are present. You will accept expenses as part of process. You must have round trip plane ticket to get you here 10th December. Aeroflot Flight 29 from JFK is good. Department to reimburse for all expenses.

At embassy show letter, matriculation paper in NYU chemistry faculty.

That is all for now.

Снаилучшими пожеланиями (Best wishes)

Irena

Elliott sat dumbfounded for thirty minutes. A blunt didn't ease his confusion, nor did several swigs of scotch, nor rereading the letter five times. On the other hand, simply looking at her handwriting stoked a tingling in his genitals. He called the Aeroflot office and asked the price of a ticket to Moscow. He nearly fell off his chair, but the extent of the larceny only served to intensify the prickling. He leaned back, laughing that he was contemplating a flight halfway around the globe just to get laid. But then again, it was Irena, and he could feel his consciousness funneling harder into his crotch. Suddenly, it did not matter if it was Irena or warm dirt—he needed it right now. With a bottle of his mother's wine in hand, he climbed the stairs to the fifth floor. Gladys had been asleep, but it mattered not to either of them.

He was especially attentive to her needs the first go, then stopped suddenly as her second climax was building to climb out of bed and grab his clothes. Though she begged him not come leave, he whined that he had to be downtown before dawn for an interview. He dropped back onto the edge of the bed, his fingers brushing her breasts delicately until her nipples became even more taut. He sucked a gentle breath between his teeth and whispered that he was being considered for a scholarship to attend a course in Moscow over Christmas. "I've got to go to the interview tomorrow morning at seven so I can, at least, get the honor on my CV. I hear I'm at the top of the list of candidates. Really a shame. I can't go even if I'm offered the place. Problem is money. Isn't it always? You have to get yourself there. They don't reimburse your expenses until after the course. What the hell. Next time. And, anyway, I would've missed you."

He stopped and waited for her to speak, but she remained silent until he touched her face with his fingers. She moaned. He brightened. "Maybe this. Could I borrow the money, I mean just until I get back? Have it to you before New Year's Eve; I promise. Maybe we'll share a bottle of good champagne."

Gladys sighed. "How much are we talking about, Elliott?"

"Eleven-sixteen."

"Eleven hundred and sixteen bucks!?"

"Yeah, but they're good for it."

"Who, the Russians?"

"This one's real, Sweet Pea. Scholarly stuff. University of Moscow. Ya know. Just like Cambridge and Oxford."

"Yeah, I'm sure."

When she became silent, just staring at the ceiling, he leaned over and began kissing her again. It took only minutes before they both climaxed, and after a final spasm, she slowly dragged herself from the bed. The next thing Elliott heard was pots and pans clanking, and seconds later, she made her way back to the bedroom with fifteen one-hundred-dollar bills in her fist.

CHAPTER ELEVEN

At six the next morning, with Gladys's largess and a couple of hundred dollars from his mother's hideaway stuffed into his jeans, he threw on a hoodie and dug around the apartment for his high school graduation certificate, draft card, social security card, junior driver's license, the nearly expired passport his mother had gotten him when he was granted citizenship, and the letter from Irena. He stuffed it all haphazardly into a ragged manila envelope then into his backpack, on top of which he tossed a couple of stale bagels, a protein bar, two packets of ketchup, and one of mayonnaise. At the last second, he threw in a razor, toothbrush, hoodie, ski cap, and a couple of changes of clothes. He scribbled a note to his mother that he was going to spend the vacation at a friend's cabin in the Poconos.

Satisfied he was fully outfitted for a journey halfway around the world into the Arctic, he bolted into the street and waited for a downtown bus. As the minutes ticked by, he remembered an English pal in his NYU physics class mentioning he always took Valium when he flew over the Atlantic, convinced the plane would ditch and he'd die in the ocean. Elliott had asked him if the Valium somehow drown-proofed a passenger, but the man had chuckled, "You still die, mate; you just don't give a damn." Elliott walked to Kingsbridge Road, bought several Valium tabs on the street, got scared that it was getting late, and hailed a cab.

An hour later, he climbed the stairs to the Russian Embassy, ignoring a gargantuan sentinel who seized him by the arm and held him until Elliott thrust Irena's letter in his face. The man grunted something in Russian that sounded a lot like "governor", then escorted him, not particularly gently, into the reception area. The secretary listened to his story, dismissed the guard, and rolled her eyes at the thought that some pimply-faced teenager had the audacity to march into the Embassy of the Soviet Socialist Republics and walk out with a visa for the asking. After several minutes of pretending to peruse the documents he had placed on her desk, she asked, "Do you have means to travel to and from the USSR? Do you have means to support yourself in a foreigner hotel and buy foreigner food?"

As he pulled out the fistful of hundreds, her pupils contracted. She explained that special consideration could be granted, though the price was steep. He peeled off a one-hundred-dollar bill and pushed it toward her face. Her fingers rubbed together until four of the bills sat on her desk. She took the money and his passport, slipped two bills into her bra, and brought the other two openly to the back office.

Minutes later, he was in a cab crossing the Brooklyn bridge toward JFK Airport. It would be the first time he'd flown, or even traveled beyond New York City, aside from visiting Sing Sing, since he was a toddler. He bought a ticket at the Pan Am counter, went into the men's room, and sat in a stall separating papers and counting what was left of his riches. He placed his documents and money neatly in the Pan Am travel folder he'd been presented with a bit of flourish by the desk agent.

When he was done, he made his way toward the departure lounge. Not thirty steps out of the men's room, he checked his back pocket for the ticket folder and realized he had left it on the toilet paper dispenser. Nervous passengers jumped out of his way as he sprinted back into the bathroom; others ran from the room when he banged on the stall, a prehistoric, Hassidic Jew flying from within, holding his pants up with both hands and chanting, "*Oy vey is mir, oy gevalt!*"

The folder was still there.

Elliott watched the passengers in ties and jackets closely as they made their way through security. When the man in front of him stepped into the x-ray booth, he grumbled, "This is a pain in the ass, you know." Elliott repeated the seasoned traveler's words, and the guard turned away and waved him through with the back of his hand. On the other side, Elliott kept trying to show his ticket to people in uniform, confused as to what came next. Most turned away shaking their heads, though one ancient housekeeper took him by the arm and led him to Gate 36. He tried to hand to her a dollar, but she pushed his hand back and clucked her tongue.

As soon as he boarded, he took two five-milligram tablets of Valium, had a glass of wine, then a second, and awoke, groggy, over the Atlantic, hundreds of miles east of New York. He stood to walk to the men's room but got only as far as the next aisle before his head began to spin, his vision darkened, and his legs dropped from under him. His next conscious thought was of sitting on the toilet in the bathroom, fully clothed, staring at a flight attendant standing in the open doorway, hands on her hips.

"And what'd you take, Einstein?"

"Wine."

"Well, consider yourself cut off, and for the rest of the trip."

He opened his mouth to protest, but a wave of nausea blanketed him, and he spun off the toilet to flip up the seat and empty his guts.

At the airport in Prague, he quickly became lost and drifted onto the line processing returning Czechs. As he was called forward, a commotion erupted around a gaggle of bewildered Americans who were quickly being surrounded by the local news media. The immigration officer popped out of his cubicle, pushed past Elliott, and joined his compatriots as they shoved and tore at the crowd fighting to enter the inner circle of foreigners where the cameras were clicking madly. Elliott shrugged and meandered through the immigration cattle chute into the main airport, walking in circles until two heavily armed police officers nudged him with their AK-47s back into the transit section. They turned him over to an Aeroflot agent, who promised to load him aboard his connection to Moscow.

The group of Americans was first to board, escorted into the premier class cabin by young, short-skirted, blond, flight attendants. Elliott watched jealously as the women guided the delegation's principal to his seat, hands roaming over his shoulders and back. But what Elliott resented most was the champagne being uncorked, and that the Americans were offered shelled peanuts and grapes while he had been handed a slice of apple and a cup of cold, bitter tea.

The delegation was also first to deplane at Moscow's Sheremetyevo Airport. Even before immigration control, a sizable assembly of paparazzi and besuited officials once again hovered around the Americans. Red, white, and blue clothed school children waved sticks tipped with paper American and Russian flags; high school kids held aloft a banner reading, "Welcome Bernie Sanders—America's Beloved Communist Mayor."

Elliott was pushed along with the Americans, and, in seconds, found himself on the other side of the restricted area, never having presented his passport. As he looked about, the back of his arm was grasped tightly. A hard female voice whispered, "Say nothing." He was jostled back toward the gaggle of Americans who were warming to the attention, posing for photos, gabbing with a new set of alluring blond women.

"Pretend you are part of group," the voice whispered harshly. He yanked his arm free and raised a fist in reflex, though hesitated when the distorted lips and nose came into focus. Her eyes followed his, and she blinked, yet recovered quickly and pushed him forcibly into the swarm of Russian officials surrounding the mayor's party. She growled again, "Stay with group, say nothing. When group is leaving, you be in middle. I rescue you outside."

As ordered, Elliott shuffled with the delegation as they were herded toward fancy travel busses. Irena gasped, alarmed Elliott would board with them. She ran into the street and waved impatiently until he wandered away from the pack. She clutched his arm again and pulled him aboard a beaten public bus. The tugging carried on until they reached the very rear, where she let go and heaved a breath, groaning, "*Privet*, Elliott Sass. I am sorry for drama. I tell you later."

He finally turned and saw her face covered with a sheen of perspiration despite the sub-freezing temperatures. Her lips twitched as if holding back tears. She appeared older and far more unsettled than he remembered. He looked away uneasily, only to witness souls he recognized from his plane pushing and wrenching at each other to seize seats. Normal appearing fellow travelers thirty minutes before, they had taken on the same hardened, faraway stare that now shrouded Irena's face. He felt as if he was back at Sing Sing.

The bus became increasingly crowded as they went from terminal to terminal. He began to feel claustrophobic but closed his eyes and forced himself to breathe slowly, diluting the fetor of unwashed bodies so poorly masked with local, cheap perfume. The cologne brought the onboard odor to a level temporarily compatible with human life, an ambience that gave him hope until another dozen passengers squeezed on at the Tsvetnoy Central Market. A man yanked at Elliott's backpack and scolded him to remove it. As he slipped it off, an old woman, so swathed in body odor even *she* had been elbowed toward the back of the bus, stepped into the newly created space in front of Elliott. Crushed against his body, the woman raised the freshly beheaded, partially defeathered chicken in her left fist and a moldy, sprouting onion in her right to her face to disguise the odd foreigner's spoor. Elliott tried breathing through his mouth, tiny sips of air at a time, but that failed miserably. The harder he struggled to limit air intake, the more he felt detached from himself, numb, terrified that he was going to die, or at best lose consciousness. He could feel his heart pounding and taste sweat dripping into his mouth.

A wave of nausea swept over him, and he exploded through the rear emergency door. As his feet slammed against the macadam, his backpack flew from his grasp, and he stood in traffic, vomiting, cars swerving, the thud of the backpack being run over a thrum beating in syncopation with his retching.

Irena tugged the stop cord and walked calmly back a block to guide Elliott into a tea shop. She sighed, "We take cab."

Outside, she raised her hand for a taxi, but the first few screwed their faces when they focused on her face and zoomed off without a second look. After ten minutes of snubs, a cab pulled around the corner and stopped in front of them even though Irena had not waved it down.

They sat in the fetid vehicle for miles, smoke from the noxious Sobranie Black Russian cigarettes the cabbie chain-smoked forcing Elliott to demand they stop to allow him to vomit once again. When he was done, he crawled back inside and snapped, almost tearfully, “What the hell’s goin’ on? Why am I here?”

The answer was so vociferous, her voice drowned his grunt as she punched him in the thigh. “You really are tired from trip! You forget we are going to chemistry professor dacha for dinner. Moscow University, Moscow University,” she repeated stridently, “want to welcome you. But first, we stop to freshen.”

They continued along the cratered highway toward the outskirts of Moscow, the sun slowly setting behind them. It was getting so cold inside the cab, Elliott began to shiver. Irena rolled her eyes and spoke stonily to the driver in Russian. “Find a black market to buy my friend a coat. You’ll get ten extra rubles.”

The driver shot into a parking lot and went to the trunk. He pulled free a used black parka, food stains on the front. He grunted, “I want fifty for it.”

Irena gasped. “Never mind. I’m not the Czarina, you know.”

“Okay, forty-five.”

She pretended to talk it over with Elliott, who asked how much that came to. “Forty rubles is ten dollars. I complain. We get for twenty-five.”

She turned back to the cabbie but spoke in English. “No. Twenty.”

With voices rising and falling like a Russian opera, the coat was thrown back into the trunk several times until they agreed on thirty. The cabbie stuck out his hand for immediate payment. Irena jammed six five-ruble notes forward. He counted with his tobacco-stained fingers several times before the howling started anew, in

English. "You say, 'Bring me to black market. I give you ten rubles.' I am black market. Give me ten more." He settled for five, and before he got back in the cab, Irena whispered to Elliott, "He can speak English. You do not say one word."

They set back off into the darkened Moscow suburbs, eventually lurching to a stop in front of a seedy hotel. Irena flipped a handful of bills at the man, turned her head arrogantly, and tugged Elliott into the dismal lobby.

At the decaying desk, she stuck her hand out impatiently toward Elliott. "Passport."

"What for?"

"I give to hotel. You get back when leaving."

Elliott eyed the greasy, pockmarked desk attendant, a Sobranie Black hanging by its gold filter to his bottom lip. Another was still smoldering into his face, its black paper burning down on top of a mounded pile of butts in a tin can ashtray. Elliott muttered, "No way."

Irena snatched the passport from his hand, slapped it on the desk, and maneuvered him past signs pointing to the elevator. The door was ajar, the cab stalled two floors above, cigarette butts stuck to the shaft's greasy walls. A long-ago-written, pencil-scribbled note hung from the quarter-open door. Even Elliott understood it—Out of Order.

In Irena's third floor room, Elliott was surprised to see her things scattered about. At home, she had always been so neat. She picked up the bras and panties, spitting as she tossed them back into a partially open drawer, "Asshole perverts."

Her shoulders collapsed, and she fell backwards onto the concave bed, exhaling as if she'd only a minute before managed to escape from prison. "Hello, again, Elliott Sass," she sighed, then lowered her voice as if speaking to herself. "This is insane. Maybe we go in morning back to airport. Take next plane to New York."

Elliott's eyes widened. "What's insane? What am I doing here? Why won't you talk to me?"

She sat up and stared at him for a moment before whispering, "Welcome to Soviet Union, Elliott Sass. In USSR you must not speak in public. Everyone listens, cabbie listened."

"What are you talking about? Guy barely spoke a word of English."

"Yes, but KGB gives him tape recorder. KGB sure to follow us from airport. Maybe state police believe you are member of stupid *Amerikanskiy* delegation. You escape group to spy. Elliott Sass, you are crazy in head to jump from bus on Moscow street?"

"It stunk in there. I couldn't take it anymore."

"You will soon be used to it. Many people live with no hot water or indoor water. Many people do not care how clean they are. In Moscow, much better than when I was child in Steppes. So clear, communist system will soon implode. But I do not care, just be careful not to be here when explosion changes Russia." She paused for a moment, tiptoed to the door, opened it quickly, looked up and down the hall, and turned to him. "We are okay here in room for now. Hotel did not know I have guest, so no need to bug room. Now, they will bug. We go for walk soon, give some time for bug to put in room…"

"Let them bug us?"

"No choice. Standard procedure, hotel, embassy, every embassy. All I can tell you now," she put her lips next to his ear, "I need special friend to come help find fortune of my father. Maybe we will find, maybe not. Probably not. It is to be here in Moscow, if it is here."

"*Maybe* we will find it?"

"Yes. If it is here, we are to be very rich, I think. If it is not, we are to be still very rich, but sometime later. It is confused story. You must trust me. I must trust you.

"Here in room, okay to talk about trip, maybe we talk about p-chem. I am sure you need to talk about p-chem; and we talk about what is for dinner. That is all. Elliott Sass, you have come into twilight zone."

They left the hotel for a walk through an almost deserted neighborhood, Irena studiously ignoring an old car with a man in the driver's seat, his head an inch above the level of the headrest. She whispered they were being followed, and Elliott was not to breathe a word. In three minutes, they arrived at an empty restaurant where she ordered two bowls of borsht. She snipped as the grubby waiter left without a word or change in expression, "At least it is boiled once, maybe once." Forty minutes later, a different waiter brought the bowls, a thumb in each. When the man licked his fingers, Elliott opened his mouth to protest, but Irena rolled her eyes. "Do not bother. He has no idea. Anyway, those fingers are now cleanest thing in restaurant."

She leaned in close and took his hand. "Pretend we are lovers." He smiled plastically, and she went on. "Good. You put arm around Irena. We whisper. Soon you will understand whole story. If people come close, speak about chemistry."

He nodded again and took a few dribbles of the borsht; sugar-cube sized lumps of beef and pork, mostly fat, floated in the center. His spoon fell to the floor. He didn't bother to pick it off the grit-covered linoleum, nor did the waiter. While Elliott wiped his mouth with his sleeve, trying not to gag, Irena looked away, took a spoonful of the soup, dropped a few bills on the table, and mumbled, "I will buy groceries in morning. Bread, cheese, wine, fruit. Okay, we go for walk."

Down the street sat the car she'd noticed at the hotel. The engine was running, black smoke dribbling out of the beaten muffler. She giggled and ordered, "Put arm on my shoulder. Okay, now we walk around block back to hotel." As they took the first steps, the car moved forward slowly. "They want us to know we are followed. That is good thing."

"What? What do you mean?"

"You did not see car at hotel, one behind us now?"

"No."

"You would not be good Russian. But who wants to be good Russian? That is local police. Hotel calls them if foreigner takes room. Police follow for hours, then they go to harassing other people."

At the end of the block, before they turned the corner, Irena whispered, "Not to look. Across street is cemetery. It is reason you travel half of world. Story is almost not to believe. I tell you when good time, sorry."

The car followed until they reached the hotel entrance. As they walked through the doors, Elliott spun around aggressively and flipped a middle finger at the driver. Irena smacked his hand down. "Get inside. Do not to do that again."

She pushed him into a worn chair in the lobby and started on him before his butt hit the cushion. "You do not behave, fine. Do not," she searched for a word, "bring in me. This is Soviet Union, Elliott Sass. You do not show respect for government, off you go to jail. No court lawyer, no bail. After three months, your name is delivered to American Embassy." Her eyes reddened. "Behave yourself!"

She calmed somewhat and walked to a hissing samovar in the corner. Holding two cups of tea, she sat down across from him and talked about NYU, p-chem, and her boss at the chemistry lab. "Pervert. Always leaning over me, chest touching shoulder. One day he just asks to go to bed with me."

"Did you?"

"*You* are pervert, Elliott Sass! No. Then he reminds, my stipend money comes out of research fund he controls."

Elliott laughed, "Big guy, bushy beard?"

Irena's face tightened. "How did you know?" Elliott looked away, and her voice hardened. "Tell me!"

"I went up there looking for you."

"Why?"

"Sort of missed you."

"Sort of?"

"You were so cool when you were teaching. I think everyone was scared of you."

"*You* were scared?"

"A little. But then I thought about how good we are, you know, when we get together."

"Yeah, yeah, yeah. If you poke Russian bear, you will not be together with Irena or any female for very long time. I say female because Russian prison not so different from USA. Maybe worse." She looked around the room with a flicker of her eyes. "Listen, we are going to room. There is bug, for sure. No talking."

"Can we do other things?"

"Maybe. You should enjoy it. May be last time. You have learned something?"

CHAPTER TWELVE

They ran to the shower; the bathroom, though, was as frigid as the life Irena had led in the tundra. She watched Elliott and scoffed as he shivered then began to quake. "Elliott Sass, this is sauna. Be glad."

"No, do something!"

She went to the window and pulled aside the molded, cotton curtain. "Ah, here is our problem." She pointed to several smashed panes, eons of dirt and spiderwebs clinging to the edges of the shattered glass. She lifted the dried-out patches of duct tape that had fallen from the gaps and tossed them through the breaks. She laughed and reached over to turn the shower spigot to full hot. After a few moments, the trickle became lukewarm, but it also stunk.

He grunted, "That's going to be like trying to shower in spit. You need to complain to the manager."

She shook her head. "So, chemistry major, what causes this smell?"

"I don't know. Borsht?"

"It is manganese. One of minerals that clog all pipes in Soviet Union. Get in before we freeze to death."

Less than a minute later, the weak stream promptly converted to a hiss of boiling yellow liquid. She twisted the spigot to add a bit of cold water, an adjustment that, while lowering the temperature, also brought a heavy whine and banging to the pipes. It was a cacophony as sinister as that of the beaten Aeroflot engines that had propelled him to Moscow. Irena smiled and spoke softly in his ear, "Ah, so we have discovered silver lining. We can talk here, but only in whisper."

He brought his lips close to her and stuttered, "I can't talk about anything until you let me touch you."

She turned the water off, bringing instant silence to the room. They giggled and ran to the bed that was more clamshell than horizontal, made love, then slept for several hours. At midnight, she shook him awake and spoke normally. "I try again for shower," but she brought her lips to his ear. "Get dressed. Take chair. We are in there for long time."

Inside, Irena turned on the water and found the setting that produced the loudest squeal. She spoke in a whisper. "Okay, Mr. Elliott Sass, this is why you are in USSR. Back in New York, chemistry dean sends note about my father. He is very ill. I want to see him before he is gone. I leave from New York so fast, I did not tell you. I am sorry. Also, probably it did not matter to you." He began to sputter a denial, but she waved her hand at his mouth. "Just listen. I find him in hell hospital in Siberia."

"Oh my God, Siberia—one of those gulags?"

"Almost. There is no more gulag. Now it is labor camp, or commune farm, both terrible. Anyway, it was total decay, father and building. I never told you whole story. He was prisoner sent to live in communal farm. I am born there, grow up there, but I have told you this part already."

She explained she had not known how prescient her father had been as the atmosphere in the Kremlin putrefied in the weeks before his arrest. He told Irena on his deathbed that he'd amassed a fortune, but she feared he was so demented, it was impossible to know what was true, and what was roiling in his imagination.

She explained that as Anatoli's reputation had tarnished, his troubles led finally to his imprisonment. He became a pariah, and so, by extension, did his wife; and by extension, his wife's family, especially her long-deceased father. "It is way they control us. Who wants to bring shame on three generations of two sides of family? Who wants entire family to be sent to gulag? They are very effective."

Her father had held out hope his first wife would try to rescue him, but in all those years, he had never heard from her, or anyone else from his past. There was one visitor from the

Agriculture Bureau, though, who sidled up to Anatoli and mumbled a few words. "Go to Yuri Yevtushenko. He will help you."

Yuri Yevtushenko. Anatoli mumbled on incoherently about the man, his first wife's father, dead long before she and Anatoli had met. Irena was able to glean only that Yuri was buried somewhere in the outskirts of Moscow, that he had been very rich, was highly placed in the Politburo, and that he despised Stalin. Over the next hours, though, Anatoli's lucidity deteriorated, and Irena understood essentially nothing. Then, out of the blue, he became suddenly coherent and pulled Irena's ear to his lips. He made her memorize the cemetery name, section, lane, row, and plot, perseverating that a fortune awaited. He repeated it over and over until his mouth was so dry, he couldn't speak at all. As Irena trickled cloudy water on his lips, she read back the numbers. He smiled, coughed, and was gone.

Irena's eyes clouded. "I was sad, but it was blessing. He was good man. You would have liked him." She remained silent for a few seconds. "I tried to pay medical examiner to find nice casket and give proper burial. He said ground is too hard, you know, permafrost. Can only do cremation."

Elliott blurted, "Wait a minute. Permafrost's there all year long. What, they never dig a grave east of Moscow?"

"More quietly, please. State usually pays for hospital and final expenses. A joke, but bastards shoved bill in my face for hospital and burial—over two thousand rubles. I negotiated, offered to pay medical examiner under table. My condition: I will accept cremation, but he must wait four days to notify central government I am gone.

"So, now, Elliott Sass, you are here to help me. We must find what is buried by grave, if anything, if such grave is here. Maybe we have some luck, find something without becoming arrested. But if we find something, *then* problems begin. We must smuggle it out of Russia."

"You want me involved? Can I be arrested if they catch me?"

"You can be arrested if they do not catch you, especially if you do not have in your bag what they arrest you for. We are taking chance. Very simple."

The water had long-since run cold, and the banging on their walls from sleep-deprived guests so thunderous, they ran into the room, jumped under the covers, and made love again.

They slept late, eventually dressing and walking the streets of the Kupnya District to buy a lunch of moldy bread, tasteless cheese, and vodka, which they took to a park across from the cemetery. When the man in the surveillance car parked thirty yards away, she mouthed a warning, "*Ublyudok* is still here. Thought he would be gone by now."

"*Ubly* what?"

"Bastard. Now please take my hand, walk with me, slowly. Maybe you can look like you are happy to be next to me. Back to hotel. Inside, you go to room. I will get key from desk. I have special job to do. You disappear."

At the desk, she asked where to find the lobby bathroom. The young clerk pushed a key across the counter. Inside, she took a bottle of perfume from her purse and touched a drop to her wrist. She opened her parka far enough that the outline of her breasts in the tight red sweater became the focal point of any normal man's gaze. She pulled free a piece of coarse toilet paper, fashioned two raison-sized nubbins, slipped them into her bra, and walked back to the counter.

She slowly slid the bathroom key across the desk toward the young man's hand, waiting until she saw the most subtle flaring of his nostrils. She straightened her shoulders. By instinct, his eyes locked on her chest.

She asked his name. He reddened and answered thickly, "Fedor," then gasped when she touched his hand and pointed to her room key.

She smiled gently. "So, you're Fedor, 'A gift from God,' yes?"

He paused, tongue-tied, but finally looked to the other guests drinking tea in the lobby and whispered, "It is you who are the gift from God. Your husband is very lucky."

She smiled, "You are sweet. And he's not my husband, just a cousin. So young, but already a great professor of chemistry. He's here to give a lecture at the University of Moscow. But that's not important.

"You know, Fedor, I have been away from Moscow for several years. Would you like to take a walk, say, when you're done with your duties? The snow is really beautiful. Ah, do you know the cemetery across the way?" She hitched her head in that direction.

"Yes, I used to work there."

"Oh, my. How scary."

Fedor harrumphed, "I'm not scared of anything."

"Really? Can we take a walk in there? Help me learn not to be afraid of the spirits of the dead. What do you say?"

"I'm done at three. We could go then, but it is much more fun at night. I'll take care of you."

And so, it was arranged.

Elliott was standing impatiently outside the room when she climbed the last steps. Her parka was still open, and his eyes flashed as if a radar intercept officer's onto her breasts. "What's going on, Irena?"

She reached into her bra, pulled the TP free, and flipped the stubs to the ground. He stood with his mouth open. She shook her head. "You know, Elliott Sass, I did not have courage three months ago to do this. Maybe I should say thank you.

"I have plan. Kid at desk. He will help us. But he does not know it yet."

"Whatta you, gonna show him your tits?"

"No more than I just showed you. But I must soften him first."

"Sounds like you're trying to harden him, and I don't like it. No rules here. He could be a rapist."

She was quiet for a moment. "You know, Elliott Sass, I am Russian. Government is toxic, but there is basic respect here that you do not always see in your country. Our terrible things are terrible, but so are yours. You can be sure there is far more rape on streets of Manhattan than in Moscow…"

His palm shot up to silence her. "Well, that's not what *I* heard."

"And where do you hear that?"

"Everybody in America knows it."

She was going to snap back at him crossly but calmed herself. "Look, this is not time or place to debate sociology. We have job to do. Now come with me."

She took his arm and led him into the bathroom to stand by the window. They looked out, breaking crusts of dry bread and cutting wedges of spoiled cheese for lunch. Elliott took a swig of vodka and handed her the bottle. "No. We have work to do. You can get drunk when we are done. It will be champagne and Baluga caviar if things work like we must make them. I think they will, *if* you do your part. Now, look out window at cemetery."

It was vast, a hundred acres of gravestones dating from the 1700s. Some were being dug that day. Irena spoke in a distant whisper, robotically, with as little emotion as if reciting from the Periodic Table. "Section 3, Lane 2, Row 49, Plot 36." She shook her head. "This is how we will find grave. We know cop will shadow us, especially because you and he are close friends."

Elliott huffed, "He wants to screw with me, then fuck 'im." Elliott's face tightened, and he spit on the floor. "I'm not scared of him. I'm an American citizen. They have no power to touch me. And I'm from the *City*, ain't nobody's bitch."

Irena shook her head. "You do not understand, do you? You are not guest here. You are tolerated, barely, only if government decides. If they do not like your shoe style, off you go to gulag. Seven years, if they do not disappear you right away. If you do not want to accept that here you are nothing, then you tell me right now. We get you out of USSR fast."

He postured childishly but finally growled, "Okay. What do you want me to do?"

"Good. Now, with goon following us, when we walk into cemetery, we are guilty of some felony. They know we have no business to be there. And, I do not have idea where grave is; we could walk for eight hours, never find it. We need someone to help. Kid at front desk knows cemetery. Worked there. He will take me for walk this afternoon. I make him use back door to get me out of hotel so your friend does not see. I will memorize path. We will go back tonight to find our future."

Elliott gasped. "I don't like this. How are we going to carry tools and not get caught?"

"I will take care of it."

At mid-afternoon, minutes before Fedor was to end his shift, Irena appeared in the lobby, smiling coquettishly at him. She waited in a corner until there were no guests at the desk then sidled up. "Fedor, could we go out some private door? I don't want people to think I have one man upstairs, one downstairs." She winked.

Fedor's hands trembled as he pulled a ring of keys from under the desk, pretending to be handing over a room key. "It's Sunday. Hotel restaurant's closed. Yeah, we can go out the back way." He picked a key and told her to unlock the dining room doors and wait for him in the kitchen. "Don't worry, I'm alone here today. All the bosses and the cooks are home getting drunk to forget tomorrow is Monday."

Inside the darkened kitchen, she headed straight for the utility closet. Hoping to find a shovel, she came across only a thick metal spatula and several heavy kitchen knives. She slid them into the sheet of congealed grease under the refrigerator then searched for heavier tools, looking into the toilet cubicle that sat between the two massive, wrought iron stoves. There was nothing but a seatless commode, no brush, not a sheet of toilet paper, a drop of soap, or a sink. She followed a corridor until coming to a second exit out of sight of the food prep area. She opened the bolt, jammed a piece of aluminum foil into the lock, and pushed the door closed quietly. In an instant, though, the wind blew it wide open. She thought of sliding a knife under the bottom edge, but that might get too tightly wedged if the wind strengthened, so she went to the cooler, borrowed a hard rind of fat from a slab of pork belly, and wedged it between the bottom of the door and the floor. She thought twice about it, but hearing the dining room door open, accepted that it would have to do.

She rushed back into the kitchen proper, kicking the handles of the spatulas and knives further under the refrigerator. As the door opened, she pulled the zipper on her parka down a bit further.

CHAPTER THIRTEEN

Fedor led her out the main kitchen exit and turned back to lock it carefully. Irena took his arm as they crossed the street. She peeked over his shoulder to check on the tail. He was asleep at the wheel, a cigarette hanging from his lower lip. Irena whispered, "Could we just walk along the outside of the cemetery first? It's so famous, I want to say I saw the whole place. But I do want to go inside in a little while when it gets really dark. Just promise you'll take care of me."

Fedor huffed, "You have no worry in this world."

She laughed nervously, "It's the next world I'm scared of."

He squeezed her arm roughly. "You must trust me."

Moscow's latitude is fifty-six degrees north compared to New York City's forty. In December, the sun sets in the Russian capitol around mid-afternoon. As they walked, the darkening sky became clouded with snow, a fine, dry layer soon blanketing the crusty remnants of the snow from two days before. By four, the sky was black, speckled only by snowflakes that added to the ground accumulation at seemingly an inch a minute. She spoke softly to Fedor. "I'd love to go inside. I'm feeling pretty safe with you."

He led her to a service gate at the back of the cemetery. She waited as he winked and lifted a paving stone to pull free a gigantic skeleton key which he jammed and wrenched until it seated in the lock. He worked it back and forth, finally breaking the ice seal. The gate creaked open. He ushered her in, secured the gate, and reached outside to place the key back under the square of concrete.

"Okay, we're finally here. Let me show you some famous graves." He rattled off a slew of names, few of which were prominent figures, but she oohed and aahed after each. Holding his arm tightly she asked, "You know, Fedor, I've never been in a place like this. I'm such a nerdy scientist. Could you explain how the cemetery is organized? Is it by neighborhoods, streets…?"

"Yes and no. But it's very easy. There are sections, lanes, rows, and plots. I'll show you." He chose a grave at random. "We'll work backwards. This is plot 43, yes?" He pointed to a tiny copper plate at the foot of the grave. "You see, 43, 31, 26, 2? So, this is Plot 43, Row 31, Lane 26, Section 2."

She brushed the snow off the crypt to the left. It was numbered, 41, 31, 26, 2, and the one directly across, 42, 31, 26, 2. "So, it's no different than street addresses, all even plots on one side of a row, odd on the other. Very clever. But how does one find an ancestor's grave?"

"Clever, yes, especially since it began three-hundred years ago. But you see, there are spaces without graves, bodies moved over the centuries, sometimes comrades who allowed their tongues to flutter harder than they waved the Hammer and Sickle. So, you can never tell where a grave is unless you go to the main office and look in the master volume. But let me show you." He took her arm and went to the beginning of a row and pointed at a five-foot high brick marker engraved with numbers."

"I see. Let's say, ah, let me pick out some numbers from the air. Say, Section 3, Lane 2, Row 49, Plot 32. I bet you can find that blindfolded!"

"No problem. Follow me." Without even glancing at the brick signs, he zoomed several rows before she stopped him.

"Fedor, wait a second. I want to look at some of the markers, just to see if I can follow the ancient plan." He looked at her askance. "Like I told you, I'm a nerdy scientist. I'm in love with numbers and arithmetic sequences."

He stared at her for a second, shrugged, then went on pointing out the numbers and how they decreased as one drifted toward the cemetery's great wooden front gates. The burgeoning snow slowed them, but many turns later, they came to Section 3,

Lane 2, Row 49, Plot 32. He pointed at the plaque, and she brushed away the snow. "You're right!" Then she skipped a grave and looked at the marker. It was number 34. "This is fascinating. How can I thank you? I will never forget this."

He blushed and helped her up. She touched his face with her gloved hand, and his cheeks warmed so with the rush of blood, snowflakes melted. He whispered, "You don't seem very scared. I did a pretty good job."

"Yes, Fedor, you did. But I'm getting a little cold. Could we look at one more grave, and then I think we should go. My cousin's probably getting worried. I told him I was going into the street to buy dinner."

His head dropped. "Of course."

She brushed the snow from the next plaque, Number 36, and smiled at Fedor, "This is really nifty." Nonchalantly, she ran her glove over the headstone to read the name. "Ah, Yevtushenko. Let's see, Yuri. Was he famous?"

"Yeah, he was. A writer, if I remember correctly. Very rich. Musta got in a lot of trouble with the Kremlin. That's why it's so overgrown. Family's afraid to come here and care for it." He paused, then blurted, "Could we go out again? I can take you to the best café around here. Real tea, not that crappy tea shop sweepings and dust the hotel buys to brew in the lobby."

"I would like that. But I have to be careful. My cousin's an American, Bible thumper. He thinks he has to watch over me every minute; my mother made him promise not to let me out of his sight. But we will find a way.

"Oh, and, also, we have to be up very early tomorrow to go to Moscow University. His first lecture's at eight. What time does the desk open in the morning?"

"Seven."

"We have to be gone by then." She pulled him close. "How can we be sure to get our passports and visas that early?"

"You can't. But why do you need them if you're only going into Moscow Central?"

"Our visas are educational. They have to be stamped each time we go into the university, so that we can keep a record of the time we were at so-called work."

He stared at her for a moment. She smiled softly. He gushed, "Look, I'm not working tomorrow, so I'll give them to you tonight. I'm not supposed to, so don't tell anyone. Promise?"

"Fedor, are you silly? Don't forget, *I* am as Russian as you. That's why I like you so much. Finally, a Russian man I can talk to who won't go off blabbing to strangers. Those Americans, they chatter way too much. Yuk. Weak, stupid."

As they walked to the back gate, she stayed a step behind him, dragging her feet, leaving a trail to follow when she returned with Elliott.

Fedor tried to unlock the door as he had twenty minutes before, but the mechanism was so frozen, he bent forward and blew warm breath into the keyhole. "Maybe it's permanently frozen, and we are trapped in here forever!" But it opened, and as Fedor squatted to replace the key, it gave Irena a chance to furtively turn back and see the highway in the snow she'd plowed.

She gave him a peck on the cheek and held his hands as they said goodbye at the kitchen door. Inside, he had her climb halfway up the back stairs as he snuck the keys into the drawer under the front desk then pulled free the passports. He met her on the landing. She kissed him once again.

He asked tremulously, "Tell me when I can see you."

"She touched his lips. "Let's plan on the day after tomorrow. When you are done with work."

CHAPTER FOURTEEN

She burst into the room hissing, but in a whisper, "Pack everything. We are leaving tonight."

"What are you talking about. Why, is that cop going to arrest me?"

"No, Elliott, he is no longer important. I have found grave. And I have tools to dig. Get dressed. We are going as soon as we pack, but we are going to leave few things lying about, especially food wrappers. I want you to bring bottle of vodka and your lighter."

"Why?"

"Just do it, Elliott Sass."

As they spoke, Irena heard rattling in the hallway, and she cracked the door a sliver, jumping back as a burly man reached forward with a key. He stumbled into the room, the reek of alcohol so powerful, Irena took another step back, nearly tripping on the tattered rug. Elliott bolted his eyes on the drunk for less than two seconds before grabbing a brass table lamp. He lifted it ferociously over his head. "You wanna fuck with me, pal, come on!" The man cowered, and Irena turned to see the bludgeon starting down toward the intruder's head.

She gasped and pushed Elliott backward. "You are crazy? It is just old drunk." She tore the lamp free and threw it to the floor. It crashed with a bang and then an explosion, glass skittering across the room. She placed her hands on the man's shoulders and guided him out the door, thought for a second, and went into the hallway to steer him to his room. She opened his door and helped him onto the bed.

She ran back snarling. "Come right now, Elliott."

"I'm not done packing."

"We are going to have visitors in one minute. Come on!"

She locked the door behind them and yanked him down the back staircase into the kitchen. She felt around under the refrigerator for the knives and spatulas, shoving them wordlessly into Elliott's backpack. With a shoulder to the service door, it swung open into the worsening winter storm. Elliott backed several steps, but she tugged him into the blizzard.

She chose a street opposite the one she'd walked with Fedor. By the time they circled several blocks, the back gate of the cemetery appeared through the veil of snow. Once again, the key refused to turn. She asked for his lighter. Heating the metal with the tiny flame failed miserably.

"Maybe pour little vodka on lock." He did, and she tried to light the alcohol, but it had frozen that quickly. On the third try, a fleeting, pale blue flame appeared, a drop of water oozed free, and the key turned.

The snow had fallen with such fury in the short time since leaving Fedor, it was if her tracks had never existed. She remembered the first few legs of the path and said nothing as she pulled Elliott along. They brushed snow from brick markers, but the wind whipped so wildly, the pillars were recovered before she could lean forward to read them. She made a tent out of her muffler and, using the lighter, slowly moved forward. As the temperature dove even farther below zero, Elliott began chattering that it was too cold to go on, then whined he was hungry and was going back to the room. Ignoring him, Irena slogged the powder, up and down lanes and rows until the lighter's flame became a last flicker. She thought she recognized the corner of Row 49 and trundled past eighteen graves.

With a deep sigh, she came to a stop, turned to her left and stood silently, hunched forward, catching her breath for a few seconds. She finally swiped at the marker with her glove. "We are here, Plot 36." She dusted the jacket of snow from the headstone. "You see, Yevtushenko."

Taking the tools from Elliott's backpack, she went to her knees at the rear of the grave and began hacking at the ivy that had grown as thick and woody as tree branches. It soon appeared the effort was going to be futile, but she dug and cut ferociously until a small area was semi-cleared. She took the vodka from his backpack, poured a bit into the earth, and waited a few seconds to see if there was one more breath in the lighter. There was, and though it burned out in seconds, she was able to cut the now semi-frozen dirt into cubes which she scooped out with a spatula. Soon out of breath, she pushed Elliott into position, and they took turns removing one-inch layers of rock-hard dirt at a time. At a depth of six inches, she plunged the knife even farther, probing for something solid.

Elliott dropped back down and nudged her aside, angrily seizing a fistful of ivy runners, grunting savagely until frozen clumps of superficial roots pulled free, and the surface area of the dig was doubled. He began excavating with the spatula, though might as well have been using wet cardboard, for the ground was that indestructible.

They warmed the earth to the flanks of the original hole with vodka. Twenty minutes passed. Exhausted, their clothing soaked with sweat, the instant one stopped digging, the moisture froze; the instant the other took over, the ice softened to run in freezing rivulets down their bodies.

Elliott stopped angrily and turned to Irena. "There's nothing here. Probably never was. Probably the wrong goddamn Yevtushenko. It's time to get the hell out of here and out of Russia. And I'm never comin' back."

She rose to her feet and whispered, "You are right."

He took the knife and stabbed it into the earth to steady himself as he unfolded his rigid legs. When he placed his full weight on the handle, the blade slid a few inches deeper, but came to so abrupt a stop, his hand slipped past the grip. His palm seared with pain, and he could feel blood oozing onto his fingers. He blurted, "I hate this fuckin' place!"

Irena shooshed him crossly, but he held up his palm. Though it seemed pitch black, she saw the blood, then the laceration. "*Bozhe moi, bozhe moi*! Oh, my God! What have you done? Elliott, make fist."

"It hurts."

"I don't care. I have to see if you cut tendons."

He slowly curled his fingers, and she resisted each digit. Not sensing weakness, she opened his backpack, took out a T-shirt, and wrapped the palm tightly. "Now tell me how you managed to do this."

"Hit a boulder, I think."

"Boulder? When grave is dug, every stone is put aside to add to cement for building. No, there is no big rock. Let me look."

She scraped and stabbed, creating a new hole that could not have been four inches in depth before the knife struck an object that clunked. It felt and sounded far more like soft metal than stone. She worked the blade along the material in a straight line until coming to a change in the feel of whatever it was. She suddenly recognized it as a corner. With that, she stabbed furiously until a rectangular perimeter emerged. The moment she paused to take a breath, Elliott dropped to his knees and scraped frenetically with the spatula. In minutes, even in the dark, they saw a change in the tone of the earth around the piece, a scattering of aquamarine dust mixed with the brown soil. Taking turns rasping and gouging, a sheet of severely oxidized copper emerged through the tailings. The dirt at this depth was not as frozen as at the surface, and Irena refused to rest, grabbing the spatula from Elliott to slide it vertically, wedging back and forth until she was able to loosen what seemed to be a small canister. Elliott impatiently squeezed in front of her and pulled at the object crudely with uncoordinated efforts that wasted dollops of energy but brought no progress. He finally lost patience, came to a squat, and grunted like a Russian Olympic weightlifter. With a grand tug, he straightened his legs, but his bloody fingers lost their purchase, and he tumbled backward into the snow. Irena put a hand over her mouth to hide a smile, but when Elliott began to laugh, she offered her hand to help him back to his knees.

"Let me." Her fingers slipped along the edges, pulling straight up, easily freeing a one-foot metal cube. She brushed away the dirt and hefted it. "Is less than five pounds, made in home workshop. Look, sides are only thin copper sheet with rivets at corners." She tried to pull the lid off, but it was so badly oxidized, it did not move a millimeter even when she wedged the knife blade between the lid and body. She began contemplating the substances a chemist could apply to overcome the oxidation. Giving up, she asked Elliott for the cigarette lighter one last time. In the final flicker, she saw the seam had been entirely sealed with solder.

Irena droned, "How far are we going to get carrying this thing in Moscow streets? What next? Let me try backpack." They stretched the material, slicing strategically with one of the knives, but it simply would not fit, squeeze as they might. "*Govno,*" she spit."

"Yeah, what does 'governor' mean in Russian? I keep hearing it."

"No, not governor, *govno*. It means shit, silly boy. Well, I suppose it will fit in my suitcase, and so back we go. You stay outside, across street, and I go upstairs. That is if kitchen is not full of cooks."

She kicked a bit of dirt back in the hole, and Elliott spread a few ivy vines over it, but they soon quit and ran to the gate. She locked it and threw the key as hard as she could back over the wall, and then they trudged through the ever-thickening snow toward the hotel. From across the parking lot, it appeared the back door was closed and that a light was on in the kitchen. She slinked to the service door, weaving in a low crawl through the randomly parked jalopies. She pulled on the door, not expecting movement, but it opened easily, and she froze before pushing it back silently, leaving it a half inch ajar. She placed her ear to the opening. When there were no sounds, she opened it a couple of centimeters. Seeing no movement, she crept down the hall toward the main kitchen. It was empty, but the door to the toilet which had been propped open earlier in the evening, was now shut. The unpainted plywood was so inadequate, a chorus of grunts and gushing gas passed through easily.

She charged up the backstairs to their room, pulled her valise from the closet, and ran into the icy bathroom. As she pushed on the window to fling the suitcase free, the entire frame fell out into the parking lot. She tensed, awaiting the crash, but it had fallen onto what was now two feet of snow. The bag hit silently with nothing but a puff of white to record its arrival. The whole thing was buried by enormous flakes in seconds.

She could not go out the front door without turning in her key, so there was only one choice. She prayed for constipation amongst the kitchen staff, but it was almost certainly the opposite. She was correct. Through a crack in the dining room door, she spied a burly, unshaven, middle-aged man emerge from the loo and walk to the prep counter. He gathered a few onions and started chopping. He had not stopped to wash his hands.

She had no choice. She opened her sweat-soaked parka. This time, she was so cold, she did not have to supplement the image. Her arm swung the door open in a grand gesture, and she sashayed up to the cook. "Were you the chef yesterday? It was delicious!"

He stood wordlessly staring at her chest. She was about to touch his shoulder but thought better of it and giggled, "That always happens when they get cold. And I have to go out to my car. Do you mind if I use your door? The man at the desk is such a leech."

CHAPTER-FIFTEEN

She and Elliott hid in a tea shop blocks from the hotel. Irena slipped the proprietor a few rubles, touched the back of his hand, and asked him to call a taxi for the Kurskiy Rail Station in Moscow. She mentioned that they were on their way to Leningrad. During the hour trip, they asked the cabbie if he was familiar with the ancient city, and where to stay. He gladly answered that he had been born there and his brother owned a fine hotel right on Nevsky Prospect. He wrote the directions from Moskovsky Station to the hotel and then added a note that these two were to be well cared for as they were close friends from England.

They made certain he saw them enter the station then went to a restaurant and had tea before boarding the underground to city center, where they took a bus to the airport. Irena explained to the Aeroflot agent that they had to leave Russia right away as her father in the U.S. had had a heart attack. The best the woman could do was to find two separate seats on a flight leaving the next day at noon. Irena pretended disappointment but agreed.

She told Elliott she was sure that by now the authorities had been notified of the funny business going on with the odd couple in Room 326. There had been trips to the cemetery, broken window frames, and horrible banging noises coming from their room at all hours of the night. "You add giving your pal finger, and we slip away right under his nose; he will take as personal affront. Thank you. That is good way to make friends of our KGB. Maybe he will ask local bus drivers and cabbies if they have seen us. Maybe he will alert the police in Leningrad at Moscovsky Station, give them passport numbers. Thank you once again.

"On other hand, they will not clean our room until noon. Maybe not even realize we are gone. Even if they realize, if they call cops, they have trouble for not watching strange guests closely. If they report we are missing, KGB friend in car must decide if he wants to make big deal. He will have many embarrassing questions thrown in face. I do not know. Maybe he will track us as far as railroad station and turn over to cops in Leningrad."

Elliott contradicted, "There's no way they'll find us—too inefficient from what I've seen. What worries me is that we won't get out of here with that box. We need to find a welder to cut it with a torch."

"No, no. If it is money or anything paper, it will become smoke. We need to cut it open. I can buy file. We find hotel. They will take passports. Eventually someone will figure out we are up to no good. We must work fast."

"Who cares? Who the hell would want to come back to this place?"

"Maybe I would."

They stopped at a hardware store. In the saw section, the shelves were bare save a single rusty hacksaw blade. Irena did not bother to ask the man to check in the back. They found a cheap hotel, and Irena paid in advance for three nights. They moaned to the desk clerk about their deathly fatigue from so many days of travel and begged to go directly to their room. Also, they had to be up quite early, at six the next morning, to catch the train to Leningrad where Elliott was giving a lecture. They showed him that their internal travel permits were stamped into the actual passports. They would need them to leave Moscow.

The clerk explained the desk did not open until seven, but, for a consideration, he would send the police the information and let them keep their travel documents until they got back from Leningrad. With three days paid, there was no hurry.

They slipped him fifty rubles, and he took back their room key and handed them one for the Prime Minister's Suite. The clerk snickered, "I don't think he's staying with us this week."

The room was a good five percent superior to the one next to the cemetery. Elliott suggested they enjoy a nip of vodka before getting to work. A bit more relaxed, they made a muffler of blankets and Elliott began to saw. In seconds, the blade snapped and jammed into the palm of his good hand. She wrapped it in a bra, took the longer fragment, and started sawing. It, too, shattered, but she had penetrated the metal to open a half-inch gap along a corner. She took the knife they'd kept, covered her hands in towels, and stabbed the hole with all her might. That tore an inch fissure in the box. Elliott placed the edge of the last spatula in the hole and worked it with both bandaged hands. As the gash grew wider, the two took turns gouging and tearing madly with their fingers. Elliott finally grabbed the box from Irena and sawed at it with the knife, a madman driving himself harder than he had at the grave site. He strained so, his eyes filled with tears.

Soon, slivers of oily brown paper sifted onto the floor. Irena picked up a scrap thinking she held cash, but it was just yellowed Russian newspaper. Elliott ripped even harder, grunting and cursing until Irena put a hand over his mouth. More newsprint came free. He pushed her hand away and, with a final profanity-laced scream, tore the box half open. Aside from more old newspaper, it seemed otherwise empty, and he dropped it angrily. The thud, though, was followed by a string of clinks as a glass jar rolled free.

Elliott lifted it to the light, twisted his lips, and grunted, "A dirty sock. It's all yours."

He flipped the bottle to her, but the lid was so rusted, she gave up twisting and tossed it back to him. "Open it, Mr. Superman!"

Contorting theatrically, Elliott managed to free the lid, but the jar opened so abruptly, a cloth bag shot out to thud on the floor. A piece of folded paper settled next to it. Irena reached for the paper first. It was covered in Roman letters, a sheet of French newsprint from a neighborhood weekly in Geneva, Switzerland. I was dated nearly twenty years before.

She shrugged and reached for the bag, but the material was so tatty, it had ruptured as it hit the ground. When she pinched the top of the cloth, the contents spread out, coming to rest in a stunted cone. Just glass shards, thought Elliott, but as Irena looked more intently at the fragments, her face reddened to scarlet. She gasped "*Bozhe moi.*"

"What?" Elliott cackled.

Irena blanched, shrieking, "*Bozhe moi, bozhe moi*! Oh, my God!"

Elliott shooshed her, picked one of the bits from the floor, perused it dismissingly, and handed it over impatiently. "What? A piece of broken glass."

Irena's hands were shaking so, the chip almost slipped through her fingers. He rolled his eyes and grasped several, even larger shards, dribbling them into a pile on the bed. He suddenly gulped, "You mean you think they're real?"

She inspected the one in her hand, ignoring his question until she asked herself softly, "Why would any person go through so much trouble to hide costume jewelry?" Her voice strengthened. "Elliott Sass, our lives are changed. Everything is upsides down." She gazed at the diamonds and the debris from inside the metal box.

Irena mused, her eyes reddening, "This must be from father's first wife. Who else could it be? But where did diamonds come from? She did not just sell everything, buy gems, and come back to Moscow twenty years ago. Does not make sense, but it does not matter. Elliott Sass, we need to get diamonds out of Russia. Quickly."

She went on in a mumble. "I have idea. Some fast work. Now, all of sudden, you are visiting professor, not chemistry, petrology.

"We write letter from my university to New York University. Letter to be signed by head of my department. He will thank NYU for sending Elliott Sass to teach new technique of oil exploration. He will write samples of shale oil you carry to be given for research with new analyzer in New York. This is part of cooperation our governments are building.

"Elliott Sass, I will take Metro to my university. Stop in to say hello in Chemistry Department. They know me. I will steal sheet of letterhead. Also make sure dean is same, and so is president. Maybe both will sign letter.

"Now, you need to do this. First, buy two black votive candles. All food markets have this, usually in back of store. I write down what to ask. Then take water glass from room, go into street, fill with dirt and pebbles, round, same size as diamonds. Get big handful. Also, go out; find old car, really old car; get under and drain oil into bottle. Do you know how to get oil from motor?"

"I think so. You undo the screw on the bottom of the engine. But I don't have any tools."

"Okay, wait here." Irena grabbed two scraps of toilet paper, placed them strategically, and went to the front desk. She asked for a pair of pliers to fix the wheels on her suitcase. She was back in the room in three minutes.

"Wait till dark, two more hours. Go to junkyard by river. No one will look at you in Russian parka. Put up hood."

"How am I supposed to do it with pliers? Don't you need a special wrench?"

She grabbed her coat and dashed out the door, calling over her shoulder, "Figure out, Professor."

Elliott cinched his hoodie and covered that with the new parka. He walked for a quarter of a mile and came to the Volga, then wandered parallel to the bank until entering an even seedier quarter of Moscow. The streets were bare save for a gaggle of alcoholics sitting around a fire. He approached and tried English but got nowhere. He tried Romanian, and a voice behind a scarf asked what he wanted. Elliott told him he needed a bottle of old motor oil and would pay fifty rubles for it and let them have the pair of pliers as a bonus. At first the man's jaw sagged, and he remained speechless until one of his brethren punched him in the arm. He babbled to his mates, "A decent meal is one ruble. Fifty rubles is a good salary for one month."

The man slugged him again. "What the hell are you talking about, Jasinsky?"

"This American says…" When their astonishment ebbed, all four jumped up, took Elliott by the arm, and dragged him over several beaten down fences into an abandoned shipyard. The ghosts of a hundred rusted cars were piled next to the rotting hulls of fishing boats that looked to have been ditched there before the Russian Revolution. Some of the rubble had been plowed into a sewage pond, the icy surface dotted with rock-hard, frozen lumps of human waste. The Romanian-speaking indigent explained that all the brake oil, motor oil, transmission fluid, rear end lubricant, combustible cloth, tires, even engine rubber seals from the more easily accessible cars, had long been scavenged to use as fuel for fires to keep the drunks alive. That meant, for this mission, they would have to climb into the contaminated, frozen water, crawl to the hulks, and get on their backs to retrieve his petroleum. There was a sudden silence, the men's eyes drifting up into the foggy night sky. The interpreter queried suspiciously, "And what's so important about dirty old motor oil?"

Elliott explained that his girlfriend's car had a leak, and he had tried to buy fresh oil, but no one in the shops had understood him, and now it was too late in the day to find an open gas station. He offered two rubles instead if the Romanian interpreter knew of a place and took him there. The men began jumping around and dragged Elliott by the arm farther into the shipyard. They stopped him before he had to walk onto the befouled ice but made sure he was suitably repulsed by the stench.

When the men returned with a bottle of what appeared to be black lard, they launched into a series of theatrical gestures reflecting the torment they'd suffered. Elliott assumed the performance was to grease the rails for more than the agreed-upon compensation, so he took the reverently proffered container and rolled his eyes. One of the men grabbed it back, opened it, and thrust it in Elliott's face. That brought on an episode of retching, the odor of his prize evocative of putrefied human remains.

His hand thrust forward the fifty rubles. When the bottle remained in the neighborhood of his face, he handed over another ten then found himself obliged to shake four hands coated in black sludge. There were broad smiles; more hand shaking; and, finally, a pause in the revelry, which he used to excuse himself.

Close to the hotel, he passed a little market and searched his pockets for Irena's note, but it had been lost in the turmoil. That didn't matter, for Irena had assured candles were in the back of all markets. He went to the rear and searched by himself until an ancient, toothless babushka waddled up and shrieked, demanding to know what he wanted. He drew a candle in the air, and as she took him by the arm, he smugly assured himself that he really had become quite the international traveler. But they didn't stop at any of the all-but-bare shelves, and he found himself in the street, the door slammed behind him.

Eventually, he found an empty restaurant in which a bewhiskered old man with only a pinky on his right hand asked, "*Amerikanskiy*?" When Elliott smiled, he pulled him inside and steered him to a chair. His face but inches from Elliott's, the man-made sounds that might have been English, though every other grunt seemed to be "fuck."

When Elliott simply shrugged, the man hobbled to the kitchen and brought back a Russian-English dictionary. He looked up enough words to form a sentence and explained that he'd been captured during World War Two. He pointed to himself and said with a bit of pride, "Igor," then pointed at Elliott.

"Elliott. I need to buy candles, black ones."

"Candle. Buy. What?" He babbled incoherently for a few minutes, every other word still sounding like "fuck." Slowly, though, the man's brain received, for the first time in fifty years, a trickle of blood to that long-fallow English language loop. A couple of minutes later, Elliott actually understood half of what was being said. It seemed Igor had bunked with GIs in a *Luft Stalag* for two years, a POW camp for captured Allied airmen. Igor's eyes reddened when he explained how well he had been cared for by the Americans during those darkest days of his nightmare.

Suddenly, the man croaked, "So, me stupid," smacked his forehead, and ran to the kitchen to bring Elliott a plate of steaming *pelmeni*, Russian dumplings stuffed with ground meat, beef, or pork—Elliott hoped—inside a dough pocket. Igor laughed and pointed to the filling. "Ah, pig." On the side were two miniature ceramic bowls, one of sour cream, the other, mayonnaise.

They sat together, the man running back to the kitchen to refill the plate constantly. He spun a tale of having had his hand partially blasted off in the Battle of Kursk, in August of 1943. He had been a tanker, and he was loading the main cannon so quickly, most of his hand was caught in the breech, his fingers sent flying in a direction opposite to that of the projectile.

Finally, Elliott groaned he could eat no more, his wife was unwell, and he had to get back to the hotel. Elliott tried again to ask where he could find two black candles. Igor rolled his eyes and pulled a box from under the front counter, riffled through the junk, and pulled free three votive candles.

Elliott extended a ten ruble note toward his new friend's left hand, the one with fingers, but the man drew his head back, affronted, and growled he would not accept a single kopeck from such a good friend. Igor touched his heart and told Elliott he was the first American he'd met since the war.

Elliott returned to the hotel, dropped off his loot, took a swig of vodka, and went into the street with a water glass. On his knees, brushing back snow to gather sand and tiny pebbles, a beat cop stopped to hover over him. Elliott looked up and pantomimed he needed the grit to clean a pan in which he had burned food. The man stood there for a few more seconds before walking off shaking his head.

Back upstairs, Elliott took two swigs of vodka and fell asleep. An hour later, he rose with a start when Irena flew in the door and collapsed on the bed next to him. She finally opened her eyes and asked, "How did it go?"

"Got everything."

"Good. I have two sheets of letterhead. Dean was there. Asked so many questions. Could not get away. Now it is late, but we have to do work. Show me what you collected." He handed her the candles and lifted the bottle of oil and the dirt-filled glass. She grunted approvingly. "We make Russian mobster out of you."

She poured a few diamonds into an ashtray. One by one she coated them carefully in hot black wax from the candle. Then she rolled them in the dirt. When all forty were done, they started on the pebbles. It took several hours to do a hundred and sixty, but in the end, there was no obvious difference between the rocks and the gems.

It was time. She opened the bottle of oil and gagged but tightened her face in determination, poured in the gems and pebbles and dirt, stirred with a spoon from the tea set, and instructed Elliott to close the bottle as tightly as his hands could twist.

"Where did you get motor oil? Sewage plant?"

"Yep."

"Okay. Customs will not want to keep bottle open. Very good. Now, you rest. I am going downstairs to use typewriter. Also, I am going to ask for passport. I will tell them we must take train to Leningrad early, staying there one night. They know we will be back. Room is already paid for."

She took the nubbins of coarse toilet paper out of her bra when she returned to the room. "That is very last time. Getting sore."

"Can I kiss the booboos?"

"Elliott Sass, you will behave. Look at two letters, one Russian to get out of USSR, one English to get into the USA. May work. If it is failure, see you in twenty years."

CHAPTER SIXTEEN

They left the hotel for the Kurskiy Rail Station at six the next morning. Inside, they laughed that they were getting to know the place as if they were everyday commuters to Leningrad, sat for an hour over tea, then took a bus to the airport and decided to wait to go through security until shortly before their flight.

"What if they ask why my passport wasn't stamped?"

Irena warned, "I will do talking. Sometimes, they do not stamp American passports. They know that can cause problems when you get back to USA. Many countries do that. I will make sure we get online with male agent. I sacrifice myself one last time."

"Are you sure I can't help?"

The agent paid little attention to Irena's face. The next step was baggage inspection, and there, an angry woman pointed at Elliott's backpack. He smiled, pulled the bottle free, unwrapped it, and placed it on the counter as if it were nothing more than a souvenir snow globe from the Moscow Zoo. Irena handed the woman both letters. The agent stared at the bottle for a moment. Finding it totally opaque, she made a circular movement with her index finger. Elliott opened it obediently, though as the stench wafted into the woman's face, she drew her head back and snapped at Elliott to close it. She shook her head and called her supervisor. He, too, made the circular motion, and, once again, the odor almost floored the officers. The male agent read the letters and summoned his superior. Several travelers began to drift over, and as the level of irritated banter rose, he began shouting at the civilians to move on or be arrested.

He asked Irena for an explanation. She pointed insistently at the letters, but the man blurted, "I think this is some sort of poison. I will not allow it."

He reached for the bottle, but Irena slowly brought her arms forward. As her hands gently touched his, goose bumps erupted on his arms. She spoke throatily. "Officer, respectfully, sir, would you please call Moscow University and ask the dean how we have worked with the Americans to develop our oil industry. This is not a weapon, sir. It smells bad, but it is harmless crude oil." She opened the bottle and took a cautious whiff. "Oh, it stinks, but it won't harm a person."

Elliott took a step forward and muttered. "What the hell do you expect 150-million-year-old dinosaur meat to smell like?"

Irena looked at him and smiled. "Elliott, shut da fuck up."

Elliott grinned and muttered, "You sound like a real American."

The agent queried Irena edgily, "You are American or Russian?"

She feigned resentment. "Russian. Do not call me *Amerikanskiy.*"

The agent ordered his underlings to keep guard over the two pests while he went back to his office to call the university, but Irena lowered her eyes and mentioned quietly that their flight time was quickly approaching. The senior officer glanced at the departure board and then his watch. He took a last gander at her chest, shook his head, and waved the back of his hand at the bottle. "Go."

Elliott pulled free the bloody undershirt from his backpack to rewrap it. The man's eyes opened as large as a radar scope. He put his hand up to stop the action and gasped, "*Amerikanskiy*, what is this, blood? You fight in my country?"

Irena explained in Russian and grabbed Elliott's lacerated hand, pointing at the upturned palm. The three officers eyed the gash and shook their heads. The senior agent asked if anyone had bothered to check Irena's suitcase, and the two dropped their shoulders in embarrassment. He tsooked and snapped the bag open. Near the top was the bloody bra. His stare shot like a rifle back to Irena's breasts; with his eyes locked there, he asked, "And this?"

Irena took Elliott's other hand and pointed to the additional laceration. He snarled, "Go now, before I change my mind."

While on the endless immigration queue at JFK, Irena leaned into Elliott, whispering. "Let me do talking," though when their time came an hour later, the man barely lifted his eyes to compare the passport photos to their faces.

At customs, nary a soul glanced at them, other, perhaps, than to stare at Irena for a humiliating instant. As they were about to exit, a foot from the hallway that led to the uncontrolled portion of the airport, they turned and smiled. "We did it!"

Their celebration was, though, one second premature. They stiffened as a German Shepherd on a tight leash came to a halt in front of Elliott, blocking the door.

The dog sniffed the air in front, to the sides, and behind Elliott, and when done, sat as stiffly as a statue. Elliott looked down at the mutt. It was smiling condescendingly. The officer demanded, "Are you carrying any contraband into the United States?"

The beads of sweat on Elliott's brow, and the visible pulsing in his neck, answered the question sufficiently for the man take his arm and lead him back, deep into the secured area and down a restricted hallway. Irena called, "Excuse me, sir, but may I come along? I have letters regarding our belongings. Everything is quite legitimate; I can promise you."

He thought for a moment and nodded. They were placed in a dirty, little grey room, on a dirty, little stainless-steel bench at a dirty, little stainless-steel table. Handcuff loops were welded into the metal. Elliott waited until there were several silhouettes hovering around the two-way mirror. He opened the backpack and withdrew the bottle, sliding it across the table. In an instant, three agents darted into the room, pistols drawn, three giants shouting for them to get on the ground. They did. They were handcuffed, pulled to their feet, and pushed back onto the bench. Their luggage was kicked to a far corner of the cell.

The agent holstered his weapon and took a seat in front of them. “Okay, what the hell’s goin’ on here?”

Elliott took a breath to answer, and the agents fixed their eyes on him, but Irena jabbed him in the ribs and snapped, “Let me explain, please.” The men tried not to smile as they turned to her.

“First, we are returning from Russia. I am chemist from Moscow University who teach advanced students at your NYU. This is Elliott Sass. He is student there. He is doing advanced studies in petrology in regard to obtaining oil from shale rock. Our department is working with petrologist in Moscow. It is all part of our joint space program.”

A new agent with captain’s bars on his collars walked in. “Well, that’s just peachy keen, but I want to know what the hell’s in this bottle. The dog alerted.”

Elliott spurted, “Dog’s wrong, but she isn’t.” He glanced at Irena.

“Elliott, please. Excuse me, officer, this is not contraband. It is nothing but crude oil and shale rock. It is new source of oil to make USA self-sufficient in fuel; that is, unless you enjoy spending day waiting to fill gas tank.”

“Yeah, right. Then, why didn’t you declare it at customs?”

“There is nothing to declare. There was no sign to say we cannot bring in bottle of pebbles and oil. It is sediment with petrified products of creation of petroleum. It has no monetary value.”

“So you say, but if you’re telling me you tried to bring it into our country, what you are importing are the remnants of dinosaurs, rotten meat; and that is a felony, patently illegal. So, either way you cut it, we have sufficient cause to hold you until we look into your story. Get comfortable.”

Neither Irena’s demeanor nor facial expression altered. “No, sir. Oil is not made of dinosaurs. It is made of millions and millions tons of tiny bacteria that grow for billions and billions years on surface of ocean. Bacteria die and drift to bottom, then covered with silt so heavy, bacteria are cooked into hydrocarbon. That is why you must dig so deep to get oil. You only need to dig few meters to get dinosaurs. Maybe you are thinking of coal. That is closer, formed from forests that die and are covered and compressed, and organic matter is cooked by pressure, but not compacted as oil. That is why you do not need to dig so deep for coal."

"Well, that's not what I learned in school."

"Sir, that is rumor began in 1933, when your Sinclair Oil Corporation sponsors dinosaur exhibit at World's Fair Chicago. They are telling everyone that world oil reserves are formed during Mesozoic Era, when dinosaurs lived. Exhibit is so popular, Sinclair adopt big green brontosaurus as company logo. Not until 1964 that we began to know better. Maybe your teacher is really old."

He peered across the table testily, but she ignored him and continued. "What I will tell you is that this stinks as if it is dead creature meat. But we are happy to open and you can test all you want for drugs or whatever your dog is good at sniffing."

"Oh, we are going to test it, but don't you touch it." He turned to his colleagues. "No one leaves until I get back."

There was silence in the cell-like room until the man returned with plastic bags and various colored test packets and swabs. He slipped on gloves and unscrewed the lid. The stench was awful. It filled the cubicle in milliseconds, and the three agents swallowed to keep from gagging. He replaced the lid quickly and ordered one of his underlings to open the door. A new officer, one wearing major's insignia, walked past but stopped abruptly, about-faced, and covered his mouth and nose but remained standing in the doorway. He barked, "What the hell's goin' on in here?" The captain pointed at the bottle, and the major went on. "That stink, I've smelled it before. Can't remember if it was toxic, a biohazard. Shit, do I have to clear the building?"

"These two are telling us it's crude oil. They're researchers at NYU, they say..."

Elliott raised an index finger. "We are. We have letters and IDs."

The agent at the desk grumbled at Elliott, "Quiet, you." He turned back to the major. "Something about getting oil from shale rock. It's bullshit. Dixie alerted. Probably just trying to cover up drugs with the stench."

"Wait a minute. Crude oil? Yeah, that's what my uncle smelled like. He was a technician out at the refinery over in Jersey, Perth Amboy. Lemme see." The agent jumped out of his seat. "It's all yours, boss."

The major opened the bottle slowly. "Yeah, that's what it is. Get me some gloves and toilet paper."

As they waited for the underling to return, Irena sat serenely, though with a trace of impatient irritation. Elliott tried to copy her expression. He could not and almost jumped out of his seat when the agent, holding a single pair of gloves, walked back in. Instead, he bit his lip so hard, he tasted salty blood trickling into his mouth. That only upped the flow of sweat dripping like a monsoon from his armpits. Still in his hoodie and parka, though, only he knew.

The agent stuck a gloved finger into the sludge, retracting a single lump of grit. Elliott felt his consciousness ebbing as the man wiped it with the toilet paper and worked the outside until there was but grit on the tissue. "This is no more a street drug than pea gravel. Lemme check another." He rolled it in his fingers and blotted it. "Same thing. Amazing that something a few billion years-old could look like the crap we sweep out of our streets. Nothing but ground up dinosaurs, that's all it is." He turned to the prisoners. "You're free to go. I hope you can figure out how to turn dirt into oil. Hated those goddamn gas lines."

CHAPTER SEVENTEEN

They stayed at Irene's place that night, so tired, they decided to wait until morning to work on the diamonds. But Elliott could not sleep and left the bed at five. He went to the bathroom and opened the jar, pouring the slime into the toilet. He did not see the few tablespoons of dirt and pebbles that slithered along with the mash. Without a thought, he flushed, and while the solids were carried away, the less viscous fractions of oil spattered out to land in a polka dot pattern on everything within three feet of the commode. He flushed once again, hoping to wash the bowl clean; however, that only turned the bathroom into a two-layer crime scene.

He went back to the kitchen and pulled free several nodules, working the wax with his fingers. It was not easy, for the coatings had hardened in the cold apartment. A much better idea was to put the dregs in a frying pan, heat it, and pour off the molten wax.

Irena awoke to the stench and shuffled into the kitchen. "What are you doing?"

"Gettin' the wax off the diamonds."

"With heat? Diamonds burn!" She pulled the pan from the fire and started toward the sink to douse the boiling slurry with cold water but hesitated and put the pan down on a cool burner. "I think if you cool too fast, can cause cracks." It was not long before a green pea omelet ten inches across formed in the frying pan.

Elliott laughed, "Calm down. Won't burn on a gas stove. Nowhere near hot enough."

"Elliott Sass, you really must study your p-chem. You are very far behind your contemporaries. Diamonds burn in air at thirteen-hundred degrees Fahrenheit. Do you know temperature of natural gas combustion in room air?"

"It's not that high."

As she poured the bottle of sludge through a strainer into a pot lined with paper towels, she called over her shoulder, "Oh, Elliott Sass, get out books. It is more than three-thousand degrees."

She sat at the table picking free nubbins from the strainer, then dried them with more paper towels. With the soaked towels and muck dumped into a baggie, she washed from the stones what she could in hot water, ammonia, and detergent. She sent Elliott into the bathroom to clean the walls, floor, and toilet, and then to the dumpster with the bag of toxins. Despite the frigid temperatures, she opened the windows, and by the time Elliott returned, the stench was more like old motor oil than sewage.

She hacked the lumps free of wax and dirt, enough to distinguish diamonds from pebbles. After an hour, she counted—thirty-six. She went through the mound of pebbles once again. She had not missed a single diamond.

"Four are gone!" She eyed him suspiciously. "Where is oil you poured off?" When his head dropped, she yelped, "What did you do with oil?"

"Poured it in the toilet." Her lips twisted, and he added, "What'd you want, I should save it for your car?"

She ran into the bathroom, sliding on a streak of oil Elliott had missed. Peering into the glazed bowl, she went pale and howled, "*O bozhe*!"

Elliott remembered that meant "Oh, God," and ran into the bathroom. Irena's face was white. "You flushed hundred thousand dollars down toilet! I could buy Rolls Royce for that! *O bozhe*!"

"Would be pretty stripped down. Might not even have a stereo."

She sighed and went back to the kitchen. "Ratio was four-to-one. How do you manage to find so many diamonds to throw away?"

She made tea, and after calming, washed the diamonds in hot water, rubbing more of the wax away. Once again, there were only thirty-six. She would not look up from the diamonds as she scraped at the remaining veneer, cautiously using a butter knife to avoid scratching the stones. She turned to Elliott. "Please, you go bring back breakfast from IHOP."

When he returned, six of the diamonds had been fully scrubbed. They sat, sparkling, in a Russian Khokhloma bowl. Elliott was taken by the hand-lacquered, translucent red, black, and gold curled leaves over which the artist had painted exquisitely daubed flowers. He reached toward it, but she softly stopped his hand.

"I am sorry. It is all I have left of mother I never saw. First, we eat breakfast. You need to rebuild strength after past week."

When the last pancake and sausage were gone, she looked up. "Elliott Sass, you will pay attention, please. I am assigning you mission. I do not care if it is legal."

CHAPTER EIGHTEEN

Papa Rueben Sassowitch listened, and when he finally fathomed his son's meandering tale, he smiled and spoke in Romanian Yiddish. His first question was direct. "How much of the take are you getting?" Elliott allowed he and Irena had not discussed that, but he assumed it would be half.

"I did not raise you to be a fool. Never assume, especially when it's a woman, and even more when it is a Russian woman. She will dump on you. You'll do the work of finding a fence, you'll do the felony, and the second the money is in her hands, she'll toss a few hundred bucks at your feet. You bend over to pick it up, she jams a shovel up your ass and runs like hell. You'll never see her again. And if you make too much of a stink, you know, threats, she'll have one of her Russian Mafia criminals call the cops they keep on the payroll. Don't worry, son, we can share a cell. Only problem is, I'll be out of here before you start your twenty years."

After half-an-hour of squabbling, Reuben groaned and agreed to help. First, he told Elliott, there were diamonds and there were diamonds. Elliott needed to take three stones to the Diamond District on 47th and 5th in the City. "Go to three stores. You only show one rock in each shop. Pay what they want for grading it. Depending on the quality, I'll decide which of the clubs here in the joint I'll hire to do the business. If they're shit, I'll give 'em to the gangbangers. Good stuff, we'll talk to my friends in the Eastern European fraternity. I'll try to keep 'em away from the fuckin' Russian Mafia, but we may have to deal with the bastards. We'll see.

"And you sit down with this girl and make sure you're getting half. Don't go one stone less. If she gets smart with you, let me know. One of my pals'll have someone on the outside pay her a friendly visit." Elliott's face flushed. "You don't care, do you? I mean, looks like she used you good. Don't worry; she has it coming."

With Christmas break over after the weekend, Elliott had only Friday to visit the Diamond District. He came out of the subway station into the freezing stink of the Big Apple, the spoor of urine hanging over the streets just a degree less than in the dark corners of the subway cars. His plan was to walk into the first jeweler's shop he came to, show one stone, get his quote, do it two more times, and be home for dinner by six. But he was instantly overwhelmed by the density of decades-old buildings lining 47th Street. The sky was typically winter grey, the pressure of the stale air heavy, depressing, and while not overtly hostile, the aura was surly. Directly outside the station was a plaque depicting the packed District as the home to over 4,000 purveyors of diamonds. A line in the description referred to the salespeople as "colorful."

His sneakers were soaked with gritty slush by the time he reached the first building. The scent of stale urine in the hallway was even more concentrated than on the subways. At the first shop on the left, the door did not budge. A bearded old man in Jewish religious garb raised glaring eyes to the glass, examining Elliott from head to toe. He continued to stare rigidly as his hand slid under the counter. Elliott imagined it was for a gun, and he backed away, but a harsh buzzer sounded, much like the ones at Sing Sing, and the door clicked open. Elliott, though, did not move toward it until the man at the counter impatiently snapped his fingers as if summoning a moron son.

Inside, Elliott walked to the glass counter and stood silently. The man, in a knitted, black yarmulke, lifted his eyes to the heavens and blurted in a European accent, "Vell, vhat?"

Elliott stuttered, "I have a diamond I want to know about. I mean, how much can I get for it?"

"Vell, vhere is it? I should guess by looking at you?"

Elliott scrutinized left and right before pulling the first stone free. It was wrapped in toilet paper. The man pulled his hands back. "Vhat is dis? I should touch shit paper from a stranger?"

Elliott looked down at the wad. "Oh, I'm sorry." He opened it so quickly, the stone skipped across the glass and rolled to the filthy floor on the far side of the counter. The man picked it off the ground with a washcloth-sized scrap of purple felt. He stared at it for a moment, as if afraid to touch it and add his fingerprints. His eyes flicked in immeasurably small increments around the perimeter of the stone before taking forceps from a drawer to continue the reconnaissance with a jeweler's loop. Elliott watched the man's face with extreme intensity as mumbles vibrated his lips.

The man looked up. "Vell, it is a diamond. That I can tell you. The quality, not the best, not the vorst."

"Could you tell me how much it's worth?"

"Vell, you have to understand, there are so many factors. Of course, you know the four c's."

"No, sir."

"Carat, cut, clarity, and color."

"I thought it was the size."

"No, no, no. It is not *size,* it is *weight.* A carat is weight. And there are ten popular shapes. Do you know them?"

"No, sir."

He spat, "Round, oval, princess, emerald, asscher, marquise, radiant, pear, heart, cushion, and some others. So, it is hard to tell you exact. And you got your color, or I should say no color, D is the best, no color at all. And you got your inclusions. None, very, very few, very few; it goes on and on. And vhat kind of inclusion? Bearding, graining, cavity, crystal, cloud, needle." He stopped and looked at the ceiling. "Vhat am I doing? Giving you gemology degree?"

"How does a person figure it out?"

"You can't. It takes an expert."

"Well, would you do that, please?"

"Vhat, I should vork for babkas?"

"Well, mister, how much is it to tell me?"

"No, not so easy. I am a master gemologist. My minimum is a hundred dollars. Higher if I have to use the tools in the back. X-ray evaluation—not so cheap. Then it is thirty dollars for a certificate. May take a few days."

"You mean I have to *leave* it here?"

"Vhat, I'm gonna steal it?"

"I don't know. I heard you guys like to switch 'em with junk. How am I supposed to know?"

Elliott was not sure if steam was rising through the man's yarmulke, but his face was red enough to boil water. "Vhata you talkin'? I been here since my father, may his memory be a blessing, bestowed this business on me and my brother." The purple in his face was now darker than on the felt rag he'd used to pick the diamond from the floor. "So, *momzer*, you get out now." He opened a drawer in which a .38 snub-nosed pistol sat on the top of boxes of hollow point ammo. "Out of my establishment, *chazer*!"

As the man's hand started toward the drawer, Elliott turned on his heels and moved quickly but caught himself and broke into a faux swagger, his head rocking side to side. His palm, though, had so filled with sweat, the diamond slipped free, and he had to drop to his knees and pry it out of a crack in the wooden floor.

On shaky legs, he decided not to chance the worn stairs and went to the next door down the hall. Here, again, the proprietor stood appraising the would-be customer before pressing the button. Straightaway, the tremor in Elliott's legs redoubled as he looked at the man, believing for a moment that he had reentered the shop from which he had just been expelled. It ran through his mind that the store had two doors, and this was the same gunman, but from the new angle he had not recognized Elliott.

This was a different Hasid. This man's yarmulke was a bit smaller, and Elliott believed he saw the slightest tinge of navy woven into the fabric of the seam. That was a good sign, for this man was, by virtue of the inclusion of a few filaments of a barely-colored thread, likely one gradation less a religious fanatic than his pal next door.

Elliott spoke up before he reached the counter. "*Shalom*. I'm here to sell this diamond." He thrust his palm forward and once again the stone fell to the floor. This shop had a carpet, one that had not been cleaned since the Hoover administration. When he picked the gem out of the rug, it came with fibers and bits of schmutz, which the jeweler blew away when Elliott placed it on the counter.

"Not so fast. It's not a pawn shop, ya know. Vhere did you get it? You steal it?"

"No, sir. It was my grandmother's, from the old country. She died a month ago and left it to me. I'm just a college student. NYU."

"Vhat, you too good for Yeshiva? NYU, a vaste of time. You learn nothing." Without taking a breath, he grunted impatiently, "Alright, lemme see vhat you got here." This man went straight to the jeweler's loop, spent less than three seconds examining it, and dropped it disinterestedly on the glass. "It's a diamond. I seen better; I seen vorse. It is from Russia, may the communist bastards drown in poison vodka; and this vun is made in the style of the Czars, but cut, maybe, twenty-five years ago. Old fashioned, not vorth so much. How much you vant for it?"

"Twenty-five hundred."

"Vhat? Shekels?"

"No, sir, dollars. It's very big."

"Big? Not so big." He pulled from his pocket a piece of folded paper in which he had a stone three times the size of Elliott's. "This is nine carats. Vhat you think yours is?"

"I don't know, three?"

"Not bad. Shape. Vhat is the shape?"

"Round."

"Very good. You know a little. Vhat is the color?"

"D."

"Vhata you talkin'? You don't know from D. Even *I* must look at two stones together to tell vhat is vhat. This is F or G, good but not so perfect. And look at all the inclusions. Not so hot."

"Can I look?"

"Vhat vould *you* see?" He paused, looked at the stone, shook his head sadly, "Look, tell you vhat, sonny. N-Vy-U, it ain't cheap. You just lost your bubba. I'll give you seventeen hundred, and that's a gift to you and your family."

"Sir, I need two thousand to pay tuition for the year."

The jeweler shook his head gruffly. "This is my Hanukah and Passover gift to you. Two thousand; but vhen you get ready to get married, you von't forget me, no?"

And Elliott walked from the shop smiling, his swagger real. He had beat the momzer at his own game.

CHAPTER NINETEEN

Well, Elliott Sass, there goes stereo system for Rolls Royce you flush away."

"What are you talking about? I made a killing."

"Did he offer you two thousand?"

"No, no. I had to fight like a dog just to get this much. The bum wanted to give me a thousand or something."

"Elliott Sass. If he gave you two thousand, it is worth forty. These people are vilest businessmen in world. You cannot beat them. Best you can do is not get hundred percent screwed, like we just did." She stared at the ceiling for a moment then turned back to him. "At least we know three carat stone worth twelve or fourteen thousand, maybe more. We look at what we have. Separate by size…"

"No, it's not size, it's weight. There's a million things you gotta know: color, clarity, and I forget the rest. Oh yeah, you know what inclusions are?"

"No. I do not need to know. We cannot do this ourself, but we should not be swindled."

When Elliott told Rueben how he'd scored two thousand for the one diamond, the man smacked his own head. "What, I raised a schmuck? I didn't tell you to sell a damn thing. You show him ID?"

"He wouldn't pay me if I didn't."

"That's the point. Now you're on record for having sold a gem. He write down your address, too?"

"I guess."

"You guess? So, now you can't take a single step into the Diamond District again. You want to sell them yourself, good, piss away a fortune, go right ahead." He shook his head and muttered, "What a waste," then turned away mumbling profanity. The guard bristled over. Rueben barked, "I'm ready to go." He turned to Elliott. "Come back when you get some brains."

Elliott sat with Irena that night and told her his father was excited he'd been able to sell a test diamond for so much. She shrugged. He went on. "Let's not get greedy. We may not squeeze every single dollar out of every stone, but we are going to do very well."

She stared at him for a moment. "What did he tell you to do next?"

"He said he was working on it. Then the guard came over and took him back to his cell. I guess I'll have to go back. Maybe a week."

He spent the next days at the public library reading about the great diamond heists of the 20th Century. What he learned was that most of those diamonds sat unsold for years, fences reticent to buy good quality, large stones. It was almost impossible to sell those jewels on the legitimate market, and that was where all the money lived. He read that the bulk of gems stolen are generic, untraceable, and mostly in the hands of junkies who get a couple of hundred dollars from pawnshops, the actual worth usually twenty times higher. Even the jewelers in the Diamond District rarely bought back a stone they'd sold a retail customer, fearful of exposing the colossal markup. His stomach soured as he began to appreciate the pitfalls in selling gems on either the retail or black markets. It was not like stealing a car or a TV.

And then there were the recent improvements in technology to establish the individuality of precious stones, essentially ways of taking its fingerprint. An x-ray of a diamond was distinct, the pattern of the beam's refraction a signature that was never exactly the same as any other gem. Then there was the growing field of laser identification, the etching of a serial number on the girdle of the diamond. That number, though, could be doctored, written over. Then it was discovered that diamonds "flash" when a laser is played on them, and the burst of light was distinctive for each diamond. Since none of their gems had ever been registered or even insured, that in itself added another roadblock. Legitimate buyers wanted protections that their investment could not be summarily repossessed when they couldn't prove the stone's origin, like gems stolen by the Nazis which were hunted down and returned to their rightful owners.

Finally, Elliott learned there were problems in legitimately owning large, high quality precious gems—insurance. Premiums against loss or theft went beyond what even the wealthy could justify. He read that Elizabeth Taylor sold one of her magnificent diamonds to rid herself of the yearly thirty-thousand-dollar insurance premium.

He left the library so depressed, he went back to Irena's apartment and sat drinking vodka until she came home. He told her about his two days of research. She stared at him for a full minute then shook her head. "Elliott Sass, are you telling me you did not go to school for two days?"

"What's more important?"

"The diamonds will take care of themselves. We can sell one by one, maybe over the thirty years. If you lose scholarship, you will never go back. What waste. You do not understand?"

"Look, there's problems, sure, but those diamonds are all two, three, and four carats. We have thirty-five left. That's way over a million. You take your share; you'll be set forever. Settle where you want. Why kill yourself working for some goddamn boss?

"You said you might someday want to go back to Russia. You invest your cut, and you can forget about ever having to ride in the cattle car on an airplane again. You'll stay in decent hotels, not crap like we just did. Screw your lab director. Who needs that life, taking orders from scumbag deans?"

She was silent for a long time. "Elliott, I did not know you want to split diamonds, go separate ways. Is that what you will do?"

It was his turn to stare at the ceiling. Finally, he spoke dryly. "You asked me to fly halfway around the world; didn't even tell me why. I did a lot of work. I deserve half, but I'll settle for forty percent."

Her voice broke. "I never said you did not deserve half. I only thought we are going to, you know, share money and time."

"Irena, I'm sorry, but I have my own life to lead. We are very different people."

She had begun to weep. "You are first man who treated me like woman, not freak. Even bastard in Russia who raped, he gags when he is finished. I am lonely every moment of my life until we were in Moscow doing something, two people together doing something for each other. Then we would hold each other at night, *together*. It is first time in my life!" She began to sob openly. "Does not matter to you. Only money and my ugliness. It is all that counts to you. ***Tell me, is it not?***" Her weeping deepened. "I will never be loved, never. There is nothing that can be done."

Elliott stared out the window silently. When it was clear he wasn't going to comfort her, she snatched a handful of diamonds, perhaps more than half, and flung them at him. He stared at her for a moment before dropping to his knees to pick them from the carpet, one by one, the pile growing in his palm. He stood, took a step toward her, hand extended, as if to return them, but his father's prediction had come true. Elliott jammed the stones into his pocket. A few fell to the floor. As he bent to retrieve them, she howled, "Leave now. Do not ever come back."

He added the loose diamonds to those in his pocket and left silently.

CHAPTER TWENTY

Elliott was aboard the New York Central commuter to Sing Sing the next morning. He spent seven or eight minutes with his father and headed right back to the Bronx. The train hit a car at a crossing, and he did not get home until midnight. His mother was asleep, but she had scribbled a message from the dean. Elliott was to appear at the administrative offices no later than eight the next morning. He thought of calling Irena, got scared, and, instead, took a few swigs of rum, smoked a joint, and fell asleep.

The meeting went quickly, even faster than the few minutes he had had with his father. It seemed there had been complaints that Elliott was entertaining a menagerie of unwashed souls in his campus apartment. Garbage had been left in the hallway, and the stink of marijuana was choking the residents. The problem was to be resolved by the next morning. He asked the dean's secretary if he could use her phone. Her jaw dropped as her head shook.

He took the subway downtown to Irena's. Though he knocked gingerly at first, he began to fume, and his banging became incessant. The same graduate student who had confronted him last time came into the hallway, fists clenched at his sides.

"You again?" he growled. "This time I'm callin' the cops."

Elliott feinted left, went right, and was out the main doors before the man lifted the phone to call the campus patrol.

Anyway, Irena could wait. She wasn't going anywhere. What he needed to do right then was cancel his sublease ruse. He should have done it months before. The seedy tenant had not once paid his rent on time, and on the two occasions checks had arrived by the first, both had bounced. If it was discovered Elliott had swindled the chemistry department, he would be expelled from the program, and worse, he might be sued for back rent. The occupant had to go quickly and quietly. Maybe he could talk to the man and explain things. He would forgive him the unpaid rent. If not, there would be months of legal jockeying to force an eviction. It was money and time he did not have.

When there was no answer at his campus apartment, he tried the door—locked. He started to walk away but remembered he'd kept a key in his wallet. Pushing the door open a crack, he stood in the hall and called with a smile, "Anyone home? It's the landlord." Silence. When he pushed just his head over the threshold, his body jerked back. By reflex, he squealed, "Jesus H. Christ! This place stinks worse than the Diamond District."

With that, there was movement on the couch. His renter, unshaven for many days, lines of cocaine on the coffee table, lay supine, practically comatose. He had peed his pants. Elliott had never met him in person, and with Plan A, to reason with the man a no starter, he simply bellowed, "New York City Narcotics Division. Get on your stomach." Elliott flipped his wallet open, pretended to flash a detective's gold shield, then put his knee on the man's back. "Okay, shit bird, your coffee table should be good for ten upstate, unless, of course, you want to help yourself."

Elliott's prisoner was barely able to choke, "Whatever you want."

"Okay, glad to see you making good decisions. First, where is your stash? And if you lie to me, you won't have to worry about prison time. My partner and I will dump your sorry ass in a ditch down by the piers. Won't we, Bender? And don't you look up at me. I'm undercover." Elliott opened one of the couch pillows and pulled the case free. He pulled it over the man's head.

The guy screamed, "Don't hurt me! Don't hurt me!"

"Shut the fuck up and tell me where to find your stash."

"Will you let me go if I tell you?"

"What I *will* do is not choke you to death. You don't wanna get hurt, play along like a good boy, and you'll walk. Understand?"

He answered with a weak, "Yes, sir, it's in the toilet tank, inside that bulb thing."

Elliott chuckled to himself as he stripped the cord from a lamp and tied the man's wrists behind him. With the leftover wire, he drew up a foot and lashed it to his hands. then pulled the telephone over and used the curly receiver wire to tie the pillowcase tight.

The man screamed, "You said you weren't going to kill me!"

"Shut the fuck up. I'm making sure you don't wiggle free. Bender, keep an eye on this prick. If he moves a single fuckin' muscle, tune up the rope around his neck."

Elliott found the cocaine, a good three ounces. The man was a dealer—minor league, though looking at lots of time. Elliott took the baggie back to the living room.

"Bender, I misspoke a minute ago. Guess who might or might not be goin' away for *fifteen* to twenty-five?" He pressed the tip of his index finger into his prisoner's occiput. "What else you got? Last chance to save your ass." The young man squealed about a bottle of pills buried in potato salad in the fridge. Elliott found sixty OxyContin but became lightheaded digging through the putrefied leavings.

He went back to the living room. "Okay, here's what's going to happen. We're gonna spare your sorry fuckin' life. If you ever get loose, gather every stick of furniture, every fork, every bar of soap, and get the fuck outta here. We'll be back in the morning to check and see what kind of housekeeper you turned out to be. Place is gonna sparkle, every fuckin' trace of you and your shit better be gone."

Elliott went silent and slipped out.

CHAPTER TWENTY-ONE

At home that afternoon, Elliott took a few swigs of rum then smoked a couple of blunts. It was too much. He threw up so hard, the vomitus was tinged red with blood. He sat in his mother's easy chair, not moving a single muscle fiber until the blasts of vomiting eased. He called Irena's apartment. There was no answer. When he phoned her lab and demanded to know if she'd come to work, the man on the other end hung up with a bang.

He took a seat at the kitchen table, his fortune spread before him: three ounces of powder cocaine, fifteen thousand on the street, more than a half-year's salary for the average American; and nineteen diamonds: two, three, and four carats, three quarters of a million dollars retail, half a million if he could fence them to the man whose number his father had had him memorize on the last prison visit.

Despite his skepticism, he made the call, the tone at the other end gruff, and so heavily Eastern European accented, Elliott understood only half of the one-sided conversation. He asked the voice to repeat itself, but there was only a thud, his second convincingly terminated call within an hour. What he thought he had heard was that he was to appear at the BMT Nassau Street Subway Station at seven-thirty the next morning, five samples in hand, and that he was to wear a black jacket.

Elliott's Soviet parka had been stuffed, unwashed, into a corner of his closet. He found it very early the next morning. It smelled worse than the day the cabbie had pulled it from the trunk. He tried to wash off some of the chunkier stains with a wet sponge, but that served only to reconstitute and lighten the color of the dried remains, morphing the smear on the jacket into a topographical map of the Seven Hills of Moscow.

He left at six, walking most of the way, thinking and fretting about the coming hours. He would sit face to face with an antisocial felon, likely a seasoned Russian Mafioso. Maybe he should turn back and forget the whole thing. Maybe he should hold the stones for a few years until he had a degree and time to better consider his future. After all, he was managing to feed himself and had a roof over himself for as long as he wanted. A little patience wouldn't hurt. He was finally old enough to understand that.

And what about the cocaine? One quick sale and he'd have spending money in his pocket for two or three years. Maybe he should have brought it along and offer it to the mafioso, be done with it. Then again, what if it got back to his father? Stealing school supplies was one thing; running drugs, dealing in *ounces* of coke, it would kill the poor man.

At seven, Elliott planted himself across the street from the station at the front window of a diner. He pretended to be reading the paper and drinking coffee. He saw a burly, dark man, beard growth several days old, come into view and dawdle fifty yards from the subway entrance. He was obviously a lookout, eyes reconnoitering without moving. He was signaling an accomplice at the subway entrance by pressing a finger to one nostril and clearing his nose constantly. Occasionally, a different message was sent, the sentry hocking up goobers of prodigious volume to dribble on top of the nasal mucus. Elliott laughed to himself. It reminded him of the old country, the dying tubercular old men sitting on the bench outside his family's apartment.

At seven-twenty-five, Elliott walked stiffly across the street, looking back up the pavement repeatedly at the swarthy gangster. As Elliott prepared to step onto the sidewalk, a black Mercedes pulled up, knocking him into the station entrance. Elliott was about to raise his middle finger but at the last second decided he didn't need the extra trouble and merely flicked his head at the driver. Nonetheless, the car pulled pugnaciously into the curb next to a fire hydrant. Elliott hesitated an instant before jumping into the subway entrance to flee. It was sufficient time for an arm to snatch his jacket from behind and pull him back into the street. Out of the corner of his eye, he saw a burly dark man, beard growth several days old, who growled, “Turn around and walk.”

Elliott, his arm now in a rock-like clench, was steered to the Mercedes and stuffed into the rear. His captor jumped into the driver’s seat, and the limousine sped off. Before Elliott could turn to his fellow backseat passenger, the car passed the unctuous man up the street still hocking and blowing.

The car smelled not unlike the busses in Moscow, and Elliott’s heart squeezed anxiously as he finally focused on the man next to him. It was yet another burly, dark man, beard growth several days old, who glared at his captive and snapped, “No talking.”

They drove for fifteen minutes, sometimes circling a block twice at the barked orders of the man in the back. When they came to a neighborhood buried in the East Village, Elliott became even more uneasy. He knew exactly where they were, Alphabet City, the area taking its name from Avenues A, B, C, and D, the only streets in Manhattan to have single-letter names. The community residing there did not thrill him in the least, for it had, in last few years, decayed into the heart of the Eastern European enclave.

“Get out.” The man yanked him into a decrepit restaurant. The lone waiter almost spilled his plate of *baniska* as the man pushed his way toward a corner booth. A dumpy, balding man flew from the back of the diner, his face losing most of its color when he saw his latest patron. “Meester Mikael Zdravkov, so good to see you again. What can I get you, sir?”

“I think I will have smoke. Get ashtray.”

The owner’s hands trembled as he shot into the back, instantly reappearing carrying a plate on which sat a small, yellowed, concave slice of material that appeared to be leather. He put it down in front of Mikael and backed off quickly. Mikael pulled a pack of Camels from his shirt pocket, jiggled one free, and thrust it in Elliott’s face, though Elliott shook his head and squeaked, “A little too strong for me.”

Mikael grinned coldly. “You take it.” Elliott did. Mikael shook one out for himself then lit both. When Elliott coughed,

Mikael shook his head and mumbled something that might have been in a strange Romanian dialect, for Elliott did not understand a single word. He was sure, though, it was not Russian. Elliott turned toward the wall as he coughed again. The label on the ketchup bottle stole his breath. It was written in Cyrillic lettering. His worst fear had been realized. He was trapped in Bulgarian territory. These folks made the black gangstas from a few miles north up in Harlem look like preschoolers. As he turned back to flick his cigarette, he realized from what the ashtray had been fashioned. His face drained paler than had the restaurant owner's.

Mikael grinned coldly. "Ah, so you see what we have. It is ear from sad little man who sells Mikael zirconium. Other one in back. You want to see?" Without waiting for an answer, he went on. "He do not need this anymore. You know what is zirconium?"

"Yes, sir."

"Good. Yours zirconium?"

"No, sir. They're real as far as I know. But I am not a jeweler. You can check them."

"Oh, yes. We check. If all well, maybe you walk out of here with two ears." He snorted ominously, shot his hand forward, and pinched Elliott's left lobe. "You show me now."

Elliott's hands trembled as he poured five stones from a test tube. One fell to the floor. He bent forward and reached under the table, shaken by the volume of hoary debris his hands would have to navigate to get to the diamond. It had not gone far, coming to rest next to an anemic *griz galuska* dumpling at the sharp tip of Mikael's filthy wing tips. Elliott gingerly picked away the dumpling to get purchase on the diamond without touching the shoe.

It almost worked, but his fingers brushed the leather, and Mikael kicked his foot out and bellowed, "What a fuck you do?!"

Elliott resurfaced holding the diamond in his fingers. "I dropped this one. It was by your shoe, and…"

"Give to me." He took a jeweler's loop from his pocket, turned away from the aisle, and examined each of the gems carefully. "They are real. Quality *dutastfishno*." It was close enough to Romanian for Elliott to understand the diamonds were sufficient.

"Now, I take weigh." He scooped the rocks into his palm and began to stand.

Elliott put his hand in Mikael's face. "Wait a minute, sir. Where you goin'? You're not takin' my diamonds away."

Mikael's pupils narrowed to pinpoints, and his face froze in a sneer. He finally took a deep breath but instead of speaking, twisted Elliott's left earlobe even harder, then grunted, "For you, I make your dick spoon to stir boiling tea."

Elliott's eyes glazed over. "I worked too goddamn hard to get those diamonds to let a stranger walk off with them." He slapped Mikael's hand away, and the diamonds flew onto the floor. "I'll get 'em...find someone else to sell 'em to."

Mikael sat back down. "So, you are stupid, eh? Commit suicide?" He stared at Elliott, whose expression had not softened a scintilla. Mikael's face opened, a rudimentary smile vaguely curling the edges of his thick lips. He nodded, "Okay, you come with me into back, watch me weigh."

As they slipped out of the booth, Elliott's eyes happened to drop, catching a fleeting glimpse of Mikael's pants. The man's slacks were tight, black satin, as wrinkled as a washboard. Elliott lifted his eyes, noticing the man's crotch was bloated, as if stuffed with a grapefruit. He imagined that was where the man carried his pistol; perhaps it was a grenade, the bulge was that obvious. He reconsidered his behavior.

Both Elliott and Mikael squatted to retrieve the diamonds, almost bumping heads. Elliott handed his three to Mikael, who was about to stuff them into his pocket but stopped, thought a moment, and handed them to Elliott.

In the back, the proprietor slipped from the room as Elliott and Mikael walked in. Mikael marched to a metal cabinet and slid out a stainless-steel shelf upon which sat an analytical chemistry lab scale. It was similar to the type Elliott had used at Isadore Goldstein, but this one was spotless. These devices could measure down to less than a tenth of a milligram. He tried to hand the gems to Mikael, but the man interrupted, "First, calibrate."

His fingers, though pudgy and calloused, delicately manipulated a pair of forceps to place a thin square of gold leaf on one of the weighing pans. He read the numbers. "Is good." Then he took a pair of forceps with rubber coated tips to place the first diamond on the platform. It was done with an unexpected delicacy. He spoke softly. "Point six-six. Not too bad. Is three-point-three carat. Asscher cut." He took a mini envelope from a shelf, wrote the weight and cut, and went through the process again four more times.

After he carefully put the packets in a larger envelope, he spoke to Elliott. "I tell you now, you have okay quality and size. I can help you, but you must not go to jeweler, like Jew bastards in Diamond District. You will lose everything. If you want me to sell, I sell. I take thirty percent."

Elliott's squealed, "Jesus! Thirty percent?!"

"You can do better somewhere, go somewhere. But I tell you now, if you try to sell on legit market, you get two thousand dollar for each stone…"

Elliott, with his reapplied game face, interrupted. "Okay, then what are they worth?"

"Maybe fifteen hundred for one carat, but..."

"So, the first one, the three-point-three, around five thousand?"

"No. You not so smart, huh? As carat get big, price become big very fast. Stone two times big maybe cost three or four times."

"Why?"

"Why? Rough stone big enough to make even one carat rare. You know, you must mine more than million rough diamond to find piece enough to cut one carat." He paused for a moment before staring at Elliott. "First stone to get near twenty thousand." He searched the messy desktop for a piece of paper but found only a picture of the owner's grandkids. He riffled through the drawers for a pen and a calculator, wrote the weights, colors, clarity, and cut of the other four stones on the back of the picture, went to the calculator, then scribbled on the picture until he finally croaked, "I take thirty percent, buyer take thirty percent, then sell for what he can. On first stone, you get eight thousand. Some of diamonds big, maybe four, five carat. No more bullshit. I give you fifty thousand for all. Is birthday present." That cracked Elliott's mien, becoming suddenly so light-headed, he staggered a step or two backwards. Mikael shoved a chair across the floor. "You sit. No hit head, blood all over. I tell you, you no like deal, go away. I give you good deal."

When Elliott's brain cleared, he began to think about the rest of the diamonds. Would this be a good time to mention them, and how about the cocaine? He could walk out a rich man, be done with the whole thing and retire before the end of the week. No more fucking deans, no more lab directors. On the other hand, he understood that even with the money Mikael was offering for the five stones, he would probably only get to the corner before a burly dark man, beard growth several days old, bashed him in the head with a two-by-four, relieving him of his gains. It was time for him to move.

"Oh, yes, yes. Good deal. Can I have my money now?"

Mikael shook his head in disbelief. "Yeh, I have fifty K in back pocket. No, Not-So-Smart-One. I take stones, shop around; when done we meet same place, same time. You call me Friday." He tossed the calculator into an open drawer, put the pen and envelope in his pocket, flipped the picture into the garbage can, and turned to Elliott. "You make problem, I make driver hit you in head with two-by-four."

He laughed heartily and marched out of the kitchen. Elliott followed slowly, thinking they were finally going to sit down and have breakfast. He worried he'd have to pick up the check, though Mikael kept walking into the street, waited for the driver to open the rear door, then snapped his fingers for the car to move on.

Elliott stood alone, five diamonds lighter. He found his way to a subway station, taking the Woodlawn Line north to the Bronx. He justified himself by claiming it was too late to go to class. Tomorrow, for sure.

CHAPTER TWENTY-TWO

It was time to start showing up for class. NYU was well into its winter semester. Elliott arrived at school early, drifting into the bookstore to buy a fistful of spiral notebooks and a top-quality NYU purple sweatshirt. At the last second, he flipped a pair of designer jeans on the pile. His p-chem course was scheduled for ten. He drank coffee for an hour trying to decide if he dared attend. With the prickling in his groin growing by the day, he accepted the need to see her but wondered how she would react when she laid eyes on him.

She had probably already heard he'd been to her apartment, and that he'd called the lab. Maybe she had even gotten in trouble because of him and was planning to go to the administration to insist they intervene and make him leave her alone. It would be the final moment of his college career.

On the other hand, she wouldn't dare admit that she'd been traveling and sleeping with an undergrad. Then again, she wasn't his evaluator; she had nothing to do with his grade in the class, and her private life had nothing to do with the university. So, she might go to the local police to file a harassment complaint. Surely, they would turn it over to the college administration, and given the inexorable left drift of the East Coast universities, his actions would beget reprisal from the institution's administration. After all, *he* had fomented an incident with an innocent, handicapped, member of the faculty. Worse, she was an exchange student from the liberal camp's darling Soviet Union.

It was better to stay away from her even if that meant another set of unexcused absences. No, he was not setting foot in her lecture hall.

He left campus to pace the streets, eying drug dealers, building the nerve to approach one and make a deal to sell his cocaine. With that money, he could stay out of trouble for several months, a buffer before he'd ask his father to find a less treacherous business partner.

He walked and walked, finding himself in Times Square, where every other soul was peddling dope. He chose the least threatening face in the mob, smiled, and came to a stop next to the man. In a microsecond, though, the pusher tore down 7th Avenue, disappearing into an alley.

That night, he sat at home smoking a joint, envisioning Irena through the vapors. He soon felt a judder in his chest as he recalled the defeat in her face when she ordered him out of her life. He phoned the one friend he'd made in class to ask if Irena had taught the p-chem lecture. She hadn't. His pal added conspiratorially, "Something's goin on, Elliott. I could tell from the guy they got to teach the class, you know, that asshole Salazar, the guy from last semester. All of a sudden, he's oh so authoritarian. None of his usual stupid jokes. You remember the one, 'I don't trust atoms. They make up everything.'"

"Guess I wasn't there for that one."

"Yeah, I know. You missed a lot of classes. How do you do it and not get kicked out? You're on that scholarship program, right?"

"Ya know, like I…"

"Uh huh. So, where you been?"

"Soviet Union stealing from graveyards."

Elliott tried to make sense of the first two chapters of physical chemistry, but there was so much tumult in his groin, it overshadowed the rest of his troubles. He called Irena from a pay phone, hoping somehow hers would ring with a tone just a bit different; after the third no answer, the machine ate his quarter. He smashed the receiver on the phone, and the plastic shattered. He looked left and right before sneaking back home.

He went through the same drill the next morning. Eventually, word would get to the dean that he was missing from p-chem lectures, and that would be the end of him. Something had to be done to break the impasse. Late in the day, he went to Irena's and slipped a note under the door, begging her to call him. He knocked quietly and then again. With his ear against the door, he was certain there was no movement.

He went to a bus stop near the building and watched her lobby door until ten, then went to the back of the building and looked up at her window. It was dark.

The next morning, he showed up at p-chem—Salazar, no Irena. He approached the instructor after class and asked what had become of the nice lady who had taught the introductory classes last semester. He was a little man who puffed his chest as he answered, "And who are you?"

Elliott stared at him before turning and striding out of the lecture hall.

CHAPTER TWENTY-THREE

On Friday, he called Mikael. There was no answer, and by Saturday night there had been no response to his message. He called again Sunday. Still no answer. All Sunday night, he lay awake deciding whether he should cut class and go to the diner where he had done business with Mikael. He'd demand the old man in the back give the gangster a call. After a scotch, he thought better of it, acknowledging a trip to the diner would likely cost him his life.

That night, Mikael called. "You so impatient. You think my work is easy?" Before Elliott could answer, Mikael added, "We make good progress. You call Friday."

Elliott did, but there was no answer. He was raving as he left a message. On Saturday night, Mikael called and told Elliott to meet him on Monday at the same subway station in the East Village, and to be there at ten this time. Elliott fussed that he had class and was already in trouble at school. Mikael shook his head. "No big surprise. You be there."

Outside the BMT Nassau Street station, he eyed the same burly dark man, beard growth several days old, standing fifty yards up the street. In a flash, a Mercedes squealed to a stop, but it was not the same one. This was a fire-engine red convertible. An arm reached out and Elliott came to rest in the backseat with Mikael. They sped to the diner. Mikael ordered breakfast, and the two sat drinking boiling tea and staring at the walls. After they ate, Mikael hitched his thumb toward the back office. As they entered, the old man fled even faster than on the last visit. Mikael snapped at Elliott, "Sit." He did. "You see, my friend, my work is very hard. Some customers not so happy with diamonds. Old style. Not so good for today luxury buyer. Yes, color, clarity, carat, *dutastfishno*, how you say in English?"

"Sufficient."

"Yeah, but cut is problem and..."

Elliott's face glowed red. "You said fifty."

"I can only do what customer pay. I make them piss at me, no more sales. I lose everything, you lose everything."

Elliott hissed, "Look, if it isn't one thing, it's another with you people. Gimme the diamonds back, and I'll go elsewhere."

Mikael shook his head and clenched a ham-sized fist. "You got big mouth," he grinned but leaned back in the owner's chair. "Big, big mouth, but maybe also big eggs. You so close to dead, but still fight back. I like that. See, you skinny, still pimples, look stupid, nobody afraid of you. Maybe you not so afraid to die. Good mixture. I give you twenty-five thousand. First time deal. Take only ten percent. Mikael know you have other things to sell, more Russian goods."

"How do you know that?"

"Ear to ground." He took two stacks of hundred-dollar notes in packets of ten thousand dollars and dropped two in front of Elliott." Elliott's eyes rose in protest. Mikael counted out another five thousand. Elliott's hand shot forward, but Mikael grasped his wrists and grunted, "In good time, Now, gotta take piss. You also piss. Come on; then I drive you to Nassau Street. I give you money soon enough."

In the bathroom, there was but one toilet bowl. Mikael marched up and made a production of unzipping. "Come, let's see what you got in pants."

Elliott's eyes drifted down to Mikael's male member. While the length was prodigious, the girth shamed many a stallion. It was as thick as a Coca-Cola bottle, maybe more. Mikael looked up at Elliott, "And you don't forget."

As the driver stopped at the Nassau Street station, Elliott noticed the burly dark man, beard growth several days old, weaving along the street. At the same moment, Mikael pulled the money from his jacket pocket, ripped off the paper bands, and began a slow, deliberate count. With each hundred-dollar note, he dispensed a serious-minded Bulgarian aphorism, then handed that bill to Elliott. Mikael got as far as four hundred when a deafening wail stopped life in its tracks. A man at the driver's window was roaring for all of them to get out of the car and onto the ground. The assailant jammed a gun through the window, slamming the driver's head so brutally, the crack shook the Mercedes. With the driver incapacitated, the man rotated the barrel toward Mikael's forehead.

Elliott remembered little of what happened next, but he did recognize the attacker as the grubby bum up the street, and he recalled flying out the back door he'd just been pulled through then sprinting the streets of the Bowery, jamming the four, hundred-dollar bills into his drawers. He fled down the stairs of the next subway station, jumped the turnstile, and dashed into the train as the doors were sliding shut. With no idea where he was headed, and not caring, he crawled into a ball in a corner seat at the rear of the car.

That night, he watched the local news. All the networks played the arrest of the Bulgarian Mafia kingpin. In the video of the capture, Elliott was seen from behind, a panicked jackrabbit fleeing into the landscape. The announcer reassured the audience that the cops had a good lead on the escaped mobster.

Elliott chugged a few gulps from a fifth of vodka and fell asleep in his clothes.

CHAPTER TWENTY-FOUR

He woke with the sun, calm for an instant but soon consumed with a sense of impending doom. His mind went first to the truancy then, after a few seconds, his innards twisted into an inflamed dread. He tried to clear his head with a violent shudder. It served only to trigger a wave of nausea. Making his way to the bathroom, he felt an irritation in his crotch, as if something was chaffing, and put his hands down there to discover four, sweaty, one hundred-dollar bills.

It all came back in a gush—Mikael's threats, the clip of him running from the arrest scene, and the announcer's assurance that the cops had a good lead on the escapee. He staggered to the living room to watch the news. It did not take long before the morning team covered the story, suggesting the gawky man in the bright purple NYU sweatshirt and designer jeans, a late teen who ran like a duck, should be familiar to somebody out there. They flashed a number to call if anyone recognized him. His head dropped to see that he was still wearing the getaway outfit.

He solaced himself that tens of thousands of students and would-be students and alumni and truck drivers and homeless wore NYU sweatshirts and t-shirts. There was no way he could be singled out, certainly not on that flimsy evidence. "No way," he grunted at the TV.

He brushed his teeth for a few seconds, but his chest clutched, and he took off the sweatshirt and jeans. He wrapped himself in a towel and carried the clothes to the hallway incinerator. As he jammed them into the shaft, a neighbor came up behind him quietly and watched as Elliott worked the hinged door to send the material down the shaft. They went nowhere. The woman nudged him and stepped forward to place two bags of trash into the opening. They also went nowhere. She grunted, "Shit. That's why you aren't supposed to put clothes in the incinerator. Gums up the works. Now I gotta go get Holtz and have him pull out your stuff. I'm already late for work. Thanks a lot." She noted Elliott returned to 2-H, then huffed into the elevator for the superintendent's basement apartment.

A few minutes later, the super banged on his door. The sweatshirt and pants were in his hands, though they now glowed with a sheen of cooking oil and cucumber peelings. Holtz snipped, "These yours?"

Elliott looked up into the face of the gargantuan, red-faced man. "No. they were in the hall. I tried to get rid of them before someone tripped."

"You're NYU, right?"

"Yeah. So?"

"Well, this is like a new NYU sweatshirt. Jeans new, too. What the hell's goin' on? You cover' somethin' up?"

"I found them, I told you."

Holtz glared at Elliott for half a minute. "Well don't put this kinda shit in there anymore. Can cause a fire in the chute. Do I need to call the cops to reinforce what I'm sayin'?"

"No, I get it."

As he turned on his heels to leave, Holtz grunted, "Don't let it happen again."

Elliott's angst redoubled; he smoked a joint before leaving for class.

He needn't have waited outside the lecture hall doors until one minute before class for, once again, there was no Irena. He watched as Salazar put his lecture notes on the podium wing to his right then wrote the next assignment on the chalkboard with his right hand. Elliott commended himself for his powers of observance and tactical prowess as he took a seat in the top row, far to the left. Out of the man's line of sight, Elliott relaxed, for he was wearing his ratty Isadore Goldstein sweatshirt, the hoodie nearly covering his face. He drew a deep, serious breath, told himself to pay attention, to start studying that day, and to resolve to get his life back on course.

The instant Salazar looked up at the class, he caught Elliott in his visual field and stared, lips pursed. When he looked away and started the lecture, Elliott had the sudden uncontrollable urge to use the men's room, and he jumped from his seat to fly through the back doors. By the time he returned, Salazar was counseling the class that the derivation he had just performed would be on the snap quiz at the end of the hour.

That evening, Elliott was home in time to watch the local news with his mother. When pictures of Mikael and his driver filled the screen once again, his mother tsooked, "Look at them. Bulgarians. What do you expect?" As they once again played the footage of Elliott fleeing the crime scene, the correspondent reiterated that the authorities had a lead on the escapee. Reminding the audience that the police could always use a hand from the public, he replayed the clip of the fugitive in a NYU sweatshirt and jeans. His mother stared for a second. "Looks very young. What a shame."

Elliott called Irena's number—still no answer. He took out his books and sat at the kitchen table trying to concentrate, but every footfall in the hallway pushed his heart that much further into his mouth. By eleven, there had been no knock. Imagining he had dodged the bullet, he rolled a joint and stared at it, but as a wave of dread rerolled over him, he dropped it in a baggie. He thought of the drug charges added to the international gem smuggling accusations.

Unable to sleep, he reopened the books. At three, there was a click in his head, and he finally understood the basic tenet of entropy, the major principal Salazar had harped on for the parts of the lecture he had attended. It was really quite straightforward were it explained bit by bit in plain English, a concept high school kids could easily grasp if presented by someone who cared a fig for his students. Salazar had padded his lecture with claptrap and jargon to fill the hour and to appear erudite. It was the way of academia, intimidate freshmen, weed out the weak early in the process, and funnel them into the social sciences and arts, courses that were far less costly for the university to offer.

It suddenly dawned on Elliott that if the diminutive teaching assistant had made clear the concept of entropy, everyone would get it, and how smart would the young scholar have seemed then? How would he control grades and futures if p-chem suddenly became demystified? All a kid had to do was put in the butt-time, go over and over the same sentence until that one magic instant it all fell into place.

That night forged two permanent lessons in his brain. First, if you stick with something, its time will come, no matter how impossible it seems at the outset. The second was as important: the power of bullshit, of purposefully complicating life's issues for personal gain. It had become clear that tactic was a basic tool employed by the toxic.

Elliott rented a panel truck and moved his things to the on-campus apartment. It took weeks to rid the flat of the reek of poverty and despair. Though he waited for his mom to call and tell him the cops were looking for him, by summer vacation, it seemed the matter had been forgotten, as were all tragedies, and usually in four days. He knew this because he'd surreptitiously followed Mikael through the court system, the case having fizzled when the DA could not prove a single allegation. Nevertheless, he had turned the case over to the IRS.

Mikael was charged with failing to claim the nearly twenty-five thousand dollars he'd been caught with red-handed at the time of arrest. He swore, though, that it was the product of a business deal that had taken place in Bulgaria, and he had just that moment been handed the cash. He was on his way to the bank to register the transaction. The IRS transferred the case to the FBI, as it appeared the crime had an international flavor, but the Feds were not terribly interested in opening yet another can of Eastern European worms. The final penalty was a simple tax bill that came to less than fifteen percent of the cash Elliott had left behind during his escape.

Elliott brought the diamonds and cocaine with him to the campus apartment. He hollowed out a space behind a cheaply built door jamb into which he secreted his loot. After he spackled and painted around the crypt, he realized there would be no easy access from that point forward; actually, no access at all without major demolition. But for the moment, he would live on his stipend, residing on this side of the law.

On several occasions, he camped hour after hour in view of Irena's, and on other nights, outside her lab. She never appeared. Then, early on a Tuesday evening, a light glowed in Irena's bedroom. Elliott trembled as he knocked. The figure of a woman materialized, and Elliott felt an inner glow, but she was in her forties and confessed she had no idea who had lived there before she'd moved in that day.

Still, Elliott called Irena's number over and over, but thirty days later, there was a message that the number had been disconnected. He sent half a dozen letters, imagining they'd be forwarded, but after several months there was no word. She was gone, and no way, ever, to find her.

Eventually, his life began to calm. He had not missed an hour of class since Mikael, and as he became more and more serious about his studies, he made the Dean's List twice. There were times he pondered his boring life but quickly decided, all in all, his present days were not terribly unpleasant.

PART TWO

CHAPTER TWENTY-FIVE

During Christmas break of his junior year, Miriam called and asked him to take her to the doctor. She had discovered a lump in her breast months before. Too scared to do or say anything, she had ignored it. Elliott hailed a cab and met her outside the front door of the apartment building. He had not seen her in many weeks and was troubled by the pallor and weight loss he saw instantly in her face.

An hour later, they were steered into a shabby exam room at Chartington Hospital. It was the only clinic at which she was able to secure an appointment, given her Medicaid insurance. The halls were teeming with patients and families, nary a word of English to be heard. Water was dripping from rusted pipes in the hallways, and trash cans in the exam rooms overflowed with blood-stained debris. The doctor was a resident, unshaven, and neither of them understood much of what he mumbled in a thick accent. He ordered Elliott out of the room and examined Miriam, though failed to recall Elliott to discuss the findings and create a plan. Miriam walked out of the exam room weaving so, Elliott had to guide her to a bench in the hallway. She handed over the sheets of paper the doctor had left on the exam table as he marched wordlessly from the room. One was a standard x-ray request, the other a prescription for Xanax. "Mammogram" was scratched on one of the orders, but there was no information as to where or when the imaging study was to be performed. Elliott sat silently for a moment but soon could not control himself and exploded from the seat to sprint back to the exam room. He opened the door viciously but came to a rigid stop when he realized a patient was on the table, topless, undergoing a breast exam. The doctor gasped and snapped a string of sounds that had the warp and woof of strong expletives in a tongue with which Elliott was not familiar. Elliott excused himself submissively and went back to his mother. She was sitting, head sagging, weeping quietly.

Before they left the hospital, Elliott dragged her to administration to file a complaint, but he couldn't understand the ombudsman. On the way out, they passed a sign that read Radiology, but after inquiring several times and not able to comprehend what the clerk was saying, she scribbled "8 floor" on the slip. The first scheduled mammogram appointment was two weeks away. He groused that it was not right to make them wait so long, but Elliott did not understand the woman's huffed reply.

They took the prescription to a neighborhood drugstore. The pharmacist was so short, he could barely see over the counter. He, too, was tough to understand, but the man spoke so kindly to Miriam, she looked about to see if he was chatting with someone else. In thirty seconds, she had told him of her symptoms, and with his gentle smile, her shoulders loosened. She spilled all of her fears. The man continued to nod and smile, listening until she ran out of breath. He warned that, at her age, Xanax had to be considered a dangerous drug, and that the fifty tablets the doctor had prescribed should last for a good forty years. He laughed, "When you come back for your first refill, I'll be long retired."

Miriam's eyes widened as she asked, "You mean, Mister, I will not be dead in a few weeks?"

"Weeks? Look at you. Healthy. Good son. You know what they can do these days? You continue eating well, lots of water, walk around the block four times a day, and watch TV so you can shake your head at this crazy world. You will be fine, Mrs. Sass."

Elliott took a step forward and asked how long it took to become a pharmacist. The man looked at him curiously. "Why? Are you interested? What do you do now?"

Elliott smiled, "I don't know, but I think you made my mother feel better. She doesn't talk to anyone. That's pretty amazing. Oh, me, I'm at NYU—junior."

"That's where I did my undergrad degree! What's your major?"

"Chemistry."

"*Joy oy*! That's my undergraduate department! Is Dean Facer still there?"

"Yep. Don't think he cares for me all that much. Kind of a Nazi."

"Ah, yes. He is abrasive."

"What did he do to you?"

"But I should not speak ill of a professor. In Asia, we are taught to respect a teacher as we do our own parent."

"Well, he threatened to take my scholarship away because I missed some classes."

"Oh, that is what he did to *me*!" He stopped and thought before going on. His face hardened and became suddenly far less expansive. "Yes, my father is still in Viet Nam. Had heart attack, so I go back to see him. His oldest son must be there when he die. A gift from Heaven to be with him and my mother. And then so much trouble when back in school…" The man's eyes clouded over, and he was silent for a moment, until his face brightened. "I am glad to help your mother. Maybe you are interested in chemistry and at same time helping people." Elliott shrugged. "If you want, you could shadow me on some weekend."

Elliott was startled. It was the first invitation he'd ever received.

CHAPTER TWENTY-SIX

Two weeks later, Miriam presented for her mammogram. The order from the doctor had not been forwarded, and, unable to contact him in the middle of clinic hours, the test had had to be rescheduled for nine days hence. The soonest appointment with a physician was two weeks after the mammogram.

A month after the first visit, Miriam and Elliott sat in the exam room for half an hour until the doctor burst in, flipped the films onto the reading box, glanced at them, and dug the radiology report from inside the envelope. He grunted, "Yes, as we thought; it is cancer."

Elliott blanched but stood. "Please show me."

The doctor stiffened as he stared at Elliott, though he turned and put an index finger on a small, cloudy mass the size of a dime. It was flecked with tiny bits of reflective calcium in a starburst pattern.

Elliott asked, "How can you be sure?"

"I attended medical school. Next is biopsy, then chemo." He pulled the films down, opened the door, and called over his shoulder, "Wait for the nurse."

The biopsy was scheduled for three weeks, and the follow-up two weeks after that. Elliott grouched to the nurse that it would mean his mother had already had to wait a month and a half for that visit; and now there was another five weeks to go, and even then, that was only to confirm the diagnosis. He asked how long it would take to schedule chemo after the next visit.

She looked down at Elliott, her expression as contemptuous as the doctor's. In clipped syllables she replied, "Two weeks. Why?"

Elliott did not answer for a moment, his face growing blood red. Still, he said nothing until an arrogant twitch of the medical assistant's lips ignited a fuming diatribe. "You make my mother wait months to help her?"

The MA glared at him. "You don't like it, don't come to a Medicaid clinic. You're lucky to be here."

Elliott leapt from his chair, his fist cocked, but his mother jumped between him and the MA. "Elliott, my *shayna* boy, come home. No, no. We go home, and I make you a nice brisket with kasha *varnishkas*. Come now."

She led him out of the tired hospital by the arm, hailed a cab, and rubbed his back on the ride home. She poured him a glass of kosher wine, let him smoke a cigarette in the living room, and spoke while touching his shoulder tenderly. "Elliott, listen, the lump, I should have gone sooner. It's not their fault. Sometimes you must accept responsibility for your own mistakes. I should never have come here to this land. It is so painful, the loneliness. I cannot tell you. But I am here, and there is nothing to be done. I did it to myself. What will be will be."

"I know, Mama, but where do they find such people? I would never be like that."

"I know that. You are my *shayna* boy. The last hope of my mother and father." She stroked his cheek. "You would never…"

On Saturday, Elliott dressed in his only white shirt and tie. The pharmacist, Twuck, was so happy to see him, he gave Elliott a white coat. Though not permitted to touch the medications, or even speak with customers, he became so fully engaged in the goings on, when Twuck's shift was over, Elliott asked, "Aw, come on, can't we just do a few more scripts?"

Twuck put his hand on Elliott's arm. "Okay, a couple. You tell me where to find the meds, what to write on label, and then we go home."

That night, Elliott chipped away at the secret hideaway in his apartment. He retrieved ten diamonds, and the next morning walked the three miles to the Diamond District. It was closed for the weekend, so he left class early on Monday and took the subway to mid-town. He went back to the second jeweler, telling himself it was better to deal with the devil you knew than the one you didn't. He levelled with the man about Miriam's cancer, and that he wanted to buy decent care for her. He did not tell him the diamonds' source, swearing they had not been stolen, were not of American origin, and had been hidden for decades in Eastern Europe.

The jeweler weighed each one this time and searched for distinguishing marks. Finally, he looked up, and allowing that they were conceivably legitimate, called Elliott into the back room to sit at a table. As he made tea, he stared at Elliott. "You're Jewish?"

"Yes, sir."

"From vhere?"

"The Bronx."

"No, vhere you born."

"Romania."

"Okay, now I tell you. If all of a sudden, by miracle, I have ten beautiful diamonds, there are going to be questions. Vord flies like *dreck* around here. Probably already got some busybody valking by the door making mental notes. May even remember you from the last time."

"You can say I'm here to buy a wedding ring."

"Vit out the girl? What are you talkin'? Listen to me. I can't sell these for a long time, maybe years. You need the money now. I vill give you fifteen thousand. You do not have to tell me that is a robbery. To you, maybe that's vhat it feels like. But not to me. I do not have a choice. Someday, I vill make money on the stones, God villing, but I am seventy-three, two heart attacks already. I take nitroglycerin all day long. The truth is, the diamonds vill be sitting here long after I am dead. Okay, enough tears. That is my situation and my offer.

"Oh, and you cannot come back here to sell a single gem. Believe me, you are already vell known, just by how long you been here today." He stopped and stared at a wall. Finally, he turned back to Elliott. "Do you know how pigeons stay alive?" He went on before Elliott could digest the question. "Vell, I tell you. They get very high on the building roof, and they sit patiently and vatch, all the time, vatching. Vhen vun bird sees a scrap, he takes off, dives in a special vay. All the others sitting on fire escapes up and down the block, just like a shot out of hell, forgive me for using that vord, all of them join in to see if it's a meal. You do that a hundred times a day, chances are you maybe eat something. Same here. These are vorse than pigeons or crows, more like vultures. They valk back and forth, checking each business. For sure I'll be getting questions about you. So, my friend, you are done here. I vish you and your mother the best, but don't come back."

Elliott went to Mount Shirls Hospital the next afternoon when classes were done. He smiled warmly but explained sadly to the receptionist how they had been treated at Chartington Hospital, and how he was literally watching his mother fade before his eyes. "And still she has not had a single drop of cancer treatment. Two and a half months," he railed, "and they still haven't told us if she really has cancer in the first place. I hate to say this, but it's worse than that damned communist country I grew up in!"

An emergency appointment with a full oncologist was carved for two days later. When he and Miriam presented to the cancer center, the doctor looked quickly at the mammogram. "Well, Mrs. Sass, there is no way to tell for sure anything just by an x-ray. If you agree, we will get a biopsy, and then we can move forward. Is that agreeable with you?"

She nodded and, within fifteen minutes, the procedure and follow-up with the oncologist were scheduled. "Mrs. Sass, we will meet on Thursday and come up with a plan. Not to worry, we will get on top of things."

Miriam and Elliott went to the receptionist to confirm the next appointment. They were first directed to the financial desk. A droll woman printed out a bill for the day's visit and pushed it across the desk without comment. It included a fee of one hundred and ten dollars for reading the mammogram. Elliott gasped until he focused on the doctor's visit bill—two hundred and seventy-eight dollars. He choked but said nothing as he peeled four one hundred dollar bills from the wad in his pocket. The woman took the money to a room deeper in the complex and, several minutes later, brought out twelve dollars in change. Elliott's hands were shaking as he reached forward for the bills.

He asked uncertainly, "Do you get a refund for Medicaid?"

"Oh, no. We couldn't cover our expenses if we accepted Medicaid. There would be no Mount Shirls Hospital."

The biopsy was twenty-three hundred, the pathology examination eight hundred, and the return visit to the oncologist only one-eighty this time. Chemo began a week later; Miriam was to get an infusion once a week for sixteen weeks. Elliott called and asked how much the treatments would cost. The clerk assumed he was asking about insurance and quoted around four thousand. When it came time to settle his account, the charge was eleven thousand. He called Blue Cross and asked how much it would have been if they had medical insurance—seven thousand. He asked how there could be such a difference between insurance and what he was being charged. She told him that was why so many doctors were no longer able to take government insurance. He asked if they could lower the bill at least to the insurance rate. The woman warned solemnly, "That would be insurance fraud." He asked her why, but she hemmed and hawed and never offered a cogent answer.

Elliott paid as much of the bill that he could with the remaining cash from the jeweler, then co-signed as a responsible party before they placed Miriam on a payment plan. Miriam's soul declined day by day; the chemo hadn't done a thing but debilitate her to the point that she could barely walk on her own to the bathroom.

She also became noticeably short of breath; the fluid in her chest from the weeping tumor, quarts of it, had to be drained every ten days. The breast also became painful, so they were scheduled for several visits to radiation therapy. She passed away before the third treatment.

Reuben had been granted compassionate leave, but only in a greasy, orange jumpsuit, his hands shackled to a waist chain and another restraint fettering his ankles. The only people there were a rabbi's assistant, Reuben, Elliott, and one of Miriam's cousins.

Flanked by two armed guards from the Department of Corrections, Reuben was not allowed to touch his son or to speak aloud other than weep, “Amen,” after the closing prayer.

Elliott owed the hospital ten thousand dollars. That did not include fees for the visiting nurse or Miriam’s final expenses. Within weeks, he began to get calls from collection agencies, each more menacing than the last. One threatened to go to NYU and report that he was a scoundrel who flouted his obligations, warning that the better universities expelled students who refused to honor their legal responsibilities.

CHAPTER TWENTY-SEVEN

Elliott stopped going to the pharmacy on the weekends, begging off with excuses that he had to cram for exams. While he hoped Twuck would try and talk him into coming, the man simply said he understood.

Elliott tightened his muscles and lifted the phone to call Mikael. There was some unusual clicking, a hum, and then silence before a computerized voice said the number had been disconnected.

That Saturday, he went back to Sing Sing. The guards recognized him and waved him through. His father still had six months before he was eligible for parole, and even that was unsure as he and his lawyer had parted ways over unpaid bills. Reuben's first question was direct. "How much you got left?"

Elliott was ashamed but had little choice other than to confess he'd flushed diamonds down the toilet, sold one for fifteen hundred, and five to Mikael, that deal netting but four hundred dollars, and then ten more dumped in the Diamond District for fifteen grand, but that was a lot more than he had had before going to Russia.

"Okay," Reuben agreed, "that comes to sixteen-nine for, what was it, twenty-six large diamonds that shoulda got five thousand each, easy." While his father did some numbers in his head, Elliott was about to correct him but didn't bother. Reuben chuckled snidely, "You're a real fuckin' businessman, aren't you? Shoulda been a hundred grand, and my college boy kid gets less than twenty k. So where is the money?"

"I spent it on Mama."

"What are you talkin'? What, you bought her a mink coat?"

"No. I paid her medical bills. Still owe a lot to the hospital."

"Miriam was on Medicaid. Not supposed to be any bills, or so the goddamn government says."

"That Medicaid hospital, Chartington, it was horrible. I wouldn't let her stay there. Bastards wasted two months and never even gave her a single pill." His face tightened, "I paid for a private hospital. That's where it went."

"Oh, now the Sass family goes first class while I'm sittin' in this shithole. So, the five-star hospital, they did such a good job? You wasted how much?" His lips twisted in disgust. "I need that money for a lawyer."

"Papa, listen, Mama took care of me for a lot of years. There wasn't enough money at the end to pay rent. I had to move back in with her and sublet my dorm room."

"What's such a big deal about that? Of course, you did. It's free money."

Elliott was silent, musing to himself that this time there would be some income from leasing the dorm apartment, for he had already collected first and last month's rent, and a hefty breakage fee. That was how he had paid the back rent on the Sass apartment.

Reuben glared at his son. "It's all gone, isn't it?"

"I'm trying to keep the apartment so you have a place to come home to."

"You don't have a penny of it, do you?"

"I have some diamonds left, and now that we are getting down to brass tacks, that Mikael you sent me to, he owes me almost twenty-five thousand. And I can't find him to get my share."

"Are you crazy? You don't get ahold of him. He gets ahold of you. Mercedes Mike? Are you shittin' me! He's the worst of the worst momzers in the world. Look, a deal went bad. Period. You were lucky to get away with your ass. I didn't want to tell you, but word on the street is that you set him up, and the feds let you get away. Only reason you're still breathing is because you were so scared of him you gave him the money to fight the charge."

"What are you talking about? I left the money behind when I escaped."

"Doesn't matter. And like I asked, how much you got left?"

"There's four diamonds, but I used my head and saved the big ones for last."

"Oy vey! You used your head?! The big ones are the hardest to get rid of. In the short run, they're worthless. Maybe even in the long run. You know, when I get out, I got no money to pay rent or buy food. Who the hell is going to hire *me*? When they open the door, you an ex-con, you got a target on your forehead. Bunch of bullshit. No one gives you a chance. Assholes."

Elliott was quiet for a moment, weighing his father's words. "Don't they help you get a job? Give you some money to get resettled?"

"What, are you nuts? You are a slave from the day you set foot in here. All they want to do is ruin your life. Pricks." He shook his head crossly. "Look, I need money right now. Period. Listen to me. You know your cousin, the one who came to the funeral? She's got dough. You see that Buick she rides up in? Brand new leather seats, air conditioning? And the rock on her finger? Maybe you could sell *her* one of the diamonds." Suddenly, Reuben's pupils narrowed to the diameter of a laser beam. "That's it. That's it. You get ahold of her and borrow money. Lots of it. Use the four diamonds as collateral. She can say she brought them with her from Romania. Nobody can prove different."

Elliott sputtered, "I don't know her. Not even sure what her name is. She came to the funeral, stayed for all of five minutes. Never saw her before or since."

"Foolish son, listen. We are landsmen, yes? She has no choice. You just tell her it is a family emergency, that Mama would have wanted it that way."

The cousin took the gems, at Elliott's recommendation, to the Diamond District. She chose, by chance, the exact shop in which Elliott had sold the eleven stones months before. The jeweler looked at them closely. "Vhere did you get these?"

"From the old country. I brought them with me. They were my mother's, her *yerisha*."

"And vhere did you come from?"

"Romania."

"Yeah, vell these are Russian, and they are from the turn of the century style. Something ain't kosher here. You part of the gang coming around trying to get rid of these? He snatched the stones and locked them into his fist. "*Alte Makhseyfe. A rud zol dir arisber iber dee gehin*! You know vhat that means? I tell you. It means stupid old lady, may a wheel run over your head. Vhat. You come in here vit stolen rocks? You vant I should be sent to a *goyishe* prison? No, you and your *drek* friends, *you* go to jail." He began pacing the room. Not me. I ain't goin'. And I'm callin' the cops."

The woman swallowed hard and tensed as if a coiled spring, then exploded, passing gas and, at the same instant, socking the jeweler in the arm with a left roundhouse that knocked him against the back wall. The gems flew across the room, pinging off a wall, three landing near the corner of the counter, and one at her feet. Both lunged for the diamonds, but the jeweler clambered to the three on his side of the counter. The woman scooped up the one at her feet and tore out of the shop before the jeweler could crawl to his phone.

As she sprinted toward the nearest subway station, all she could imagine was spending the next several weeks, maybe years, on Riker's Island. And she ran even faster, darting onto the platform just as an arriving train was emerging from the tunnel. Skidding to a stop to keep from falling in front of the train, one of her heels snapped, dropping her to her knees. As her left hand jammed forward to break the fall, the diamond flew free, skipping along the platform, finally arcing over the edge to land in a wad of grease on the third rail. With the subway car pulling into the station, the diamond became part of the 625-volt circuit that powered the line. The dazzling flash of light as the stone vaporized drew oohs and aahs from the awed commuters. One clapped.

She called Elliott that night and screeched she wanted nothing to do with him, his father, or the hot merchandise. She said the jeweler kept three of the diamonds, surely as proof of a theft ring. She shouted that Elliott and his convict father were both plagues on the Romanian community, and she was going to take matters into her own hands and call the cops herself. She'd see Elliott sent to prison to join his jailbird father.

When the crash of the receiver burst into Elliott's earpiece, he went to his mother's armchair and pondered a plan to divest himself of the last of his largess. There was the bottle of sixty OxyContin, 80 milligram tabs from his former tenant, which could be arsenic for all he knew; and what remained of his mother's Percocet, 10 milligrams, twenty-two pills left in the bottle. The OxyContin, he had been told, was going for eighty dollars a tablet on the street, the Percocet for twenty. He would sell the lot, willing to accept fifteen hundred, and then be done with his old life for once and all.

At class the next day, he asked some of the grubbier students where he could score OxyContin. They turned away scornfully. He went to the sociology building between classes. Standing in the foyer, he was treated to a parade of the university's, and perhaps the city's, supreme unwashed. He asked bashfully where he might buy a single joint. No one stopped.

That night, he sat back in his mother's recliner. Maybe he would just use the pills himself over the next couple of years, an occasional cocktail at night to relax, clear his muddled mind, before cracking the books. While he had tried only a few granules of the meth he'd manufactured back in his high school chemistry days, he'd never imbibed in anything stronger than weed since. Clearly not addiction prone, he believed, as did everyone he knew, that marijuana was not a drug at all, and in fact, was less toxic than an Oscar Meyer hotdog.

He sat over a glass of vodka, then a third, and pondered what the attraction was to crushing a pill and snorting the powder, and how that could be worth the thousands of dollars addicts everywhere he turned were spending each month. Assuring himself once again to be genetically safe from getting hooked, he took half a seven-point-five milligram Percocet, used his mother's meat cleaver to mash it to dust, sat back down, and sucked it into his nose. It burned like hell, but it was not the oxycodone that hurt, for that was water soluble and dissolved quickly. The Tylenol, the acetaminophen portion, did not go into solution and just sat there, an acid corroding the overly sensitive mucous membranes lining the nose. He was quite unhappy, but only for the minute it took until the oxycodone was absorbed and the fire ebbed. Seconds later, he was blanketed by a euphoria he had not before imagined. His problems shrank in front of his eyes, soon evaporating completely, life now good, silky smooth, and bright.

But the bliss was gone soon enough, and he crushed the second half. Life was again lovely, but not *quite* as rosy, and he considered trying one of the OxyContins, the real thing. He decided he'd first have to think about taking that next step, and he lay back in the recliner. The next thing he sensed was morning sunlight flooding the room. He was dizzy, hungover, and ashamed. He had used his mother's bare hope for a sliver of peace and freedom from pain in her last days to cover up his failure as a son, as a friend to a good woman, as a man. He began to cry and thought about wolfing the dozens and dozens of pills and be done with it, all of it. Maybe that would bring the relief he so desperately sought.

Too late for class, and certainly not prepared for the scheduled quiz that morning, he got a glass of seltzer from the kitchen, a pillow from the bedroom, and his mother's blanket from her hideaway bed. He dropped again into the recliner, pushed the chair back as far as it would go, and covered himself. In a few seconds, her scent wracked his conscience, and his tears flowed as hard as the day she'd died.

When he calmed, he opened the OxyContin bottle and stared at the pills, revering them for the simple relief they promised. He smiled wryly that the solution was so easy, right there, clutched in his palm.

He had nothing to lose, no one to leave behind, not a single warm, joyful memory to cherish before the candle flickered out. He filled a fist with OxyContin, then took a mouthful of the seltzer.

The sudden ice-cold carbonation, though, shocked him awake, and he jolted forward. Anger with his weakness built shockingly faster than he could have imagined, and a string of profanity issued from him so boisterously, it had to have been heard on Jerome Avenue. He ran to the bathroom and flushed away the thousands of dollars in opioids.

CHAPTER TWENTY-EIGHT

Elliott went to the pharmacy that afternoon and asked Twuck if he could come back. The gentle man smiled. "It would be my pleasure."

That Saturday, when the two took lunch, they sat in the break room rubbing elbows with deli counter attendants still in baggy plastic gloves; cashiers, whose fingertips were forever stained dollar-bill green; and maintenance men with decades of dirt ground into their hands.

When most of the staff drudged back to their labor, Elliott whispered, "I was going to quit school, but I don't want to end up like them. Minimum wage, living paycheck to paycheck. God, no."

Twuck thought for a moment. His perpetual smile faded as he looked up at the ceiling and formulated a response. "It is not ideal life, I know. Back in Viet Nam, my family are workers, every day of week, every week of year, only two days off for Tet. That is our New Year and Christmas all in one. Not a good way to live, but you think about where would our world be without them? We could have doctor do stocking of produce shelves. Better, congressman slicing ham. I heard they always talk about pork. Maybe better world if we, the lucky ones, know more about the not-so-lucky ones. I am glad you choose to stay in school. What plans do you have?"

"I think I am going to apply to pharmacy school. I hear it's good money, and you don't have to work all that hard." Twuck's expression did not alter a trace, even when Elliott spurted, "Oh, yeah, and Twuck, by the way, what do you make a year?"

Still the man remained straight-faced. He eventually answered, "Good question but not so simple. Everyday pharmacist make maybe forty-five, maybe near fifty, but whole range depend on where you work: hospital, if you own store, or you are in Safeway pharmacy."

These were numbers that made Elliott's head spin; forty-five thousand was enough to buy a small house in Yonkers. He could hardly contain himself. "How long does it take?"

"Twuck is PharmD. That take four years at NYU for chemistry degree bachelor, then four more at NYU for PharmD. Still owe so much money for student loan. Maybe pay off when Twuck is fifty, if all go well. So, you see, when you take off from salary for loan, it is whole different story. But Twuck is very okay, thank you." He stretched and hummed, "Now, Twuck must get back to his easy work."

Elliott spent the rest of the afternoon dissecting how he would spend his forty-five or fifty thousand dollars a year. Before he left, he strolled the aisles of the store checking the prices of real food, not the Ramen and Sugar Pops on which he had subsisted for the past five years. On the way home, he took a bus to Fordham Road and went through the big-box stores, inspecting stickers on furniture, refrigerators, and good TVs. Fifty thousand was over the rainbow, even more than a million, for *real* money was just a fairy tale, a lesson he had already learned the hard way, several times.

On Monday, Elliott went to the NYU Medical Center after classes. He identified himself as a chemistry student in the special program for disadvantaged scholars, put a copy of his transcript on the counter, and asked to speak to an admissions counselor. The receptionist perused it quickly, an eyebrow raised, took it into the back, and returned with a raven-haired woman in her forties who showed him into her office. She scrutinized the transcript carefully and asked, "May I make marks on this?"

He nodded, and she put light checks next to the grades in General Chemistry, Organic Chemistry, and a double check next to the A in Physical Chemistry. "You have done well in the important courses."

He looked down at the marks "I'm surprised you consider General Chemistry important. It was easy."

"Not for most people. All of sudden, there're lectures flying at you several times a week, and then there's lab. You have to keep a professional notebook. First time most students are graded on their understanding of the scientific method. Second semester's worse: acid-base, electrochemistry, lots of competition. It begins to show us who's who.

"Organic's next. This is the killer for the pre-meds. So much memory. The who's are percolating to the surface. You get through organic with an A, you've made an important cut. And p-chem. You get some p-chem in General Chemistry, but the full p-chem course in your junior year; well, I don't need to say much about that. It's the final cut. Get an A in that maze, and you're a pretty high number in the draft. Means you know your calculus, which you need for pharmacy, certainly any research position.

"Your transcript is strong. Do you have any experience in the field? Many of those we accept have done things like working on a volunteer health team in Third World countries. You do any of that?"

"I'm shadowing a pharmacist here in the City. His name is Twuck."

"Twuck! He's one of our graduates. A wonderful man. You would need a letter from him and several chem profs, especially the p-chem instructor. We also do a background check. I'm sure you don't have any legal record."

He flushed then responded a bit too quickly. "Of course not."

She eyed him as if secretly tallying the seconds before the color was fully restored to his face. "Well, now would be a good time to submit an application. Come on with me." They walked to the front desk where she took a packet from a file drawer. "Let's get these back to me in a week. We will write to your choices for letters of recommendation, but you should let them know they've been listed."

Elliott pretended to think. "You know, there was an instructor who I really thought was great. Believe she was Russian." His eyes gazed upward. "Irena, if I remember correctly.

She's not here anymore. Really like to ask her. Do you know how I can get an address?"

"Oh, I know who you're talking about. She was a gem. Just list her name, and we will get her a letter request. Now, any other questions?"

"Do you know where she went? I'd sure like to personally ask her for a letter."

She stared at him once more. "You know, that's sort of classified. We try very hard to protect everyone's privacy."

Elliott's head slumped a few degrees in contrition as he acknowledged, "Of course. I'm sorry. I forget that we are here in the USA." She squinted at him. "Ah, I grew up in Romania. Awful place. No privacy at all, not for anyone, except the Party. It is so good to be here. I am blessed."

She relaxed and smiled. "Well, Mr. Sass, I hope we can move forward on your application. Thank you for stopping by."

CHAPTER TWENTY-NINE

Elliott applied to the School of Pharmacy later that week then went to the chemistry department offices to drop off notes to three professors asking if he could use their names as references. He did not know why, but he had chatted up the receptionist a week before when he had come in for a copy of his transcript. She was a chemistry major, a junior, and known to be overly studious; so much so, she kept a text open on her desk, as if a Bible, to which her eyes shot in between answering Elliott's questions. She was, from twenty-five feet across the room, quite pretty: a luxuriant, dark bob cut and crystal-blue eyes. A little closer, though, and the picture faded. To be gentle, her moustache was fuller than the feeble attempts he had made over the years. The hair on her chin was long and coiled. He wondered if she was a virgin; he wondered if she'd ever been on a date.

When she looked up and seemed to recognize him, she returned his smile sparingly. Speaking softly, he moved his left hand, the one holding the requests, over her desk, close enough for her to get a trace of the cologne he'd so carefully applied to his face and wrists that morning. By now, it had mellowed subtly, as if the scent was *him*, not from a bottle. Before she turned her face away self-consciously, he caught a glimpse of her pupils dilating. The color in the cheek facing him blushed before his eyes. It was if she had just come out of the sun.

He chatted with her for a moment longer, finally asking, "Seems like you're here all the time. Don't you ever get out?"

She whispered feebly, "Yeah, it does seem like it," and her eyes quickly went back to her textbook.

Elliott filled the silence with a secretive, “Can I stop by and say hello again?”

She smiled for an instant but said nothing as her eyes shot even more rapidly back to her book.

His letters of recommendation had been done quickly. The secretary called him and spoke officiously, “Mr. Sass, your letters are ready. All of the professors agreed to let you see their comments. I can mail them to you. Do you want them sent to your campus address or your home of record?”

“Could I stop by and pick them up? Give me a chance to say hello.”

She did not answer for a second then caught her breath and stated almost formally, “I’m sure that would be acceptable.”

With the cologne applied even more subtly, he arrived at the office an hour later. He sensed her head move forward to capture his scent. That was problematic, though, for it would have been difficult for her to appreciate anything other than the bargain Woolworth tincture in which she had apparently saturated herself after he mentioned he would be coming by. It was worse than being stuck on a streetcar in Moscow.

She pressed her head forward to bring the reek even closer to Elliott. He felt his head begin to extend in reflex but caught himself and pretended to draw in a lungful of her aura, letting his eyes weave in circles of forbidden delight. And once again, her pupils dilated. Elliott’s contracted to pinpoints.

He asked her softly if she would like to get a cup of coffee after work, downstairs in the new shop called Starbucks, but she screwed up her face and grumbled, “I can’t drink coffee. It gives me such gas.”

“Well, do you like tea?”

“Actually, I’m allergic to it unless it’s really, really weak.”

“Okay, after work, meet you down there.”

“Okay.”

At 5:05, they sat for a few moments before Elliott rose and asked, “What’s your pleasure?”

"Ah, jasmine, I guess. Please remember it has to be very, very weak."

"Tell you what, I'll bring hot water and a tea bag. How's that?"

"Okay, I guess, if it's very weak." His eyes rolled surreptitiously.

She dangled the bag and examined it. "This is jasmine-mint. I'm allergic to mint. Could you take it back?" He did and, in an effort to avoid a crisis, simply ordered and paid for a new cup of tea. This time it was oolong. She held the bag up to the light and read the tab. "Oh, my, I can't drink this. It's Chinese. Way too strong."

Now that they had two cups of boiling water on the table, he asked if she liked "white tea."

"Never had it,"

"Well, it's just hot water. When Mao Tsetung was on the Long March during the Chinese Revolution, they would eat on the move, raw grains of rice and 'white tea.'" He laughed. She stared out the window.

He sipped the water and asked nonchalantly, "You know, there was one more professor I wanted to ask for a letter of recommendation. That was Irena Ledderova. Do you remember her?"

"Yes. She had that awful thing on her face. I think she got married or something and moved to Switzerland."

After the knot in his stomach relaxed, allowing him to speak, he smiled plastically, "Really. So glad for her. I hope she continued her studies."

"I'm pretty sure she did after she took some time off. I think it was at the University of Geneva. Yes, that was it."

Elliott's chest tightened again. "Good for her. Hey, well, I gotta go crack the books. Sure was nice talking with you."

He rose and stretched. She looked up at him. "Are you going to call me again?"

"Of course. Real soon."

That night he sat in his mother's recliner smoking a joint. Had Irena been able to sell the diamonds, travel to Europe, and start a new life? Was she really married? If she was, did she already have a kid, maybe two? He smoked another joint. Was he going to call the University of Geneva? Was he going to send her one of the new-fangled emails? Would she write back? What would he do then? Get on a plane and find her? And if he did, what did he expect, that she would pack up that night and return to the U.S., to the teaching appointment at the Graduate School that was no longer hers? What then? Maybe she would call the cops if he showed up and tried to touch her. He smoked yet another joint, became nauseous, and went to bed.

CHAPTER THIRTY

The offer of admission came two weeks later. It was a thick manila envelope, and Elliott excitedly pulled free the papers he assumed outlined the next scholarship he'd been awarded. Instead, it was a slug of loan applications. At best, he would graduate in four years with a PharmD, along with between one hundred fifty and two hundred thousand dollars in student loans. Though the interest rate was not draconian, on the salary he expected, both he and Twuck would be paying off loans into mid-life, maybe longer.

Every night, he promised to wake at three A.M. and call the University of Geneva, imagining nine AM there would not raise eyebrows. And every night he got up at three and found one excuse after another not to expose his vulnerability.

On the other hand, there were certain needs that were going unfulfilled, what with his studies and lack of money. He considered his little black book which, when pondering only the entries still readable through the pen gouges, Elliott was basically bereft of all but two names. The first was Gladys, his mature friend from upstairs. He had seen her a few times over the years in the neighborhood supermarket and had thought about approaching her, but, in the harsh light of day, realized she'd become quite wrinkled and stooped. And there were also the fifteen hundred dollars he owed her for the trip to Moscow. He'd handled the situation with what he felt was aplomb; he hid a few aisles away until she left the store. The other entry was the secretary from the Chemistry Department, and *that* was a non-starter. He had written only,

"Sec'y Chem Dept." For the life of him, he could not recall her name.

When the edginess in his groin intensified as the days warmed, he found himself less averse to the most convenient solution—an elevator ride up to the fifth floor. He calmed himself with a beer and mulled that alternative for a minute or two. No, no, no, the fifth floor was utter capitulation, final proof he was no longer in control of his wits. With a splash of cologne, he hurried to the Chemistry Department downtown.

He stuck his head through the door of the secretary's office and searched her desk for a nameplate. No joy, but she did return his smile with an uncertain twist of her lips and, this time, did not reflexively look away. In fact, she closed her textbook.

"Hey, kiddo, you look great, ravishing! What's goin' on?"

She blushed deeply, and Elliott took a single step into the room, put a finger to his lips, and whispered almost inaudibly, "Same time, same place?"

She craned to gather what she could of his cologne and, once again, her pupils expanded larger than nickels. She looked about the room and allowed herself a conspiratorial grin. Now he was sure and turned optimistically to leave, absentmindedly pushing the door open right into the face of the Chemistry Department dean. Rather than being aroused by Elliott's scent, the man's head jerked back, and he spit a reflexive, "Oooooff."

Before leaving the floor, Elliott walked down the hall and knocked on another administrative door. He stuck his head in and asked the woman at the desk, "Hi. Hey, I'm fourth year chem. Need to ask the head secretary to send off my request for letters of recommendation. She really helped me last week. I'm such a dullard. I forgot her first name. I just don't want to be impolite, I'm sorry to bother…"

Before he could burp another line of drivel, she smiled broadly and hummed, "Francine. I'm certainly glad we have at least one well-bred undergraduate. Good for you!"

He met her at Starbucks. She asked for "white tea" then awkwardly punched her hand forward and tapped his forearm.

He brought two cups of steaming water and mumbled, "You know Francine, I don't even know your last name!" He was going to touch her arm, but it was quite hairy, and he stopped himself in time.

"Wilson."

"Is your grandpa's name Wil?"

She thought for a moment and answered more as a question, "No, it's Ben."

Then you should be Francine Ben-son."

She paused for a moment and half-giggled. He shook his head. "This place is pretty plain, don't you think? Do you ever go out and have a glass of wine?"

"Not really."

"Well, would you like to try? There's a cool place right down the block. Nice thing is, chemistry majors never go there. Too exclusive. I mean not for all of them; I mean not us." He waved his hand over his shoulder. "Come on!"

Perhaps Francine had never had a glass of wine, or maybe she'd had a lot of glasses of wine. Either way, she guzzled the merlot so quickly, he hardly had time to pay for the first before she asked for a second and then a third. Her face scarlet, she took his wrist and rubbed it against her cheek. "I want to remember this forever."

Though he tightened, worried he was about to light a stick of dynamite, she seemed not to notice and bent forward to touch the scented area of his forearm with the tip of her tongue.

She lived in a tiny flat not far from campus. She led him into a corner of the room in which her futon was unfurled, the bed sheets scattered over the floor. She dropped onto the mattress and sat there staring at him. Elliott, assuring himself there was little need for foreplay, grabbed her breasts and massaged them a few rotations before lifting her sweater. She did not respond, and so he felt authorized to proceed with step three of the algorithm—he reached around and clumsily unsnapped her bra. While this was a moment he had, in the past, anticipated hungrily, tonight, it became at once sobering. Her chest was matted with more fleece than his, so he skipped the prescribed next step and moved to her slacks.

That, too, was a bit of a shock, unearthing a region more luxuriant than the National Forest. He slogged, not without difficulty, through the tresses, and dawdled there until the engine was primed. While Elliott was ready to shift into high gear, she remained utterly inert, and he paused, retreated a foot on the futon and whispered, "Do you want me to leave?"

"Oh, no. It's just that…" She began to bawl. "Okay, I'll tell you the truth. I haven't had that much experience. Okay, the real truth, I'm a virgin. I promised Father I would keep myself pure until marriage. He told me only God had a right to touch me down there, you know where I mean, until I was wed."

"You promised your father?"

"No, no, of course not. Father Sheridan."

Elliott shook his head. "Francine, why were you talking to the priest about *that*?"

"He told me that boys were going to want to do things down there, and a lot worse than just touching. He wanted to make sure I understood what they had in mind, and how to stop them."

"But how did that even come up?"

"He told me his holy duty on Earth was to protect me from the forces of evil."

"What forces?"

"Boys."

"What do boys do?"

"I told you. He said to me in the confessional that boys were always going to try and touch my private parts."

"How old were you, again?"

"I think thirteen or fourteen. I mean, I didn't even know what he was talking about. Then he asked me if I knew where my clitoris was."

"Did you?"

"I wasn't sure."

"Then what did he do?"

"He told me to come into his office."

"Then what?!"

"He showed me."

"Showed you what? Not his thing?!"

"No, of course not. He's a priest, for goodness' sake. He showed me this vibrator, not that I knew what it was at the time, but it was big, a golf ball at the end of a tube."

"Did he have you use it on yourself?"

"No. He wouldn't let me touch it. He said it was safe for *him* to use it on me, but I mustn't do it to myself. That would be a sin."

"What happened?"

"It was unbelievable. I never felt that before. I couldn't stop."

"Stop what? Like he didn't put himself inside you, right?"

"Oh, no. *That* would have been immoral. He said his responsibility was to protect me before marriage, that it was part of a priest's obligation to his flock, and that God allowed him, his representative on Earth, to let me see what it's like to be intimate. It was okay if *he* used it, but only because just the tip of the vibrator touched me. I mean, he never really contacted my flesh with his. But that other thing, I mean inside, that moment would be decided by God, and only when God was ready, and God could only be ready when I had gone through the sacrament of marriage."

"So, why did you let *me* touch you?"

"Well, Elliott, I'm not an idiot. I'm a thinking person. He was kinda old, ancient ideas. Touching the outside is not such a sin. I mean, I'm not obsessive or anything. You can't get pregnant that way. And I thought you might give me the feeling I had that day. I've waited a long time."

"You remember you said you couldn't stop?"

"It was something!"

"Well, what if I had gotten so aroused that *I* couldn't stop and tried to come inside you?"

"Oh, I would have screamed, 'Elliott, no means no!' And I would have marched right down to the police station and had you arrested for rape."

"Even if I didn't, you know, go all the way?"

"You boys don't have to go all the way with a girl. You can take care of yourselves. I've read all about it. It's unholy, but that's what boys do. You will pay in the end, and *that's* just the way it is."

The wave of ice water that gushed over Elliott silenced him for a moment. He stood and looked down at her. "You are very nice, Francine, and I respect your purity. I'd love to move forward, but I have to be honest, just like you were. I don't have any experience at all, either. I would never trespass on your feelings, I mean lead you on, but my plate is pretty full right about now.

"I didn't tell you, in fact I haven't told anyone at the faculty, but my father is being held captive in Iran. He worked on an oil platform out at sea in the Persian Gulf. They arrested him as a spy. Wasn't even in their territorial waters. So now, I have to care for my mother, at least until this whole thing is over. She's real sick. I cannot think of myself right now, especially for a long-term relationship." He paused and sighed. "I'm so sorry." He reached out to touch her shoulder, searching in the meager light for a square inch that wasn't covered with a generous patch of fluff.

She lay back on the bed and covered herself with a sheet. Elliott calmed, dressed slowly, and started toward the door. She gasped. "You're not leaving, are you?"

He shook his head, whispering to himself, "What the hell did they put in that merlot?" then aloud, "Well, I just can't promise you what you want. Like I said, I respect you, and I would *never* lie to you."

She began to weep. "It's the hair, isn't it?"

Elliott was blanketed with a sense of dread. He tightened, glanced over his shoulder at the door, and readied himself for escape, but his confusion got the better of him, and he blurted, "What do you mean?"

"I have PCOS. That's why you won't make a commitment. Do you even know what that is?"

"Ah, no."

"Polycystic ovarian disease. It means I have a hormonal imbalance. It's what makes the hirsutism happen." She cried harder. "Not like it's my fault."

"No, of course not."

"And it makes you gain weight, gives you diabetes. It's a curse, and I will never get married. You men are so shallow. Can't you see through the outer shell?"

He hemmed and hawed for a moment, so she went on. "Well, just to let you know, I finally found a doctor who is helping me. But, of course, you wouldn't know anything about that, would you?"

Elliott remained speechless a little longer. "Would you mind if I used the bathroom?"

She did not respond, and he walked to the tiny room. On the sink was a blister pack of pills. Two had been used. He read the label: Ethinyl-estradiol and norethindrone. He recognized these as birth control pills, the ones they often provided at the pharmacy. He did not, though, understand why she was taking oral contraceptives when she was so adamant about remaining a virgin. "Of course," he mumbled to himself, "priest probably told her if she has sexual thoughts, decides to touch herself, she'll get pregnant." There was also a bottle of metformin, which he knew to be a medicine to lower blood sugar in diabetics. She did not look like the diabetics who came to the pharmacy in droves, most of whom were considerably overweight and much older.

As he finished in the bathroom, he did not take a step toward her. He called softly, "I'm sorry Francine, I can't give you what you want."

As he walked through the door, she sobbed, "Oh, Elliott."

Just weeks before graduation, he relaxed, knowing there was no reason for him to return to the Chemistry Department offices, ever. Then came a letter from the dean that he had done so well on the Graduate Record Exams, the department had a certificate to present. They asked him to make an appointment for the ceremony—everybody would be there to honor his achievement. He drank a beer, then a second, and a third. After a joint for good measure, he tossed the letter in the trash, threw on a pair of sweats, and took the bus downtown to the travel agency where he'd bought the documents for Russia years before. The ticket to Geneva essentially drained him of what he had saved from the rent on his

NYU apartment. He packed as he had for the USSR, bare beyond the bare necessities, and shoved all of it into the same tattered backpack he'd carried through junior and high school, the trip to Moscow, and the four years at NYU.

At the airport, he wrote a letter to the Chemistry Department begging off graduation, explaining that he was off to the Middle East to seek the release of his imprisoned father.

CHAPTER THIRTY-ONE

The University of Geneva was founded by John Calvin not that many years after Columbus discovered the New World. Many of the structures date from the beginning; some have been built quite recently. The Faculty of Science was housed in one of the more historic buildings, the third floor dedicated to the chemistry labs. Elliott, still toting his backpack, walked the stairs to the doors of the lab. He stuck his head in and asked a woman if he was allowed to enter. She told him no and then asked why he was there.

He had to think quickly, this part of the plan even more poorly thought out than the rest of it. Somehow, the truth blew through his lips. Even he was surprised as the words formed. "I'm looking for Irena Ledderova."

"May I ask who is calling?"

"I am Elliott Sass. Dr. Ledderova was my chemistry professor at New York University. I just wanted to tell her about my graduate school plans."

The woman hesitated but stood and walked into the lab proper. Elliott looked away from the swinging doors, steeling himself for the sound of their steps. He was unsure of how he would react but swore to himself he would not peek at the deformity, not even for a millisecond; he would focus wholly on her eyes.

A moment later, he heard the swinging lab doors open. He drew a deep breath and turned back. The woman was alone. "I'm sorry, she isn't here today. Why don't you leave your number? I'll have her call you."

"Well, ma'am, you see, I just got here from New York. I don't have a phone number, not yet at least."

"Please write down on this paper where you are staying."

"Well, ma'am, I haven't even gone to my hotel yet. I came straight here."

"But what hotel is it?"

"Well, it's the Hilton."

"Which Hilton?"

"What?"

"Which Hilton, Monsieur?"

"Ah, the big one."

"I don't know which you mean. There are several." She wrote on a slip of paper and handed it to him. "Please, you can call this number when you are settled, and I will make sure Irena gets it."

"Oh, that's too much work for you. I'll just come back tomorrow."

"Monsieur, please, these laboratories are off limits to the public. It is better if you do not return here."

Elliott hesitated, and the woman's hand crept ever so slowly toward her desk phone. Elliott nodded. "Okay. No problem. I'll call. Thank you, or should I say, *merci*?

"As her face turned away, she grumbled, "Thank you is fine."

Elliott found a hostel close to the university. He was stuck in a room with six men, several of whom snored away the spring night so loudly, others threw shoes at them, some of which barely made it over his bed.

Having scarcely slept an hour, he dragged himself to breakfast in the canteen before sunrise. When he tried to engage a table of sciencey-looking students, they quickly placed his distinctly New York accent and studiously ignored him. He took a corner seat by himself, sipping thick coffee and gnawing on a twist of *zopf*, a butter-drenched, challah-like bread. Since all Swiss meals are simply an excuse to jam cheese into your mouth, when Elliott started on the bread, leaving the Emmenthaler on the plate, his audience rolled their eyes and snickered in unison. Finally, when one pointed unambiguously to the cheese then at the *zopf*, redoubling the roll of his eyes, Elliott spread some on the bread. There were nods of condescending approval. It was suddenly all he could stand, and he wrapped what was left of his meal in a paper napkin, snarled, and made a spitting gesture on the ground as he passed the xenophobes.

Parked at a table by the front window of a café across from the entrance to the chemistry labs, he hid behind a copy of the *International Herald Tribune*, keeping watch as swarms of students arrived for class. How would he recognize her from a hundred feet away? He decided to evaluate the women by ranking their bodies, so neatly wrapped in tight jeans and even tighter tops in the burgeoning warmth of the season. Most were fives or sixes, a few sevens, but he smiled that he was waiting for the TEN. Then, again, what if Irena had married, had kids, or she had sold the diamonds and was living an opulent lifestyle, having gained a kilo here, another there? Best not to think about that, he warned himself, and went back to his surveillance. By nine-thirty, the best he had observed was an eight-plus. Two minutes later, the waiter bent over Elliott's shoulder without an apology and began moving the silver and condiments about.

Elliott stood arrogantly, chest puffing as he threw a few francs on the table. Ready for battle, he marched across the street as if on a suicide mission, charging the stairs two at a time. Though short of breath, he pushed through the door, mouth foaming. The room was empty. "Screw it," he hissed louder than he'd intended and hurtled through the swinging doors. The bang as they slammed against the walls raised the ambient energy from a hum of gurgling, whirling chemicals into a frenzy as voltaic as that inside a lightning cloud. All eyes in the lab locked on him, the intensity of the stares from the associate professors working closest to the door, to the not-so-eminent scientists in the far corners, gave off an aura of negative ambiance as if he'd encountered an energy shield. There were also gasps, the loudest issuing from his left. By reflex, he turned that way and saw the receptionist, her face as crimson as the Swiss flag. When she began taking backward steps toward the wall phone, he stiffened and began turning to bolt.

But the gasp had not come from her. A different woman, face partially hidden by a clear plastic protective mask, started toward him. Elliott scrutinized her carefully but quickly gathered it was not Irena, for even through the shield, he saw no hint of the wildly thickened features. The woman was in a loose-fitting lab coat, her figure concealed from the world. No, it was not Irena, but whoever the creature might be, she was closing on him quickly, and with such determination, he keeled about and blew through the doors.

The woman followed, calling in heavily accented English, "Elliott Sass. You stop right here."

He did. As he turned, his chest filled with a sense of shock and dread and excitement, his balance now an issue. She walked up to the weaving man, lifting her shield, her face as close to him as it could be.

"What the hell are you doing? You have no right to come here. You have no right to jeopardize my life. I never cursed you before, but this moment I do. I once told you to leave and never come back. I am not your toy. I am no longer plaything of you, you loathsome person. Do you understand me?"

Elliott's head slumped to his waist. He could not speak, for it was as if he were having the most intimate, intense conversation of his life with a soul upon whom he had never before laid eyes. Who was this? It shook him to the point that his heart was smashing against the inside of his chest. He could not draw a breath, but his eyes reddened and then began to tear. When his quaking slowed, he was able only to whisper, "I'm sorry."

She did not respond but turned and walked through the lab doors, leaving him in sobs. He begged God, if there was such a spirit, to stop the pain, but it did not, and he dropped to sit on the cold concrete stairs. It was better than to die standing.

CHAPTER THIRTY-TWO

Elliott Sass sat in the hostel common room staring at the ceiling fan. In rare flashes of lucidity, he deduced he was simply in a dream, that he was at home, drunk, in his mother's recliner, and that he had to get up and make his way to school, an exam scheduled for which he had not read a single chapter. Upsetting, yes, but not as terrifying as reliving how brutally Irena had rejected him.

And then his mind began to clear, his eyes met the cigarette-smoke-stained wallpaper, and finally the television in the corner blaring French. It was real, and he began to anger, soon furious that Irena had made such a fool of him, taken advantage of his vulnerability. He cursed her, uncaring, mean, fricken nuts. He tried to think about what he had done in life to make God loathe him so. Nothing came to mind.

He pushed himself out of his chair and marched to the lab, planning to charge right back up the stairs and confront Irena, demand to know why she had assaulted him so wrathfully. As he walked, his calor waned, and he weighed if the time in a Swiss jail was worth another encounter that would certainly be worse than the last. He went back to the café across from the lab and hid behind a French newspaper he'd picked from a trash bin. Now, at least, he knew what she looked like, and again his mind fogged trying to understand how it had all changed, how a miracle of that enormity could have transpired on this blighted planet.

At a few minutes past five, she walked from the building, two women on either side, an escort surveilling the environs for threats. An insinuation of warped features emerged when the afternoon sun played directly on her face. She paused at the top of the stairs and looked furtively in both directions before descending the worn marble steps. At the bottom, she looked again, hugged her colleagues, and turned left, walking briskly, faster than he remembered.

He followed at a distance and hid behind a car when she halted abruptly and turned to scrutinize the street behind her. A few blocks later, she entered a four-story set of flats. He watched the windows closely to perceive the slightest movement, but there was none. Assuming she lived in a rear apartment, he went to the front door mailboxes and looked for her name. It was there—405.

He thought he might stand behind a parked truck and see if she left again to go shopping, a perfect excuse to run into her by chance. He did not have to wait long. The front door opened. A comely, mature woman emerged, then a toddler, a boy, who turned and screamed, "Mama, *allez*!" to the woman who next appeared—it was Irena in short shorts and a brief top.

After the two women embraced, they spoke for a bit, Irena's hands gesturing busily, as if relating a story. They hugged again and kissed cheeks, the older woman shaking her head. They started down the street holding hands. The little boy followed a few steps behind, soon to run forward and grab Irena's other hand, holding it to his chest hungrily.

Elliott's exhausted mind clouded even further, his chest gripping as various scenarios played out in the miasma. Was she really married? Why was she living with another woman? Oh, my God, was she gay? When did she discover it? He spoke aloud, "Was she seeing a woman while we were together?" Jesus, what diseases did that mean? Elliott wondered if he was harboring Russian venereal infections, the ones he had heard were yet to be detected in the West. And the child. Was it hers or the other woman's? Was it artificial insemination with, like, a turkey baster, or did she just talk a guy into it? After all, who the hell would have slept with her in those days? He, alone, had seen through the obscenity. He had traveled the world with her. Who the hell did she call when she needed help with the biggest problem of her life? Didn't she appreciate a damn thing?

His fury built, not in a slow burn, but by quanta. He cursed her infidelity. He had thought of her for years, long before she had, somehow, transformed the curse. She knew that. Of course, she did. A woman had that sense; Irena knew he had been thinking of her.

It had been her responsibility to contact him. She was the one who left without a word. Bitch! The second she got her filthy communist hands on a little money, off she flew to live with a woman, to be what she really was. Of all things, a woman!

The angry clouds swirled for so long, the three had reached the end of the long block. The woman continued straight as Irena and the boy turned the corner. They waved to each other. Irena called out in French, the child threw kisses, and the other woman blew them back. Everyone was bubbling with happiness, save Elliott.

He found himself, yet again, at a crossroad. Given her lewd proclivities, he was probably not going to win this skirmish, and not likely the war, but he badly wanted her to know what she had done to him. Maybe he would sleep with her one more time and then disappear. He'd send her an awful letter when he got back to the US, maybe before he left Switzerland. Yeah, he would fuck her one more time, and she would never see him again.

He would go back home. Maybe one of his fellow pharmacy students would introduce him to a cutie, a young thing interested in a man who was on track to make something of himself. But this time he would play hardball, first make her chase him, train her from the get-go how to treat a man.

Armed with that resolve, he waited in eyeshot of Irena's front door for an hour. When the two turned onto her street, he started forward, planning ever so precisely for the exact moment to spring. At the last second, as Irena put the key into the door, the little boy looked up, saw Elliott, and waved. The smile was so innocent, it stopped Elliott in his tracks. Irena reached behind her and gently pulled the child forward into the foyer. As the door closed, Elliott stood frozen, hoping for one more glimpse of them. It was not to be.

PART THREE

CHAPTER THIRTY-THREE

As course work came at the speed of light in the first year of pharmacy school, Elliott had little time to cultivate his anger over Irena's rejection. But it was there all the time, simmering in the background. He dated, sometimes even seeing a woman a third or fourth time, but he spent intimate periods comparing them to Irena, deeming them frigid and not worth his time if they could not climax twice or three times in an hour. His friends began to run out of fodder for blind dates.

At the beginning of Elliott's junior year, a senior pharm student introduced him to his cousin, not, however, without imparting a good-natured jibe: "Elliott, try and get this one right."

Bridgette Dankins worked in the administrative offices of the NYU Medical Center as second secretary to the CEO. Not directly involved with pharm, or any other health science students, she was technically datable.

While Elliott had heard the adages, "Don't get your meat where you get your bread," and, "Don't dip your pen in company ink," he was as immune to that levelheaded life philosophy as any fourteen-year-old. And off he went on a first date at a local watering hole. His initial words upon seeing that she was not a dog, were, "Hey, Brooklyn Bridgette, nice to see you looking so good. I was kinda scared, you know, you know what I mean, a blind date and all that."

She watched him quietly, though optimistically, waiting for that glint of humor in his eyes, the sure sign he was just a jabbering, fun-loving, New Yorker. But no such signal issued from Elliott Sass. He did eventually begin to tell jokes, lots of them, bing, bing, bing, each racially more thoughtless than the last. He rattled off Polish jokes, Jewish jokes, Black jokes, and blond jokes.

This kept him cracked up for an hour or so, until she feigned a migraine; cursed the music, a juke box at the far end of the bar; and stood without another word to cut and run.

Elliott finished his drink and asked rhetorically, "Was it something I said?" Apparently, he had forgotten, perhaps never noticed, that the friend who'd set him up with his cousin was a quarter Black, a quarter Polish Jew, and that Ms. Dankins was a bottle blond.

The hospital pharmacies to which he was assigned as part of practical courses were structured completely differently than where he'd shadowed Twuck. He was shocked at the panoply of exotic medications, ones he'd never heard of or seen in retail stores, or even in his textbooks. Especially interesting were the anti-cancer drugs, many of which were so toxic, they had to be handled in hermetically sealed workstations through which the operator stuck unwieldy rubber gloves to amalgamate the poisons. Masks, face shields, and gowns were often required, even though the pharmacist was never supposed to be any closer to the venoms than the imperviable, three-eighths inch Plexiglas that surrounded the prep workstation.

No one on the pharmacy admission board could have known that Elliott Sass was less than adept at the fine motor skills required to practice in a hospital setting. He simply did not have the dexterity to draw infinitesimal amounts of precious medications from a rubber-sealed bottle and inject them, via hypodermic needle, into just the right type of plastic bag containing just the exact amount and type of dilutant. And who knew his powers of concentration might not be up to carrying that bag onto the correct hospital floor and transferring it ceremoniously to a no-nonsense, sterile, space-suited oncology nurse, who would formally go over the patient's name and lots and lots of numbers to ensure the right toxins were shot into the right cancer victim?

The next problem was his sterile technique. Why it was so awful was never diagnosed. Try as they might, the instructors could not get him to keep his supplies aseptic. They warned him over and over that the slightest mistake, the smallest brush of a contaminated glove with a needle drawing up cisplatin, might carry bacteria or viruses into the patient; that those suffering with cancer no longer had the immune capacity to fight off even microscopic inoculations of usually benign microbes.

Finally, one of the technicians took it upon herself to file a formal complaint, warning that Elliott was, to put it bluntly, dangerous. Unfortunately for Elliott, the whistle-blower was another cousin of the senior pharm student who was the cousin of Brooklyn Brigette. The matter came up at Thanksgiving dinner, and Bridgette saw the opportunity to use her position to funnel the complaint to the Dean of the School of Pharmacy.

Elliott was summoned to the dean's office. The visit was fairly benign. All the woman could do was compel Elliott to attend remedial glove-use classes at night and over the weekends, all summer long, until he was considered safe to proceed to his senior year.

He fought back, pleading that he would never need those skills, that he had no intention of ever working in a hospital or research lab when he graduated. He was interested in doing retail, earning enough money to do volunteer pharmacy work in Third World nations. That's where, he told her, his heart lay. As he stood to leave, he feigned bitterness toward the process that accused him of a deficiency without revealing the accuser. "And, Dean, I'll tell you this. I'm as proficient with sterile technique as anybody in my class."

A compromise was reached. He was to take a practical exam to see what a real pharmacist, not a tech, thought of his skills.

In fact, there had never been a single formal class given in sterile technique. It was something one learned on the job, and from nurses and techs who were themselves only marginally competent but loved to sabotage the efforts of young professionals. They took glee in manufacturing situations in which students were forced to contaminate entire sterile fields, surreptitiously knocking arms into walls, pushing over goose-necked floor lamps that the student had no choice but to catch to prevent a smashed bulb, and a panoply of other tricks of the trade perfected over decades.

Elliott spent the weekend before his practical reading about how to keep your gloves away from everything then went to the surgical suite to ask for tutorials from surgeons. It worked—beautifully. His examiner told the dean Elliott was as adept as a non-surgical student needed to be, so she called him in for an apology and offered any elective he wanted to start his final year. He chose forensic pharmacology.

That was a fairly new field, one paralleling the explosion in DNA testing. Gathering the scientific and technological skillset to enter that line of work was as arduous as for any discipline in medicine. Elliott had taken quickly to the computer and advanced so far that his peers and professors often came to him begging for help with difficult programming questions.

The professor who taught the forensic pharm course, Dr. Sanford Barron, was a dapper fellow who had graduated from NYU with a PharmD before attending law school. He drove a Mercedes, and while that was not, in and of itself, terribly uncommon amongst the health sciences faculty at NYU, one incident made it clear that this was a man whose lifestyle had percolated above that of his colleagues.

First thing each morning, Elliott and the other student taking the course were to present themselves at Barron's office for a tutorial before starting the day's lab work. During Elliott's initial week of the course, Barron blew into the office thirty minutes late, apologized quickly, and held up his palm. "Hang on gentlemen; this'll only take a minute. He thumbed through the Rolodex and pulled a card free. As he dialed, he winked at them.

"Charles, this is Sandy Barron. Hey, real busy, but just wrecked the S500. Skidded to miss a dog on Tremont Avenue. Wrapped it around a telephone pole. So, look, got any midnight blue in stock?" There was a pause, and he winked again at his students. "Yeah, good. Let's upgrade the stereo this time, and can you clean it up and get it ready by the end of the day?" Yet another wink. "Good, I'll call campus parking and tell them to let you in; just leave it in my usual spot. Send the driver up to my office to leave the papers and keys…Good. Thanks, and just use the card on file. See ya."

He turned to his pupils. "Well, that's all taken care of. What a pain in the arse. *Okay*, let's get started."

Two weeks later, Dr. Barron walked into the lab and asked Elliott to come by the office later in the afternoon, "And, no, you're not in trouble. Need some help on a project."

Elliott approached the man's office, tail between his legs. Barron greeted him with a smile and offered a seat. "Elliott, you're doing a good job, really taking to this material like you been doing it for years."

"Thank you, sir. Just basic computer stuff."

"Maybe," he raised his fingers in air quotes, "'just basic computer stuff' for you, but it's very useful. And that's what I want to talk to you about. You see, I still do some legal work. I represent pharmaceutical corporations and retail pharmacies in court when they get sued, which is constantly. Think about it. These companies either create or dispense poisons that some doctor in the field does not understand but quickly writes a prescription for, so he can look like he's on the cutting edge. That's important when the hospital board evaluates him for privileges every few years. Gonna be some nasty side effects in a certain percent of those cases. We're all different, physiologically. One med helps Douglas, lays his twin brother Donald low. It's more than just the genes you were dealt. Almost as if the environment doubles back and changes how the exact same gene expresses itself depending upon what the patient was exposed to in life: diet, exercise, smoking, alcohol, even stress, all that stuff. Unbelievable. Who woulda thunk it? Called epigenetics. Mark my words. This is the future of medicine.

"Anyway, all the FDA testing does is make sure the level of complications is in line with the percentage of people who die of surgical or medication errors, which is not all that high a bar to hurdle. There's a level of collateral damage we tolerate as a society. How else can you treat the ill? One bad outcome for a great drug, and it's off the market? Doesn't make scientific or humanitarian sense.

"On the other hand, and there's always another hand, the dead patient's family ain't havin' none of it. These pharmaceutical companies are going to court around the clock. Unfair, you say? Hey, you want fair, go to Hester Street." Elliott looked at him curiously.

"Hester Street Fair? Lower East Side?" Elliott" shrugged.

"Sounds like you need to get out more often."

"Okay, here's what I need. I'm representing one of the giants in court. There's a lot of research that goes into my testimony. I want you to help me prepare the case. Go to the med school library, use one of those new search engine things...maybe you could tell me sometime what the hell a search engine is...find everything there is to find about valdecoxib. It's one of the new-fangled, non-steroidal, anti-inflammatory drugs. Still can't tell you what was wrong with plain old aspirin, or if you have to get exotic, ibuprofen. Anyway, it's a selective cyclooxygenase-2 inhibitor. Used for everything from menstrual cramps to rheumatoid arthritis. Hype is that it does not cause as much stomach upset as the non-selective NSAIDs, like my friends' aspirin and Motrin. And that means less intestinal bleeding, or so the company claims. Sounds like an okay drug, but the maker of the *other* cox-2 inhibitor is scared to death of losing market share and is suing, claiming that the new kid on the block causes strokes and heart attacks.

"You do a thorough job on the research, and I'll have you help me in court. Throw a few bucks your way. No problem with the administration. They tried to tell me, because I'm on a contract with NYU, I couldn't use my expertise anywhere else unless I turned over all my fees to the university. Fought 'em like a mad dog. We compromised—half and half. But since I can charge what the market will bear, I just upped my hourly fee. I also bill for pretrial research, but not as much as for court testimony."

Elliott asked quietly, "May I ask what you charge for testimony?"

"No, you may not, but let me assure you: if you learn how to do it, a few years out of school, I'll introduce you to some of my contacts. You can ask *them*."

Elliott did a good job. Professor Barron bought him a suit, seated him at the defendant's table, and taught him to produce documents when he, Barron, wished to make a formal point, or when he needed hard copies of evidence for the court record. Barron slipped him five hundred bucks for his efforts.

CHAPTER THIRTY-FOUR

Elliott graduated toward the top of his class. He could have done post-doctoral work at NYU, or Columbia, or anywhere he might have chosen, but all he could think about was being done with school and making a living. Reuben had been released from Sing Sing but not before maxing out, repeatedly denied parole over the years for his lack of remorse. "Victimless crime," he croaked at each parole hearing.

He was back in the City, living at home and purportedly looking for work but, truth be told, happy to be exploiting Elliott's student loans. He marched around the living room shaking his head in disbelief, "My son the doctor!" But what made him even happier was contemplating his son the doctor making a full salary as a health professional. And he wasn't inhibited in providing vocal encouragement.

So, Elliott took a position as a junior pharmacist at Twuck's pharmacy. He would wake each morning with the sour feeling, "'Nother day, 'nother exam," but after a few seconds, he'd smile. He was done with the professors and the snooty lab techs and the snooty medical students with whom the pharm students had done hospital rounds each morning and afternoon; and the snooty nurses, the snooty nursing students, the snooty physical therapists, and the snooty respiratory therapists.

Occasionally, Dr. Barron would throw a bit of research Elliott's way. The money was generally gone in a week, much of it spent on Reuben's growing appreciation of aged scotch and smuggled Cuban cigars. Though he had been madly opposed to recreational drugs before going to prison, his attitudes had matured in the joint. He'd learned to enjoy a little weed before lights out and perhaps a snort or two of cocaine on the weekends, all paid for with money Elliott had added continuously to his Sing Sing commissary account. Reuben even had a few disparaging words to say about the quality of the dope Elliott had lying around the house. As he became more demanding, Elliott spent increasing hours away from home, even working an extra hour or two off the clock learning the ropes at the drugstore.

Toward Christmas of Elliott's first year at the pharmacy, Reuben developed a hacking cough that kept both of them awake. He had no medical insurance, and Elliott finally dragged him to a local emergency room, though remained outside as his father checked in, fearful of being coerced into co-signing on Reuben's promise to pay. In fact, Reuben listed a bogus address and telephone number, telling himself it was to protect his successful son the doctor from greedy medical bill collectors. It hardly mattered, for after a sentence or two from Reuben, the clerks knew well they would never see a penny of the final bill.

The x-ray showed a quarter-sized opacity in the right lung. It was so obvious, a janitor sweeping the hall stopped by the reading box outside Reuben's room and pointed to the abnormality. Reuben's attending PA laughed and quipped, "We'll make a radiologist outta you yet, Achmed."

Reuben was referred to a pulmonologist at Sydenham Hospital in Manhattan. A biopsy was ordered and, post-op, Reuben was placed in a private accommodation, the same room in which Eddie Cantor, the famous singer and actor of early TV, had been hospitalized when he passed in 1964. The staff tried to convince Reuben that it was quite an honor to be given that room, but he grouched the entire night, trying to finagle a bottle of beer from the nurse. By morning, the biopsy had been read. While there had never been any doubt, Reuben collapsed when the nurse delivered the diagnosis of lung cancer. He cried to her that he would stop drinking if a reprieve could be arranged. The woman smirked that he could drink as much as he liked; it was the cigarettes that had done him in. Reuben shook his head and allowed that would be more than he was willing to sacrifice.

The hacking cough was driving him crazy—Elliott, too. The oncologist gave him codeine cough medicine, the opioid usually successful in dampening the cough reflex. But by this juncture, Reuben was inured to the effects of such a mild narcotic. A friend found him oxycodone on the street, and that helped, but only until Reuben ran out of allowance for refills. For several nights, Reuben drank rye until he passed out and could not feel or hear the cough. Elliott, though, could, and at work the next day forged a prescription for OxyContin and delivered thirty pills to his dying father. When those ran out, Reuben waited until Elliott left for work then went to the pawn shop half a block up on Jerome Avenue to sell Elliott's TV and stereo. Elliott wanted to throttle his old man and actually started toward him, arms outstretched, fingers spread, but stopped himself, pulled money from under the floorboard in his bedroom, and bought the stuff back from the broker at a premium. He took the subway and returned to the pharmacy that night to falsify a second prescription.

He had been careful to use two different patients' names, from two different doctors, Gordon Anvil and Hershey Heroff. Both were widely known as "hot pencils," physicians who were comfortable prescribing narcotics in quantities sufficient to sedate the Budweiser Clydesdales. Yes, there had been some grumbling about doctors fueling a burgeoning opioid predicament, but at that time, doctors unafraid to treat patients in pain were considered courageous and noble. The argument was that because doctors were not very good at curing disease, but fairly proficient at treating symptoms; and because pain was such a noxious symptom, ameliorating agony was simply another wrench in the toolbox. In fact, controlling pain was so important, it became the fifth vital sign, after pulse rate, blood pressure, heart rate, and respiratory rate. At each office visit, a nurse used objective instruments to determine the first four, but only a chart upon which the patient pointed to his level of pain that day, the day before, and an average since the last visit. It took longer to do the pain evaluation than to gather the real vital signs.

At the same time, and in cahoots with the push to make pain a four-letter word, the pharmaceutical giants were hocking prodigious quantities of their opioid wares by seducing trusted neighborhood doctors across the country to attend lavish meals at expensive restaurants, where paid speakers put on elaborate multimedia presentations. The take-home messages were that *their* narcotic was the most powerful tool available in the armamentarium to afford patients godsent pain relief. And, best of all, if used correctly, their medication was no more addicting than white toast.

From these cozy dinners, local medical movers and shakers, the "thought leaders," were selected. The next step in the corporate marketing plan was to invite the key local players to join celebrities and professional athletes on cruises, and, for the city's' most revered medical voices, all-expense trips to Europe. From there, the drug companies built a stable of nationwide spokespeople, respected MDs who were injected into smaller communities to stand before even larger groups of doctors, albeit at lesser restaurants, and lecture them on the safety of long-term opioids. The only caveat was that the patient had to be suffering from real pain. When asked by these minor-league doctors how to define valid pain, the expert speakers said simply, "What the suffering patient tells you." They spoke so assertively, it seemed to community docs that these physicians had deciphered the answer to the unanswerable enigma of what was treatable pain. The bottom line was that very strong narcotics, that is, legal heroin in pill form, was appropriate and safe as long as the patient said he needed it.

The two patients whose names Elliott had chosen for his father's scripts were a shopping cart away from a pauper's grave, their body odor evocative of the nastiest potions he'd created back in junior high. No one cared about them, about their desperation, or even about the doctors who were dragging in mountains of money from Medicaid to keep them coming in for their two-minute, weekly opiate visits. Treating the indigent was good business, both for the wayward MDs and the pharmacies. Mum was the word.

By summer, Reuben's demands were so interminable, his cough so unceasing, Elliott stopped coming home after work, staying behind to rearrange shelves and streamline the computer program. He came and went as he pleased after hours, stopping off at Sarge's Deli for corned beef or pastrami, then back to the pharmacy for a cup of coffee in the break room. On a late Friday night, he entered quietly through the back door. One of the pharm techs, James Prince, was bent over a desk, writing so intently, he did not realize Elliott was standing right behind. Elliott grunted playfully, but the young man looked up with such shock in his eyes, Elliott jumped back a step and gushed an apology. As he looked past the man, he saw two prescriptions next to each other, one fully filled out, the other only partially. Both men were silent until Elliott asked softly, "Prince James, what's going on, my man?"

Jimmy dropped his head and whispered in a thick Irish brogue, "Elliott, I'm going to be straight up with you. My old man's got cancer. It's in his liver. He itches all day, all fuckin' night. I'm just writing a script for Vistaril, cover the itching, the anxiety, let him sleep."

For a moment, Elliott did not speak. Then, slowly, without emotion he warned, "Jimmy, you know that's a felony." He paused and let his own shoulders droop. "Funny, well, not so funny; my old man has cancer, too. Doctor ain't doin' shit to help 'im. So, I know where you're coming from. Now, I'm not going to say anything, but you need to be more careful."

As Jimmy began to look up, Elliott turned and left the store.

Reuben's and Jimmy's fathers died within a week of each other. During the memorial gathering at the pharmacy, Jimmy and Elliott did not look at one another, but they spoke for a minute at the door and decided to go to a bar that evening.

The first few minutes were uncomfortable, but after a drink, their shoulders relaxed. After a third, they were talking about the girls at the store and then, after the fourth, about one of the two notorious narcotic-prescribing doctors who had approached Jimmy Prince. Jimmy looked to the sides warily and went on in a Gaelic whisper. "You know Heroff, yes?"

"Of course."

"Well, listen to this shit, Elliott. That old, fat bastard was standing outside the store at the end of the day last Tuesday. In the fuckin' rain if you can believe it. Walked right up to me, said he wanted to talk about 'some pharmacy ideas.' So, we come here to Donovan's; took a seat in that dark corner over there in the back. I'm lookin' around. Holy shit, Little Jimmy Prince's rubbin' elbows with one of the local big shots. But then, I mean, what's wrong with talkin' to one of our clients? I mean, that's what they are, the doctors, aren't they?

"Anyway, he's tellin' me that medicine is a changin'. Nothin' but a business anymore. Says everyone's gettin' in on the revenue, even pharmacy workers. He says, 'Fuck your employer. Just usin' you. Even usin' the pharmacists. Think about it.'

"Makes sense to me as I'm sittin' there, so I says, 'I'm listenin''. Second beer, he tells me he knows I got a bit of a spotty past, if you know what I mean."

Elliott lifted his palms. "Whoa. What spotty past? You never 'shared.'"

"Very funny. Look, I had a little problem with a fuckin' Protestant back in Belfast. Me mates got lifted for a minor assault on a bigmouth Protestant called Nicholas Howland. Nothin' much. Bumps and bruises, that's all. Bloke deserved it—got all what was a comin' to 'im, stinkin' hun. Coppers blew it out of proportion. I had to get out of town. Left the next day. Flew here. Cousin in the East Village took me in."

"How the hell did Heroff find out?"

"He didn't say, but I'm guessin' it was through me cousin. He runs a janitorial service. Heroff's one of his accounts. Cousin introduces me to this wagon. Turns out she's also from Northern Ireland. That's good, right? Maybe. Then turns out she's workin' in Heroff's office. That's the connection, but still neutral.

"Then out of the blue, third date, she starts askin' questions, sensitive shit 'bout leavin' Belfast. Gets steamin', six, seven beers. Wants to know if I was still in Belfast when they murdered that hun Howland. Shit, what's it to her? She's a Catholic, like me. And, anyway, when I left the bastard, he was still cursin' and spittin' at me and me mates.

"Had to break it off quick with the girl. Ain't been answering her calls. Been lookin' over me shoulder ever since. But there are certain pressures in life, and a man has to do what he must, so I found this new one, right here at Donovan's." He pointed to a table near the front. "Right there. Angel. Gorgeous. Crazy in bed. Was outta me mind. Who's to know she also works for Heroff? I never asked; she never told me. I don't know shit until she invites her pals out to meet me. No need to tell ya the rest of the story.

"So, Heroff's got me by the short hairs. Can have me shipped back to Belfast before the sun goes down. Gotta kiss his ass. Tells me OxyContin from the manufacturer ain't cheap, but since a legal pharmacy can buy it in quantity, and he writes for it in quantity, he could get a good price, two-thirds of what the small guys pay, *if* he can dispense it from his office. 'Good for you,' I says. Then he levels with me. Tells me doctors can't order OxyContin directly for their practices, not openly in New York State, at least. He tells me it's stupid, because a simple pharmacist, no disrespect intended Elliott, just repeatin' what the jerk tells me, can order it if he opens his own dispensary. Now, if that dispensary happens to be a space in a doctor's office, all's good. Hospitals and bigger clinics do it all the time.

"Now, the pharmacist has to get a new Drug Enforcement Agency number for the corporation, a few regulations here and there—easy to get around. That's all it takes. He says it's all legislative corruption up in Albany anyway. Bureaucrats don't give a shit who orders what, as long at the drug company lobbyists keep the politicians' wheels greased. The more Big Pharma pushes product, larger the bribes. So, in the end, no one's watchin' for illegal sales, only for sales.

"He says if doctors could dispense *directly* after each patient visit, they could set a lower price, and that would accomplish three things: first, more affordable the product, greater the pool of customers; two, greater the number of consumers, more product ordered from the manufacturer, lower the wholesale price. The precious cycle grinds on. And last, but not least, fewer patients sent out of the office with prescriptions bearing their signatures, less chance for some goody two-shoes local pharmacist to get suspicious and alert the state board, not that the goons up there would do anything to upset the apple cart.

"He convinced me that docs these days were businessmen first, always an ear close to the ground for opportunities to increase profits. No different than anyone else. But just like every other businessman, they gotta dance around idiotic government regulations, especially those that could wind them up in Sing Sing.

"So, he starts to go into the details, like getting quantities of OxyContin from the manufacturer by pretending he's a big pharmacy. This requires more than a couple of phony signatures on an order form. First thing he needs is a pharmacist. Then there have to be records of the pharmacist having a pharmacy; you know, finding a place to open a drugstore, proof of paying rent, on and on. In this case, it's easy. He lets space in his office. Next, this pharmacy has to have employees: workers' comp, withholding tax forms, all sorts of business crap. Bottom line, Heroff needs a computer guru, ya know, cover all the picky details, soup to nuts.

"If he just goes out and finds a computer hack, it's not long before the guy gets nosey, figures it out, and next thing you know, blackmail. Guy like Heroff won't pay it, too cheap. So, off the bloke goes and sends a fax to the Pharmacy Board. They don't do dick at first, but he sticks with it, and some cocksucker on the Board sees opportunity, pushes for indictment, gets a doc thrown in jail, likes the power and attention, and it's a run for congress. I mean, that's who gets themselves appointed to the Board, isn't it? The piousest bastards of them all.

"So, anyway, back to Heroff. I, one Jimmy Prince, remembers who's the good guys. Didn't use your name but told him I had a trusty pharmacist friend and also a genius on the computer. Kill two birds with one stone. The man was interested. Whata you think?"

After a fifth drink, Elliott was drooling. He mused to Jimmy that at this point in his life, he had not an obligation other than to pay his rent-controlled apartment once a month and buy a sandwich at night from Sarge's.

"There is not a single human being on Earth who knows, or cares, if I live or die. Prince James, it's time to amass a fuckin' fortune." They high fived, had one for the road, then wobbled toward different subway stations.

CHAPTER THIRTY-FIVE

Two days later, Elliott took a sick day and journeyed north on a reconnaissance and fact-finding mission. As his train sailed through the New York Central Sing Sing station, he forced his eyes closed to avoid even a single glimpse of the massive institution. He exited in Albany and took a cab to the New York State Board of Pharmacy offices. In a tie and jacket, he introduced himself to the receptionist, explaining that he was considering seeking a spot on the commission, hoping someday to be involved in keeping the profession he so loved on the straight and narrow. As she showed him through the premises, Elliott commented about the outdated computers. She explained that the commission was far down the technology food chain, at the bottom, years away from upgrades. She added, "Actually, we all complain, but, really, what do we need cutting edge computers for? We only use them to make sure you guys pay your license fees and do your continuing pharm education every four years. If we did it faster, more efficiently, I'd be out of a job, and so would the commission—whole thing could be run by a robot."

Elliott asked, "Well, you do need to keep your eye on us pikers down in the trenches."

"Oh, that. All done by hand. Complaint comes in, I copy it, snail mail it to one of our three investigators, and wait. Our so-called 'detectives' are overwhelmed. We send them thousands of complaints a year, mostly nonsense like, 'Pharmacist gave me pills spelled different than the doctor wrote.' Investigator looks it up and tells the patient it's just the generic name."

Elliott shook his head. "But there's some serious stuff; doctors over-prescribing, right?"

"Yes, of course. But that has to come from a patient or a pharmacy, and usually several times. If it's a doctor, we forward it to the medical section. We don't go out looking for violators. Barely able to open the envelopes on all the complaints as it is. There are close to twenty-five thousand pharmacists in the state. We aren't the FBI, you know."

By the end of the week, Elliott and Jimmy had met with Hershey Heroff twice. He ordered them to show up in Yonkers after dark, in out of the way taverns. The pudgy, balding man in his fifties wore a threadbare hoodie which he only pulled tighter as the seedy patrons filtered in. Elliott felt the man was as unctuous as his old friend Mikael, but Heroff started throwing around big numbers of both pills and dollars. Jimmy would get one percent to massage the paperwork to and from the manufacturer, and five percent would go to Elliott for the use of his DEA number and the purchase and delivery of the OxyContin. Elliott's head swam with the numbers, far more than enough to retire in five years. Heroff promised to pay them at the end of each month. The two shook their heads in semi-concurrence, but then came the caveats: the biggest, that Heroff would deduct a thousand a month for so-called rent in his clinic. "Gotta make it look good."

Despite his negative credit card balance, Elliott ran out that Saturday and bought a hot new computer. The machine, driven by a Pentium II chip, included an upgraded Windows 97 suite. It was years ahead of the junk the Pharmacy Board, or even the DEA, was using.

For the next month, he spent his time away from work creating a corporation out of whole cloth, one that intimated ties to his day pharmacy. Since it was customary that pharm techs were assigned medication stock monitoring and ordering, Jimmy had become an expert in the fine points of purchasing scheduled medications like OxyContin. He and Elliott worked together to hack the store's ordering software. It took several days, but they were able to transfer a copy to Elliott's laptop. With that in hand, the appearance of their requisitioning documents would reflect the sophistication of one of the country's largest dispensing pharmacies.

Elliott added a few lines of virulent code to dance around the Board's tracking software, a few more to fool his pharmacy and the manufacturer, and hundreds of lines dedicated to misleading the DEA. His goal was to fashion, before the end of the year, an endless loop that fed back upon itself. The closer you analyzed his creative accounting, the more tightly you were drawn into the delusion that all the dispensing was done by the store. Bottom line was that Elliott's personal corporation was nothing more than one of the many delivery companies licensed to carry scheduled medications to large, commercial pharmacies.

When he did try to sleep, he lay there ciphering in his head; if he put in six hours after work per day, and the whole weekend, his sweat equity would harvest a thousand dollars an hour in two to three years. He would stash that money overseas, in Romania, use his computer skills to hide it, and then retire.

He laughed to himself that would be his fourth retirement: two from the drug trade, and one from smuggling and moving hot diamonds. But this one was certain; it was underwritten by a filthy rich, New York medical doctor who'd been raking in grotesque profits for decades. This wasn't some smarmy goon. This man was unassailable, a doctor, American nobility, *and* a brilliant businessman, the contemporary ideal.

Thinking of the diamonds brought back images of Irena. He refused to admit he was still hurting over her loss and managed to cull sham bravado to convince himself he was far better off without her. She was still deformed; better, yes, but not great. And she was a lesbian; and she had a kid, the latter a millstone around her neck, one he refused to hang about his. The child had his mother's smile, though, and he bet Irena was a good mom. As hard as he tried to block it, a wave of melancholy swept over him. Too bad it hadn't worked out. On the other hand, he heartened himself by repeating that there wasn't a soul in New York City that couldn't say, "Too bad it hadn't worked out." Not one. Put on your big boy pants and get over it.

The cabal met again the next week. Eying Heroff surreptitiously, Elliott hinted he had put a lot of money into new technology for the project. Heroff nodded. "Very smart of you. Protect yourself. Always stay one step ahead of the momzers in Albany. And don't forget; you have to spend money to make money."

Over the next months, Elliott wound up putting far more time into the initial computer program than he'd planned. Even the basics took weeks, and he spent another month petitioning the Drug Enforcement Agency to get a separate DEA number to open a supplier pharmacy and to order and carry scheduled drugs commercially. Then there were legal fees for incorporation, a business license, and, since crates of OxyContin delivered to his apartment day after day didn't seem prudent, he had to find a secure, temperature-controlled warehouse. That cost him first and last month's rent as well as a security deposit before the landlord would even take his name. By the end of the month, his credit cards were maxed out. He had only enough in his checking account to pay the rent, nothing left for electricity and water.

He dusted off his suit and let it hang in the bathroom, the hot water from the shower turned on full for hours. In the morning, the suit was dry and wrinkle free but shapeless. On the street, he discovered he did not have enough for carfare and walked miles to his Chase Bank branch. The loan agent wanted surety, Elliott's job far from underwriting the fifty thousand he wanted, so Elliott walked to Heroff's office and asked to meet with the boss behind closed doors. The receptionist told him to return at noon and bring lunch, reminding Elliott that Dr. Heroff kept kosher.

Elliott went to a Jewish deli and brought a tub of matzo ball soup and two pastrami sandwiches, all the time chanting, "You need to spend money to make money."

Heroff did not stand when Elliott entered his office. The old man spent the first fifteen minutes carping that the matzo ball soup was too salty. "Don't you watch your blood pressure? And the pastrami. It's loaded with salt and nitrites. How about the cholesterol? You really don't take care of yourself, do you?"

Heroff finally growled, "Better if you and I aren't seen together, especially in my private office. What is it you want?"

Elliott explained that the program was ready for testing, and he had to install a small bit of it in the office computer. Heroff's face took on the hue of the pastrami. "I don't want anything on my computer. Nothing in this office."

Elliott spoke calmly, though his voice trembled. "Dr. Heroff, I understand your concern, but this is how the process has to flow. Nothing suspicious, not a single bit of evidence left behind. It'll be simple logistics and accounting. I mean, how do you expect to justify my rent payment? How 'bout hiding what you make? If it shows up on your standard books, that's a problem for you, not me. How 'bout my share of the utilities? Gotta account for all that. The good stuff, that'll be on my books, not linked to yours; but, come on, don't you want to know how much you're paying me, and how 'bout what you've collected from your patients? Don't you want to watch for employee theft? I create my own set of books, ones that your staff has no idea exist. It's the way things are done."

"Okay. But right now, I want to know about when we're getting deliveries."

"Coupla weeks. And how do you want it delivered here."

"I want *you* here with it every morning, including Saturday, by eight- thirty."

"What, I just drive over, pull into the alley, and drop the stuff off? I don't think so. We need to hire a delivery service."

"No! Fewer people involved, the smaller the footprint. That's why I'm paying you and that Irish kid to figure out all the ways to keep us safe."

Elliott surprised himself as he stood abruptly and pushed aside his bowl of greasy soup. He snapped, "Doctor, I'm not your step and fetch it. You wanted someone with a DEA license and computer skills. You got one."

"Don't raise your voice to me, young man!"

Elliott snatched his briefcase and pastrami sandwich from the table as he about-faced and marched toward the door. Heroff grunted, "Wait a minute. I just don't want anyone in my computer, and I don't want the product delivered by a stranger. Surely you understand that."

Elliott's voice raised. "Of course, I do. But first, the system doesn't work unless we have access to each other. You need to tell me what you are moving day by day. How much you need for the next week. How 'bout when you're on vacation? Christmas week. You want baggies with a thousand oxycodone sittin' outside your door?"

Before Heroff could answer, Elliott conceded, "Tell you what; you go ahead and put all your sensitive stuff in a locked partition. You know how to do that, yes?"

"Of course."

"Good. I'll only have access to the very basic logistics; band aids, B-12 injections for old ladies. We'll call these, instead of pills, let's see, here you go, we'll call 'em Xerox paper. List it by the number of sheets. You just keep enough money in the till for me to do the ordering. Check it every day if you want. I don't care."

Heroff thought for a moment. "You're telling me that my financial files will be secure? You can't touch my accounts?"

Elliott's shoulders sagged theatrically. "Yessssss, and glad to hear we are trusted partners."

"Yeah, well, you read what's happening all the time with on-line theft. I had a self-destruct program added, but I hear you computer hackers are getting very good, can even beat that." Elliott didn't answer. Heroff finally replied distrustfully, "Okay, but I'll be watching."

Elliott was given a desk in a back room and allowed to enter the office records under the eyes of a nurse. Heroff warned over his shoulder as he left the cubicle, "She's thoroughly computer savvy, so watch yourself."

Elliott set up the partition, gave the woman the passwords, and explained how to change them. He had her sit at the computer and talked her through the process, turning his back to her as she chose her birthday for the new password. They shook hands as she stood, and he retook his seat. He told a few jokes as he worked and asked for a cup of coffee. It took only seconds for Elliott to disable the seventh grader's self-destruct function and worm into the private files. With a few more keystrokes, he connected his laptop to Heroff's most sensitive records, even finding a link to his cell phone. It was so easy and quick, there was time to slip a few sheets of the doctor's letterhead into his briefcase before she returned

When Elliott was done, the two drank coffee and flirted. At the end of the day, they met at a bar, had a few drinks, and she invited him back to her apartment for the night.

After work the next day, Elliott sat at home over a scotch and just scratched the surface of Hershey Heroff's private life. There were files clumsily hidden, porn downloads, and blackmail notes received and written. But for the moment, all he needed was a way to secure a loan from the bank, so he pushed out of his head notions of raiding the man's personal coffers. Elliott found his salvation when he discovered Heroff owned a waterfront summer home in Tarrytown on the Hudson River. He nearly fell off his chair when he saw it was valued at six hundred and fifty thousand. Elliott used one of the sheets of letterhead to make it appear as if Heroff had sold it to Elliott, free and clear, and that the document would have to serve as a temporary deed until Westchester County finished processing the transfer papers.

Though the dark web was in its infancy, Elliott found an address in Chinatown that would notarize any document for one hundred and fifty dollars. The papers were to be dropped off, along with the particulars and the cash, in a mailbox that hung by the door of a slum on Canal Street. He was to return exactly three hours later and retrieve the finished product. Elliott followed the instructions to a tee and pretended to leave but hid in a greasy chop suey joint across the street. He was sure no one had even approached the letterbox, yet three hours hence, he reached inside and retrieved the bogus deed. It had been stamped and signed by Arlington B. VanHouten, III, Notary Public.

The bank agreed to lend him fifteen thousand. He spent the next days filing corporate documents, listing phony persons for the president, secretary, and board of directors. Watching reruns of *Hogan's Heroes*, he jotted down names of actors and producers to fill in his corporate leadership. He even used his parents' Social Security numbers to open credit card accounts from New York to Michigan.

It took a few weeks, but he woke one morning to find the first shipment of OxyContin had been approved. Elliott called Heroff and asked if the goods could be brought to his office the night before they were to be dispensed. Heroff spit that it was too dangerous to store the drugs in his office, that after the first day of business, everyone within ten miles would know his practice dispensed opioids. If there was the slightest hint the drugs were stored there, the building would be robbed before midnight.

Elliott asked, "Then, can it be shipped to your house?"

The man cracked that addicts were smart; in two days they'd figure *he* was bringing the dope to work on his person. His throat would be slit by the end of the week. "Look, all you need to do, Mr. Sass, is act like a professional pharmacist and order some meds online and drop them off at my office. It's monkey work. A clerk could do it. I'm the one doing yeoman's service here. I do all the gathering of customers, sales, collections; all the corporate thinking and decisions; and most of all, the money-making. You're going to be a very rich young man in a few months. Don't blow this, Mr. Sass." He thought for a moment. "No, the deal is you get the stuff to me every morning before nine."

A week later, Elliott received a fax from the pharmaceutical supplier setting a date for the first delivery. Elliott was to coordinate with FedEx. They agreed to deliver the sensitive medical supplies from the airport to the warehouse but would need a signature before they could release the packages. Elliott called the owner of the storage building, who barked, "I ain't some kinda fuckin' notary. I ain't signin' nuthin'."

Elliott called FedEx to ask what time the meds would be delivered. "Between 8 A.M. and 6 P.M." Another day of work lost. He called FedEx back and asked if the packages could be left without a signature. No, the manufacturer demanded a chain of custody. Elliott considered calling the drug company, but that meant discussions and explanations, ones that certainly did not ordinarily take place between authentic professionals. He would simply have to be at the warehouse all day.

The packages came at 5:45 P.M. He sat in his cubicle and marked "VETERNARY ANTIBIOTICS" on each box. Considering his audience, he added, "FOR ANIMALS ONLY". He carried it aboard the subway. Gangs of unhappy young boys poked at him, demanding to know what he was carrying. He told them to read the label, but they could not. He asked a fellow traveler to read it for them. Still, they didn't understand, but by the time they tired of his rubbish, the train pulled into his stop.

He donned rubber gloves and spent the evening repackaging the goods in new Ziplock baggies and small cardboard boxes which he'd bought furtively at a small grocery in Yonkers. It had taken all Saturday to find a market that did not have cameras.

Before the containers were sealed, he wiped them with Lysol to remove fingerprints, hairs, and DNA, anything that could conceivably be tracked back to him. He marked Heroff's clinic address on the box and chose a sender's name and return address pulled randomly from the page that opened when he tossed the Brooklyn White Pages onto the kitchen floor. At 2 A.M., he sat back and smoked a joint, satisfied there was not a scrap of evidence left behind that could conceivably link those pills to the batch from which they had come.

Though the weather was balmy, Elliott dressed in a stocking cap, his old hoodie, and Elton John sunglasses. He took the New York Central to Yonkers to a Mailboxes Etc. and spoke in a grunt as he answered the clerk's questions about the contents. Elliott told the man these were his medical records, but the clerk shook it and heard the pills bouncing as loud as maracas. Elliott paid the freight for next-day, early A.M. delivery, never removing his gloves, which he had wiped of trace evidence with Clorox sheets several times. The first thousand pills were moving toward their commercial destiny.

At nine the next morning, he called Heroff to ensure the merchandise had been delivered. Heroff was apoplectic, not only about the failure of the package to arrive, but because Elliott had called him at work. Apparently, the phone had also become strictly verboten. The old man barked, "Just do it!" The phone slammed down.

As Elliott's shift did not start until one, there was time to hand carry the day's stock to the clinic. He went through the front door and explained to the receptionist, in veiled babble, the nature of his business. She rolled her eyes and curtly ordered him to leave the box on the floor behind her desk. He asked if the nurse he'd met the other day had a minute, but the woman snapped, "She's busy. Is there anything else, *sir*?" As Elliott turned to leave, Heroff came out of a room and, with a sixth sense, looked into the waiting area. His eyes penetrated Elliott's, the vitriol verily thrusting Elliott out the front door.

There was not time that day to work on a different delivery strategy, and Elliott found himself approaching the clinic again at eight-thirty the next morning. He could not, though, believe his eyes. There were already echelons of the Big Apple's most tarnished radiating from the door to the bus stop at the end of the block. The clatter was as earsplitting as in the men's room at Yankee Stadium between a doubleheader, the mob whirring with excitement. As Elliott looked more closely, though, he realized no one was nattering with the next soul in line; it was mostly distinct organisms mumbling to themselves. He worked his way to the front of the queue, pretending to ignore the invective spewing from the enraged who felt an intruder had pushed them back a single slot in the logjam.

At the door, he was stopped by a large man, a bouncer from a local security company, he assumed. Elliott became confused when he took a better look and realized the man was clad in a Westchester County Sheriff's Department uniform. The deputy put his palm on Elliott's chest. "Where *you* goin'?"

"I'm delivering medical supplies, sir."

The cop walked him to the receptionist's desk. The woman raised an index finger to stop him until she finished processing two young men, clearly brothers, both thrusting hands packed with crumpled, one-dollar bills into the woman's' outstretched palms. Their eyes were as remote as a shark's until the receptionist finished counting the money and looked up in acknowledgment.

With that approval, the men began to shake and writhe like backup disco dancers, their gyrations not ebbing until a rumbling sound shook the walls. The sudden odor was awful, and while Elliott assumed it was but errant bowel gas, it was actually one of the boys pooping his pants. The receptionist's eyes opened, not in shock, but in disgust, recognizing the daily fare had begun so early. She barked orders, sending the tramps to the far corner, took a breath through her mouth dramatically, held it, and withdrew into the treatment area. In thirty seconds, Elliott's nurse friend marched into the waiting room, arms outstretched, thumb and index fingers gingerly holding two small paper bags. She, too, took a deep breath through her mouth and stepped up to the boys quickly, shoving the pills forward into trembling hands. Failing to hit the moving targets, the bags fell to the floor. Her reflex was to kneel and retrieve them; after all, these were still patients, but at the same second, the pair threw themselves forward with such abandon, they knocked her backward. Elliott's jaw dropped at the intensity of the crack as her spine hit the ground. He waited for the boys to pause their grasping and apologize to the poor woman, but they ignored her, arms still flailing toward the drugs, football linemen scrambling for a fumble.

Elliott moved forward to help the nurse to her feet. Though he had added a fake mustache to his disguise, she recognized him instantly. The look on her face went from disgust for the two addicts to loathing for the man who had been afforded such opportunity in life and summarily pissed it away to wait in line at a drug clinic. She hissed at him to go away and never come back. "If I ever see you in this office again, I'll have the guard beat you until you'll wish you had died in childbirth."

That left Elliott with no choice but to take yet another day off work and find a local delivery service. He visited several offices; only one could guarantee delivery that early in the morning. He would pay a premium—up front. The contract, however, lasted but two weeks before one of the service's vans was ransacked by a throng of Dr. Heroff's more observant, frantic clients. It was almost as if the dopers could smell the goods through the walls of the panel truck.

The delivery company failed to inform Elliott of the attack, and he was woken by a blistering call from Heroff at nine-fifteen. Elliott explained the threat he'd gotten from the nurse and, therefore, couldn't do the deliveries, but Heroff cut him off. "You get that shit here within the next thirty minutes, or I'll have an associate deliver something to you, make it hard for you to get it up—ever again, if you know what I mean?"

For the next weeks, Elliott was in the alley at the clinic's back door by eight-thirty with a Safeway shopping bag, the now twelve-hundred-tablet daily delivery sandwiched between a stale loaf of Wonder Bread and a head of daily wilting iceberg lettuce. He'd bang on the door and wait, usually for five minutes, sometimes ten, before a female hand shot out and seized the goods, nary a word exchanged. On the last day of the month, an envelope was passed through the door. The cash was nowhere near what he'd expected, but it was still a lot of money, so he said nothing. After several months, he was able to pay off the bank loan and his credit cards. He started to rebuild the stash under the floorboards in his bedroom.

Adapting to his new world as a delivery boy, the work became rote. He began to show up a few minutes late, and then later. On a stormy, October morning, Elliott decided not to wait in the rainy alley. Instead, he marched arrogantly to the front of the building, dodged threats from Heroff's ragged legions, and strode past the cop at the door. He flashed his pharmacy license and store badge in the man's face. "Medical delivery."

Pushing through the inside queue, he sidled around a cachectic woman tendering a fistful of soiled dollar bills into the receptionist's face. He snapped, "Where do you want this?"

The receptionist, who he had not seen before, looked up and glared. "What?"

"Look, lady, I don't have all day. You want this or not."

The woman gasped, "What the fuck," as she vaulted from her seat and ran into the treatment area. She emerged behind a large, heavily bearded man in dirty scrubs who took Elliott by the arm and led him into the back. Elliott did not resist, assuming he was going to meet with Heroff. The next thing he knew, he had been driven out the fire exit.

Seconds later, Elliott's cell phone rang. It was Heroff. "I don't give a shit about the rain. Don't come *into* this office again. Is that clear? You stand out in the alley until we get time to open the fuckin' door. Got it?"

Elliott shouted before he figured Heroff could pull the phone away from his ear," "That's enough. If you want today's supply, you're gonna give me my salary before I let you have the goods. You're not holding my money anymore."

"I told you, at the end of the month, and if you know what's good for you, you'll wait by the back door until we're ready."

"Will there be an envelope today?"

"Are you deaf? At the end of the month!"

Elliott's shoulders sagged. But as he entered the alley, he was stopped short by an unfiltered wrath that had been roiling deep within his gut from the moment he laid eyes on the momzer, Heroff. It hurt so bad, he worried it might be the angina his elderly customers with heart disease so feared. He had had enough. There was excess cash under the floorboards of his bedroom, more than he could spend in the next year.

"Fuck 'im!" he called aloud, "No soup for you." He turned and left the alley, walking dejectedly toward his subway station, the plastic shopping bag filling with rainwater. As he stopped to poke a hole in the bottom, he was blown into the street by a gust of wind. It wasn't, though, of meteorological origin. The jet was generated by a crush of rain-soaked degenerates leaping into traffic, streaming helter skelter as if hounded by the FBI. And an instant later, there was, in fact, a squad of tactically garbed police chasing the inglorious. Elliott was frozen in place as the cops ran past.

It would be hours before Elliott learned that three minutes after he'd left the alley, that same rear door had been battered open by a platoon of screeching police, weapons drawn, infiltrating Heroff's back office.

When Elliott went in for his afternoon shift, Jimmy Prince pulled him out the fire door into the smoking area. “Holy shit, Elliott, did you see the news about Heroff? Shit bird got busted this morning?”

“What? I was just there a few hours ago. Chewed my ass, prick. I’m done with him. Sorry, pal. Enough is enough.”

“Hey, mate, we are done no matter what. DEA got wind of the drugs. You missed the cocksucker being led out in cuffs, crying, perp walk, whole damn thing. Shoved his ass into a grey Chevy. I’m here to tell ya, I never trusted that scumbag, not for a second. Now, I’m sure the asshole has enough in his pocket to make bail, and quick. And he’s smart enough to keep his mouth shut until he lawyers up, so you and I have a little time to go on the offensive.”

“Ah, offensive
”

“That’s right. I’m not takin’ no fall for this prick. Way I see it, cocksucker’ll be back on the street in two hours. Look, Elliott, I’m gonna leave now, and you’re gonna cover for me. I’ll follow him on my Yamaha. Wait ‘till he gets home, have a little talk with him and his wife, kids, too.”

Elliott flushed. “What are you gonna do, Jimmy?”

“Blow his muther fuckin’ kneecaps off. Muther fucker’ll never take another step in his life. Wife might not either. He came up with this, used us, and he’ll try again if we don’t get creative, get the family involved. This is the way it’s done in Northern Ireland. Just like I told you about that hun, Howland. Fuck with us, you get a visit and a six pack.”

“Six pack? Beer?”

“Jaysus, Elliott. Six shots, and not goddamn whiskey. Thirty-eight. Two in the shoulders, two in the kneecaps, and two in the ankles. Very persuasive.” Elliott began to shake. Jimmy waved his hand. “Listen man, this is life and death. You ever heard of Sing Sing?”

At home, Elliott guzzled three shots of bourbon and stumbled into his bedroom. What the hell was he going to do with the thousands and thousands of OxyContins in the warehouse for which he was contracted to pay rent for the next eight months? And more immediately, what about the baggies of two thousand pills under the floor three feet away? He thought and thought. There was only one course; he'd sell them himself, slowly, a few at a time, and get what he could. He had no choice but to become a street dealer.

As he cogitated and drank bourbon, a sense of de ja vu overcame him, as if this was not the first time he'd found himself slipping into noxious territory. Through the alcoholic haze, he intuited the outcome of those previous forays had not been positive. His mouth became dry, and his sweat soured to a malodorous syrup. No, there wasn't any choice. He dumped all but one packet of pills in a black plastic garbage bag and stumbled west toward the Jerome Park Reservoir. He got as far as Goulden Avenue when a gaggle of Hispanic teens sauntered across the street and surrounded him. With what he saw in their eyes, there was but one option. He threw the bag at them and sprinted home.

Jimmy called a few minutes later. "Elliott, that dick ain't goin' to be making any trouble for us after all."

Elliott screeched, "Oh my God, you didn't *kill* him, did you?"

"Fuck no. Better than that. You ain't gonna believe this shit! He got busted for sexual abuse. Been doin' little boys for years. Finally got enough on him to arrest his sorry ass. He took pictures and put them on his office computer, of all things. Apparently, asshole had a secure partition on his main drive. Supposed to self-destruct or some shit if anybody tried to get into it. He musta disarmed it, forgot to secure it again. Jerk off.

"I talked to him. He was happy to forget the whole drug thing, not wantin' his shit pool stirred up. He did ask me for a favor. He wants the rest of the pills delivered to some Russian Mafia dude, a Mikael. He gave me his number."

CHAPTER THIRTY-SIX

Elliott lay low for a while. He and Jimmy hardly spoke, and then only about pharmacy business. After not hearing a word regarding Heroff for several weeks, Elliott began to relax and asked for his old, early-day schedule back. He was soon promoted to shift lead and rarely saw Twuck, save for meetings in which the corporate officers came to the store to lecture about the growing abuse of OxyContin. The suits spun the tale of the pharmacist in New Orleans who had raised red flags about three unscrupulous local doctors who were writing OxyContin scripts as fast as their fingers could fly. When the police ignored him, the druggist contacted both the DEA and FBI.

"Terrible, terrible, lost their moral compass, these doctors," the corporate officers moaned, but in the next breath cautioned the audience that the poor pharmacist down South had had his license pulled for coming to work with alcohol on his breath, among other breaches of social and professional etiquette. "Lascivious comments directed toward customers," read the list of additional charges listed on the Louisiana Board of Pharmacy's website. "There's a lesson here, Ladies and Gentlemen," the corporate administrators counselled, "these physicians had been pillars of the community for decades. All were highly trained professionals who, no doubt, had their patients' welfare in mind. So, while we need to keep our antennae up for forged scripts, you need to be absolutely sure of wrongdoing by physicians or customers before making a fuss at the counter, calling the cops, and so on. From this moment forward, if you have a question regarding a doctor's handiwork, you will report it to your supervisor and to no one else, including other staff. Don't forget, legal exposure attaches to pharmacists who blow the whistle prematurely. Be careful out there."

Jimmy and Elliott eyed each other more closely than they had for months. Jimmy tipped his fist toward his mouth, and an hour later, they met at Donovan's. Jimmy laughed, "Those fuckers at corporate must be making a hell of a profit on OxyContin. I don't know about you, but they said we were to accept any script, no matter where it comes from. That what you heard?"

"Yes, my friend, you hit the nail on the head. I wondered why that goddamn OxyContin drug rep was sniffin' around last night. Corporate must be kissin' ass again. Guy says our sales of Oxy are down. Asshole's pushin' me to tell him why, *and* to get on the phone with the docs and tell them everybody's usin' it. Gave 'im a big smile, told him I'd do just that. Flashes me a shit-eatin' grin and shoves two Rangers tickets in my face. Wanna go?"

They went, and before the evening was over, discussed the boxes of leftover OxyContin Elliott still had stashed in the warehouse. Jimmy offered, "May be time to off-load that shit. How much is left?"

"Oxy 80s, about two thousand count."

"Jaysus, Elliott. That's a hundred and sixty k on the street. I could call that Mike guy that Heroff told me about."

Elliott flushed, fearful that if Mercedes Mike heard his name, it would remind him to take care of unfinished business. But he also did not want to tell Jimmy of the diamond debacle. Jimmy already knew too much about him. "I don't know. Those guys fuck people like you and me. They do a lot of shooting. Can't trust 'em. Tell you what, why don't you take some of the stock, let's say a hundred, and see what you can get for it. If it works out, we'll get rid of it all and be done. Split everything fifty-fifty."

They high fived and turned to walk to their respective subway stations. Jimmy called in a loud whisper over his shoulder, "Hey, Elliott, no phone calls, mate. Cocksuckers tappin' everybody these days."

"I got you, my man."

Jimmy and Elliott worked different shifts, but when they crossed paths, all Jimmy would grunt was, "Life's slow."

Elliott finally let it go, relieved there were no felonies percolating with his name umbilically attached. He felt neutral for the first time in months as he got home that evening and sat down to go through the mail. There was a thin, blue airmail letter postmarked Geneva, Switzerland, but no return address. It could only be from her. He began to shake as he tried to peel the glued edges apart. Getting as far as pulling free an inch of one flap, he cheated and looked inside. Reading the first words, "Mr. Elliott Sass," his fingers began to tremble so, he lost his dexterity, tearing free ragged pieces of blue tissue paper, shreds fluttering to the ground. He began to lift himself from the chair to fetch a steak knife, but, halfway up, the old landline phone blared, jolting him back into the lounger.

It was Jimmy. He was yammering so loud, and in such a grinding brogue, Elliott barely understood. "Man, get rid of those fuckin' pills. DEA just busted into my house. Said they had information I was dealing. Bullshit. Musta been Heroff. Shoulda killed the hun. Probably fingered us in a plea deal. Don't matter right now. Just get rid of your shit." And with that, he was gone.

Elliott threw the letter to the ground. He sprang from the chair, running first to the bedroom, then to the kitchen for a baggie, and back to the bedroom. Up came the floorboards. He took the money but stared at the plastic-wrapped OxyContin he'd pulled from the warehouse, threw the money down, grabbed the pills, started for the door, dropped the pills, went back for the money, started to jam bills into a baggy, stopped as a wave of dread tightened about him, spilled the cash onto the floor, and ran to the bathroom for a piece of dental tape; but reaching into the medicine cabinet he yelled, "No, the drugs first."

He sprinted back to the pills then into the bathroom to flush them away forever. He froze in mid-toss, fearful that if the bowl was swabbed for trace signs of contraband, an accusation of tampering with evidence would be tacked onto his charge sheet. Instead, he swung open the door and dashed blindly for the incinerator chute, though had to brake to a skidding halt to avoid crashing into the neighbor lady he hated. She had been tossing bags into the furnace briskly, but the instant she focused on him, her movements decelerated as if she were in an NFL replay. Sensing his impatience, she spoke over her shoulder. "Just wait your turn, mister."

"My ass." He nudged her aside with his hip, careful not to let his hands or his crotch touch her, then forcefully jammed the bag down the chute. The heat of the incinerator flare drove him back so strongly, he bounced into the woman. With flames now licking up the chute walls, she bellowed, "What the hell did you put down there this time? Gasoline or somethin'? I'm callin' the super."

He shook his head as he closed and locked the door behind him, bewildered that such a mass of emotional overload had been squeezed into less than two minutes. He caught his breath but abruptly remembered the bundle of cash. He jammed it into a baggy and raced back to the bathroom for the thread of dental tape, which he tied to the bag and let dangle out the window. He tied the free end of the floss to a screw sticking out on the underside of a fire escape rung.

After another panicked breath and, "Oh, shit, the grass," he rolled a final joint, stood by the window, and sucked on it so fiercely he burned the tip of his nose. It was gone in seconds, and so was his grasp of reality. In a stupor, he rolled the last quarter inch of hot paper and weed between his fingers. Instead of tossing it from the window, he absentmindedly took it back to the living room, where he slumped, deeply intoxicated, into the recliner, drew a long breath, and bent forward unsteadily to pick the envelope from Geneva off the floor. As he reached for it, he realized he had been unwittingly rolling the compacted joint nubbin between his fingers as if a prayer bead. Now less than a sixteenth of an inch in diameter, he flicked it toward his ashtray but did not see it bounce off the rim of thick glass and arc into the gap between the edge of the seat cushion and the chair's arm. After a few seconds of rest and another breath, he took the letter from his lap, slit it partially open with a steak knife, and focused on the decidedly European cursive.

The ireful static steaming from the first few words muffled the buzz, so he lifted himself from the chair to go to the kitchen for a drink. The empty mason jar in which he kept his stash of marijuana was sitting in the sink. He slapped himself in the forehead and washed it out well, allowing the last dust of grass to wash into the drain. He let the faucet run to get rid of the tailings while he poured his drink. With a tumbler of scotch finally in hand, he returned to the recliner and sat for another few moments thinking about a life without constant tsuris. He could not imagine it.

With the alcohol slipping into him, he lit a cigarette then closed his eyes. Rather than a pall of pleasant tranquility, there remained a disagreeable pressure in his chest, the jumble of chemicals igniting uncomfortable spasms in his legs.

It was time to deal with the damn letter and face the music. He bent forward to restart reading, for the third time, but his hands froze as a sharp rap at the door startled him. For an instant, he feared the mean neighbor lady had come to beat him to death. Then he realized, from every crime show he's ever watched, it was a cop knock. It was followed by, "DEA. Open the fuckin' door."

A fraction of a second later came a second bang, this one decidedly not a person's fist. It was a hard object, like a bat. In fact, it *was* a bat, and the next thing Elliott saw was the "big red key" smashing through the metal door, taking with it three locks and the door handle.

The cop wielding the battering ram had culled such strength for the breach, he lost his grip, sending the hunk of hardened steel whooshing on autopilot into the living room. Before bleeding off its thrust, it crashed into the side table by the recliner, taking the ashtray and goblet of scotch with it. As it came to rest, a smog of stinking ash and dozens of Marlboro Lights smoked down to the filters drifted about the chair.

Four men in DEA vests pushed past Elliott. The next to the last had a German Shepherd on a tight leash. The dog turned immediately to Elliott, bared his teeth, and growled. The handler smirked, "Dog don't like you. You're already guilty."

The final officer, a sergeant, spit, "You Elliott Sass?" Without waiting for an answer, he bellowed, "Federal warrant to search for opioids and illegal weapons. Step aside."

The goon pushed a stack of papers into Elliott's gut. When Elliott caught his breath, he looked at the tall man. At Elliott's eye level was a name tag engraved G. UVEGES. Lifting his eyes all the way up, he came to a face that weakened his knees. Agent Uveges had had awful acne as a kid, and there were still plump whiteheads on his cheeks and forehead. The nose had swelled with the years of inflammation to a bulb, giving him the look of a pockmarked W.C. Fields. His face was so cratered, there were tufts of hair he was not able to get to with a razor. Elliott's stomach churned, and he wanted to look away, but a patch of bright, white-colored hair, a circle wider than a silver dollar on the man's right temple, caught his attention. It stood out harshly from the otherwise jet-black hair.

"Fine, knock yourself out," Elliott sneered. "I don't touch that stuff."

The thug handling the dog rolled his eyes, "Yeah, right. Okay Cruiser, find the dope, dope, dope!" He unhooked the lead, and the dog flew into the bedroom, right for the hole in the floor. He sat down at rigid attention, but all the cops found were his mother's and father's wedding rings, his old passport from Romania, and his naturalization papers.

One of the feds got in Elliott's face. "Well, wise ass, we'll bust you for smoking dope. Smelled it as soon as we walked into the lobby. Place stinks of it. Where's your stash?"

"Not me. Don't have any of that either. Everybody else is doing it, but not me. Look for yourself."

One of the squad pushed his way past Elliott, sputtering, "You knock over the butt-can? Try to fool the dog?" He took a pair of tweezers from his tactical vest, donned rubber gloves, and dropped to his knees. Watching the troglodyte sift through the detritus on the floor with the fine forceps reminded Elliott of Mikael placing the wisp of gold leaf on the scale. Then his reverie vaporized, and his face glowed as red as the battering ram still lying in the corner. The agent sensed the fear, looked up, and laughed knowingly. Elliott, thinking the vestige of his joint had fallen into the ashtray, not bounced back into the chair, imagined seeing the scrap on the floor inches from the agent's tweezers. He stared at the mirage until the bit grew magically to the girth of an apple. There was no way to miss it, and as Elliott's head collapsed in defeat, he took a deep breath to man up, hoping his admission would buy a dewdrop of compassion. The cop on the ground, however, called for the dog, who barked loudly at the sound of his name. Elliott's opportunity to whine his penitence had been harshly drowned out.

The creature skidded to a stop a foot from the cigarette accrual. It began sneezing wildly, mucus shooting from its mouth and nose to land on the cop and the chair and the shattered tumbler of scotch. The excretions mixed with the splatter of booze, the heap of butts, and the ash to form a puddle of toxic mud. The dog backed off a step and lurched into a fit of coughing, the likes of which Elliott had not heard since hospital rounds on the TB ward at Bellevue. When the animal caught its breath, he sprinted to the bathroom to suck water from the toilet. Finally, the handler releashed the dog and pulled him away wordlessly. The three remaining cops glared at Elliott as they marched past him into the hall. "Don't worry, asshole, we'll be back, over and over," the unsightly sergeant mocked over his shoulder.

There had been sufficient noise and barking, both human and canine, during the failed bust to draw neighbors to their doors. Elliott's old adversary saw the DEA vests and jumped into the hall. She was moving quickly, breathing like a racehorse, and the lead cop extended his arms to stop her. When his palms collided with her breasts, she jolted and lost her balance, falling backward, her robe flapping open as she struck the ground. She had nothing on underneath. She screamed and jabbed at the cop's legs, bellowing at the same time, "I was gonna tell you what the fuck was goin' on, but now you can kiss my ass, MALE COP PIG!" When the woman started to rise, the second cop pushed down on her shoulder, so she grabbed his leg, her teeth bared, jaws wide, trying to latch on. He seized her wrist and twisted until he could slap on a pair of cuffs. She flipped around on the ground, kicking, trying to get in a good bite. Another officer put her feet in restraints.

That, however, begat the woman's partner from their doorway. She began swinging before breaking into a string of profanity that stood up even the cops. This lady, though, was not a skinny waif. Far from it. She was at least five-ten and two-twenty-five, so the cops backed off and sent the dog to work.

The blood spatter evidence was sufficiently arrayed on the hallway walls to carry a two-hour episode of *CSI*. Someone called 911, and with New York's finest on the scene, there emerged a sibling rivalry between the two law enforcement agencies. Senior officers from both departments were soon in the hallway. They ignored the screaming from the various camps and retired to Elliott's apartment. The door, what was left of it, slammed closed, the council rematerializing after some minutes to order the two women uncuffed. They advised the gaggle of witnesses that it would be in their interest to forget what had happened, as this was an undercover, anti-terrorist operation.

As the last of the New York cops took a step into the elevator, he turned back to growl, "And don't forget, we know where you live."

There was quiet for a moment until Elliott turned to the angry woman, her robe still not closed completely. "Ma'am, I am really sorry for all that's gone on. But if you need a witness to what those asshole *men* did, I will take as many days off work as necessary to get justice for you. My partner, he was watching and listening from inside. I'm sure he heard what those thugs were saying behind our backs. He's so shy. But he'll testify under oath for you. I promise."

Both the angry woman and the angrier woman looked at Elliott inquisitively until the big girl sputtered, "You are…?"

Elliott smiled, "Of course. Isn't everybody?"

Now the women smiled, and the neighbors smiled, and there were "Good nights," and "Sleep wells," from around the horn.

CHAPTER THIRTY-SEVEN

Elliott jammed a chair against the broken door. Perhaps he was safe for the night, but he had not the slightest notion of how to protect his home the next day. He left a message on the pharmacy's HR hotline that he had been broken into and could not be at work in the morning. He took one of his mother's extra thick bath towels, ones she'd saved up for over several years, and sopped up the remains of the DEA's visit. As the mucous, scotch, cinder, glass, and years of grit soaked into the towel, it became so stained, he peeked into the hallway, saw the coast clear, and dumped it into the incinerator. He poured himself a fresh glass of liquor and, as he was about to drop into the chair, his hand landed in strings of mucous on the recliner's arm. Another towel was sacrificed, its smoke and ash quickly added to the entropy of the universe, all that it once represented to his mother instantly vaporized to disordered gas.

He fell into the recliner gulping two ounces from the tumbler before his back hit the chair. As the harsh alcohol was drawn through the lining of his empty stomach, it charged into his brain at warp speed, restoring some of the buzz lost during the assault. The day was finally over; he shook his head. Nothing more could happen. Then his chest clutched; there was still the letter from Switzerland. He started back to work on the glued flaps with a steak knife. The letter opened with chunks carved out by the blade. It did not matter. There were few words to read.

Mr. Elliott Sass,

You will please give me your email address. Mine is iledder@unige.edu.

I must discuss with you. It is important.
You must ***not*** *come here.*
Irena Ledderova

Elliott sat, paralyzed, until he unthinkingly gulped the last half-inch of his drink. "What next?" he slurred at the TV. He reread the letter and realized he had never sent an email overseas, imagining it would probably take days to get there. Finally, he lifted himself out of the chair, poured what was left in the bottle into a fresh tumbler, and sat down at the computer.

What should he say? Should he tell her he thought about her all the time but had not had the balls to write? Should he accuse her of cheating with a lesbian? Should he even write back? Over and over, he mulled the questions until he opened his mail account and wrote:

Irena,

You want to know my email address, but I want you to know some things. I think about you all the time, every day, the fun we had in Russia, how I made you feel so good in bed. Why did you hurt me the way you did when I traveled all that way to tell you that? I can never forgive you.

If you are going to write back and be mean, torture me some more, don't bother. I'm already beaten, defeated, if you must know.

But if you are going to be kinder, you may reply.

Elliott

There was an answer when he awoke at four AM to chuck up what he had not had for dinner the night before.

Mr. Elliott Sass,

Thank you for writing back promptly. I am contacting to tell you that I am moving back to

USA, New York. I would like you to help me with paperwork, that is, MY son, Aaron's paperwork. I want him to go to school in USA. You can arrange for him to enter Isadore Goldstein? I will not ask for money to raise him. He thinks his father is Soviet soldier killed in Afghanistan. That is way I want, also, as I am sure, is your deep wish.

I write again when I find out what papers are require for immigration.

Irena Ledderova

When he digested the meaning of Irena's words, he ran back to the bathroom. It took an hour before he was able to sit in the recliner and think through this latest bash in the gut. He wished he had kept a few of the OxyContins, but had he, this nightmare would be going on in the Tombs. He settled for a Sleep Eze and, after an hour, fell off. He awoke at ten, shaken by his dreams, though he could not evoke a single scene from even one.

That morning, he got the super to repair the door and replace one of the locks. Walking about the apartment as nervous as a cat, he called the pharmacy and offered to work the late shift.

Being there, though, was worse than being locked at home. Beyond the headache and volcanic gastric spasms, his fear of the future rendered him unable to count pills accurately, and he found himself redoing prescriptions several times over.

Normally, when a customer came in with a prescription, a tech entered the request in the computer at the counter. The pharmacist then took the information off the computer at his prep area. But they had gotten so busy, Elliott just lifted the next paper prescription from the pile and went to work filling it. It was for quite a slug of oxycodone: ten milligrams, with what looked like "60 tabs" next to the letters "TID,", three times per day.

Elliott glanced at the counter to see a little old lady, a customer he remembered as suffering from worsening dementia. She was waiting quietly, her left arm in a fresh plaster cast. Ah ha, broken arm, so she needed *something* for pain, but he shook his head that the doctor had written for so many of the powerful narcotic pills. He assumed this was simply an everyday quantity blunder, so he checked the amount written in words. The chicken scratch could have been "forty" or "sixty". This was a mistake as common as writing the wrong year on a prescription on the 2nd of January. It wasn't even worth a call to the physician, but he called anyway. While he was on the phone, a tech entered the paper script into the computer.

When he finally got through to the prescribing doctor, Elliott told him he'd had a bit of a problem reading the number of tablets to be dispensed. The man, far too busy to retrieve the chart, muttered, "Yeah, whatever."

Elliott made a note in the computer that he'd called to ensure the doctor wanted a batch of that size supplied and that the doctor had refused to clarify; so, as a happy medium, Elliott had dispensed fifty. With time wasted on the call, he was getting even farther behind, so he counted out fifty, handed the pill bottle to the tech, said the patient's name and birthdate, and grunted "fifty" after he had turned back to his workstation. She placed the waiting computer label, upon which she had entered a pill count of what *she* had read as 60, on the bottle. It would be a long time before he found the number of pills in the bottle and the number label did not match.

Elliott started on the next script but was uncomfortable and went to the counter to warn the frail woman to break the pills in half, or even a quarter, so that she would not become light-headed, fall, and break a hip. He knew well that would be the end of her, for she would be admitted to the hospital, contract pneumonia in three days, and die in five from one of the new, bizarre infections making the rounds at New York's Medicare wards. He suggested she not even use the oxycodone—better, a Tylenol every six hours.

The woman became teary, lamenting that the pain in her arm was terrible, and that she needed something strong. Elliott reached across and took the casted arm into his hands, checked to see it had not become too tight as the arm had naturally swelled, then touched her shoulder. "No problem, Mrs. Smith. I'll make sure everything is just fine." He took the bottle back and hurriedly split the tablets into quarters and eighths and told her he had replaced the full tablets with a size that was quite safe, as long as she never took more than one of the nubbins every eight hours, and then only if she had pain not relieved by a single Tylenol.

Jimmy came in an hour later for his shift. Elliott told him about the absurd number of oxycodones a woman of eighty some years and eighty some pounds had been prescribed. He also mentioned splitting the pills.

Jimmy laughed sourly. "Be careful, Elliott. You know about those guys got busted over at Med Direct Pharmacy on Canal Street."

"No, I don't."

"Yeah. Breakin' pills for the demented. Script for forty, take out five, put 'em in your pocket, split the rest into eighths. Who's gonna know? You just made four bills on the street. Not that I'm suggesting it. Surprised you didn't know.

CHAPTER THIRTY-EIGHT

A week later, Elliott received a concise email from Irena.

Have you make progress to get Aaron to Isadore Goldstein High School of Science and Math?

His answer was as terse.

Working on it.

That night, he sat in his mother's chair smoking weed, pondering how to approach Goldstein for a favor. Considering how he'd left things with Vice-Principal Arthur Julian, he was afraid he'd be tossed off campus before he reached the front doors. But there was no choice. He wobbled to the bedroom and picked his white shirt from the floor, the one that had lain there untouched since his foray to the bank. He started into the basement to wash it but, so unsteady from the dope, threw it into the sink and rinsed it by hand. Waiting for it to dry in front of the open oven door, he sat in the recliner and smoked two more joints, became impatient, and decided to dry it by iron. Scorching a one-inch triangle on the collar, he put it back in the sink and rubbed the burn away so hard, the collar frayed. He clipped the protruding fronds of polyester with his mother's old sewing scissors. That left a divot.

Disgusted, he threw it back into the corner and pressed one of his blue pharmacy shirts, figuring he would keep his jacket closed to hide the store logo. Next, he wobbled back to the bedroom for the suit Dr. Barron had bought him years before. It had not been hung up after the bank, spending eons draped catawampus on the back of a wooden chair next to the bedroom window. The patina of dust barely hid the uneven penumbral fade reflecting the path of sunlight and shadow diffusing into the room. Then again, the dwindling of tones at the edges might pass as a purposeful pattern to match the tie that had been tossed, askew, on top of the heap. At least, that is what he told himself as he left the apartment the next morning and tossed the ruined white shirt into the incinerator.

In the main hallway, stopping at the directory of school administrators, he sucked in a thankful breath to find Mr. Arthur Julian was no longer Dean of Men at Isadore Goldstein High School of Science and Math. But the reprieve was short-lived as he scanned up the list. Mr., no, now Dr. Arthur Julian's name sat atop the register of institutional staff. He was the principal.

Elliott walked deferentially into the office. He asked to see Dr. Julian, explaining that he had been a student there years and years before when Mr. Julian was but the Dean of Men. The secretary eyed him suspiciously, noticed the unusually highlighted suit, and the even more oddly colored tie, but rose guardedly and knocked on her boss's door.

A man stuck his head out and stared. It was not Arthur Julian—this man was soft, chubby, balding, and the fringe of hair that endured on the sides of his head was dull white. Nevertheless, the man's jaw dropped, and it was that expression that Elliott recognized. It soured his gut.

A moment later, while Elliott could not be sure, there might have been the most minimal smile forming on the principal's lips. He motioned the visitor forward and extended his right hand warmly. Elliott hesitated a fraction, worried it was a ruse to sucker punch him in the nose, but had little choice, and so took the man's hand.

"Well, well, well, Mr. Elliott Sass! You look great. This is quite a surprise, to say the least!"

"Thank you for seeing me. Been a long time."

"It has! Tell me about you."

Elliott recounted the decade-plus since graduating from high school. Julian listened in rapt attention, shaking his head subconsciously in disbelief as Elliott told him that he, too, had the title doctor etched next to his name. They congratulated each other.

Finally, Elliott explained the reason for his visit. Julian listened as politely as if he was conferring with a colleague. He explained that attendance at Goldstein was by invitation only, and that invitation was eighty percent based on test results and teacher recommendation. He thought for a moment, "That sure as hell doesn't have a whole lot to do with who's actually walking, I should say trolling, the halls around here. On the other hand, your young Aaron has quite a bit of life experience, living in Europe, speaking several languages. I'm sure you can get testimonials from his teachers. Go ahead and gather up what you can and get it to me. Let's see what we can do. You have made a success of yourself, and I, for one, am proud to say you are a product of this school. Good job, Doctor."

While still dressed for success, Elliott made a long put off decision and took the subway to the NYU School of Pharmacy. He knocked on Professor Barron's door. It was Elliott's second warm greeting of the day, a personal record, considering a single soul delighted to see him was not an experience he could recall. Barron motioned him to the seat across the mahogany desk, one twice as large as Julian's.

They exchanged pleasantries and caught up. Barron leaned back in his plush chair then shifted around uncomfortably. Elliott sagged, realizing the man had already tired of him. Barron, though, grumbled, "This goddamn chair, James Executive, best on the market, or so they say. You ask me, it's a piece of shit. Hurts my back. Three thousand plus for this thing? Tell ya, Elliott, everyone's out to fuck the next guy. Now, what can I do for you?"

"Dr. Barron, you remember when you said I might do legal work in the future, you know, testify in court about pharmaceuticals? Have a little practice on the side?"

"I do remember. You did some research for me. Top drawer stuff as I remember." He leaned back and grimaced,

"Goddamn chair. Look, I can talk to some of my lawyer friends. You need to start slowly. I mean, don't expect to make big bucks, not for a few years, but you stick with it, may turn good. Who knows?"

"Would I need special training?"

"Now, that's the sixty-four-dollar question. I came into it with a law degree. I knew the ropes in the courtroom, knew who was on my side, who wanted to grill my balls for breakfast. That takes a long time to learn, figure out what a lawyer is doing when they ask you this question or that. Attorney's job is to set you up with a situation that you agree is reasonable and then bang, ask you the final question, which you have no choice but to answer in a certain way because of what he's already pulled out of you. And when you give him the answer you must, you realize, as it's rolling off your tongue, that you just lost the case for your client. Guy'll never ever call you again, and the word gets out fast. So, what I guess I'm saying is that yes, you need some sort of training.

"You know, you can take law school in night classes. Much less competition from your fellow students. Night kids are married, most of them, in shit jobs, barely able to make tuition. Not a good situation. Lotta stress. Hardly any time to study. But as they say, what do you put after your name if you finish last in your law school class?"

"I don't know?"

"Esquire! But let me talk to some of my friends. Start you off with research again. If there's a need for testimony at a deposition, maybe you'll get some work. On the other hand, do well, remain patient, and let's see what happens."

Elliott collapsed in his mother's chair that evening and told himself to sit and rest and stop moving for a minute before opening the liquor bottle. As he watched sparks from the Jerome Avenue elevated, he nodded to himself that it had been a good day. He would forego getting sloshed—he had work to do.

He opened the email on his new laptop and began to write.

Dear Irena,

I have spoken at length with the authorities at Isadore Goldstein. There are several steps we need to take to get this done. The principal told me the request is quite unusual but not impossible.

Here are my suggestions:

1- *A list of Aaron's most recent marks. If they grade differently than in the States, we will need a way to compare the two systems.*
2- *Three letters of recommendation from teachers. I would suggest they be in English, as flawless as possible.*
3- *A way for Aaron to talk on the phone with the principal here, or whoever the principal chooses to represent him.*
4- *Proof of citizenship, or proper immigration status.*

We need to get started as soon as possible.

Look forward to working with you on Aaron's future,

Fondly,
Elliott

As Elliott pushed the send button, a flash of Aaron's affectionate smile washed over him like a warm blanket. But that was followed by a chill harsher than the night in the cemetery outside Moscow. Elliott had no idea what Aaron looked like, not even the color of his eyes or if he was short or tall. He began to cry; he didn't know his own son's full name, not even his birthday.

CHAPTER THIRTY-NINE

Elliot met with one of the attorneys Barron had called. He agreed to do research and soon became quite facile at using the National Institutes of Health collection of medical resources. He even convinced his pharmacy to pay the subscription fee as a means of delivering better information to his colleagues during staff meetings. His work was so good, the attorney introduced him to several of his partners, and Elliott's workload exploded. Finally, a lawyer invited him to testify at a deposition.

Elliott asked for a primer on how to answer questions, so the man invited him to come in after hours.

"Now, Elliott, I can't ethically tell you what words to use in your testimony, but I can warn you what the plaintiff's attorney believes is the harm done by the drug they are suing over. You look at their specific accusations and build your research and testimony around their false claims. And then we'll whittle that down to diamond-tipped spears. When you look at how these malpractice suits are structured, plaintiffs' attorneys don't look at the facts as much as who has the deepest pockets, insurance wise, and then tailor the case to go after that hapless soul, and with a vengeance.

"Bottom line is that the drug company almost always has the biggest insurance policy, and also the most to lose if their drug is proven, at least in the public eye, to be dangerous. Makes the manufacturer willing to accept settlement to keep things under the rug, particularly if it's an old drug, no longer raking in billions. Newer drug, they might fight like madmen.

"We're not talking about a lot in this particular case, couple hundred thousand dollars, chicken feed. If I can build a solid case that the drug is far more important to mankind than the oddball side effect in an oddball patient, and don't worry, we'll make the patient look like the oddest ball of all, and a felon. If we can twist the facts, I can get a quick resolution. Fine, the plaintiff'll get a few bucks for their trouble, and my client'll write it off as an annoyance, just the cost of doing business. Not a mortal wound for the corporation if we can make the jury believe any drug can cause any side effect. No point in throwing the baby out with the bathwater. Who knows, we could even win—no award. Next plaintiff's lawyer'll think twice before putting a year of his time and a hundred grand of his own money into attacking our client.

"So, boiling it all down, what we need from you is research and testimony that this quite effective drug *may* cause so and so side effect, yes, but it is so rare it cannot be predicted unless certain exotic, exorbitantly priced genetic tests are done before the doctor writes the prescription. We will show the jury that the package insert makes it clear this medication should not be prescribed without those tests. Why weren't they done? Maybe the doctor who wrote the prescription should be included in the suit. Maybe the pharmacist who filled the script could be added. Sorry 'bout that. My understanding is that, in this case, the plaintiffs like the doctor very much and refused to sue him. But that sure is going to be one of the factors I'm going to bring up. Don't sue the pharmaceutical corporation; put the blame where it belongs, directly on the doctor's shoulders."

Elliott interrupted, "But that's throwing the doctor under the bus. He'll never use that drug again."

The attorney eyed Elliott for a moment over his half-readers. "The doctor will have his own legal team if the family suddenly gets even greedier and forgets how much they loved him. Yeah, loved him until it looks like he's the only one they're gonna be able to squeeze bucks outta."

He paused for another few seconds. "I mean, you're on board, or you're not. The legal profession is a business, not a church. It's simply the way it is and always has been. I imagine you're just like everybody else, you know, need to find a way to pay the rent, keep the kids fed."

"I understand completely."

"Good. Now, the deposition is in this office next Wednesday. Suit, starched white shirt, conservative tie, none of this cutesy hand-dyed stuff. Shine your shoes until they glow. Clothes make the man."

During the hearing, Elliott was questioned for only a few minutes before being excused. The lawyer handed him one hundred dollars. It worked out to five bucks an hour, and that did not take into account the new white shirt, the can of spray starch, taxi fare, and the loss of a sick day. No matter, when the attorney called again, Elliott was happy to take a cab back to mid-town.

CHAPTER FORTY

Elliot relaxed for a couple of days, avoiding the booze and marijuana as he worked on the next case. But the dilemma of Aaron's entry status into the U.S. diverted his attention until he went to an immigration attorney. The lawyer outlined the miles of barricades they'd face, given that he and Irena were not, and had never been, married. Most of all, there was no proof of Aaron's parentage.

Elliott emailed her that evening. She wrote back telling him that, actually, Aaron had been born in New York at Sydenham Hospital. Since she had listed Elliott as the father, and Aaron had been born on American soil, Aaron was an American citizen, and it would not be as hard as the attorney had warned. When Elliott realized the lawyer had not even asked those questions, he wanted to demand a refund of his four hundred dollars, but the man had been recommended by Barron, and he thought better of it.

The letters of recommendation and grades, with interpretations, dribbled in over the next few weeks, but Elliott had been up against deadlines for the coming court testimony, and had not forwarded all of it to the school. Or, at least, that's how he justified his laziness. Irena had sent Elliott the letters in sealed envelopes addressed to Dr. Arthur Julian at Isadore Goldstein. Elliott was to hand deliver them or put US stamps on them and send them through the mails. He was not to open them. But he did, then scanned them into his computer and sent them as attachments to Dr. Julian.

The letters and Aaron's grades were glowing. Julian called Elliott and confirmed that a place in the school had been carved for the boy. He did, however, want the staff to meet with Aaron during the summer to welcome him and help design a study plan to orient him to American schools.

Elliott emailed Irena with the news. She wrote back sparingly.

> *Elliott Sass,*
>
> *Thank you. I will deal with school by myself in future. You need not do anything. Elliott Sass, you must not tell Aaron you are his father, for you are not.*
>
> *Irena Ledderova*

Elliott paused and wondered for a moment what Irena was implying, but soon understood. Whenever he saw a glimmer of hope, Irena dashed it. Though he had hours of research ahead of him, he dipped into his stash of grass then drew two Xanax from a bottle of the anti-anxiety meds he'd forgotten to leave at work. The pills came from the prescription a patient had returned, complaining the medication had made him so dizzy, he had hit an elevated subway pillar on Jerome Avenue. He wanted to know why Elliott had not warned him the pills were so dangerous. Elliott went to the computer and showed him an image of his signature agreeing not to drive or operate machinery while taking the pills. The man growled that his name had been forged, and now he was going to sue for that as well.

Regulations stated returned medications be counted then discarded, a witness selected from the staff to authenticate the process and fill out limitless forms. It was an hour of work that could be done at the end of the shift and claimed as overtime. "I'll do it later." The bottle had dropped into Elliott's pocket to keep it separated from the pristine stock.

He washed the Xanax down with a beer, sucked through two joints, and minutes later, closed the computer and turned on the TV, soon falling asleep. He awoke in the morning, hungover and so ashamed, he used his dejection as an excuse to skip any research that morning before work.

At the pharmacy, it was as it had been the day before, and the day before that. It seemed so hollow an existence compared to life in the genteel, opulent law offices, sitting atop skyscrapers that hovered over his grubby pharmacy. Though he could easily send his research to the attorneys via email, he began to get up early, don his suit, and drop off the work in person, just to draw a scent of the young receptionist's perfume.

And then he would head south, his high wearing off with each step closer to the pharmacy, where he would spend the next eight hours facing one unhappy customer after another. No matter what he tried in his head to spruce up the gloomy encounters, to cast himself as a health professional doing God's work on Earth, the more disgusted he became having to serve the steady parade of angry, demanding contemptables. By breaktime, his attitude on most days soured the staff so, they began to avoid him, turning away when he came to the microwave. Finally, after a morning of bitter encounters with newly arrived immigrants, someone snuck into the back and called Twuck, who called Elliott. Twuck suggested Elliott request a replacement for the rest of the shift, take a few hours off to relax. Elliott snapped back that he was fine, and that it was the ever-increasing flow of miscreants, not *his* attitude, that had precipitated discord in the store. "Neighborhood's getting worse by the day," he growled before ending the call abruptly.

Twuck showed up half an hour later and sat with Elliott. The gentle man allowed he was concerned Elliott was working too hard. "A month ago, you also work too hard. Then you get better. I do not know what make you happy, what make you sad, but my good friend, if you have problem, you tell to Twuck. Maybe make workplace happier."

Elliott impatiently brushed aside the need to discuss his ire but agreed to take the next two days off and consider slowing down on his study of just-released drugs, the assignment given him by corporate to keep the pharmacy up to date with the exponential introduction of new medications. Of course, this was an extra duty for which he received no compensation. He used that as a justification for his most recent request to dip into the staff enhancement coffers. While he declared the funds were for continuing pharmacy education credits, the six hundred dollars actually went for a subscription to Westlaw, the premier legal research website. Though available at the NYU Law School Library, and free to alums, it was far more convenient to do his research at home. He was able to find lists of questions plaintiffs' attorneys might ask a supposed expert pharmaceutical witness during cross-examination. He began to structure possible testimony and scientific conclusions based upon what to expect, and then present that to the lawyers who were considering Elliott for deposition or trial.

It worked. Elliott became facile with legal jargon, occasionally able to speak intelligently with attorneys. A percentage of lawyers, though, were affronted that a person not formally trained in the law could possibly fathom the complexities of legal concepts such as burden of proof and due process. It torqued their jaws that this fledgling professional had the temerity to use terms like admissible evidence, tort, and voir dire. In the end, things sifted out as only the less supercilious lawyers hired him. One even asked him to appear at trial as an expert.

For a time, he was less angered by the constant flow of the gritty into his pharmacy. He began to see them for what he believed they were, mindless masses, as replaceable as worker bees; no, not as elegant as bees, more like meaningless ants. They rose every day to do as they were genetically programmed: mill about searching for dinner; mill about doing daily chores; and crawl like caterpillars to his counter to pick up prescriptions, the first syllable of which they could not pronounce even if they could read English letters, or any letters, for that matter. But he would keep his day job for as long as he needed the income, until he could escape the tedium of life amongst the brackish.

Keeping in mind the coming opportunity to make a name as an expert witness, he steeled himself to work hard during the day and study harder at night. It was worth it, for just gazing at the law office assistants' fine scarves and skirts blunted the constant stab of thoughts of Irena.

Slowly, cobwebs began to appear around the cap of the Xanax bottle. It found its way to the back of the medicine chest, forgotten, at least for now. He was smoking far less, drinking sporadically, staying up later, getting far more done. Before work, he began taking breakfast and reviewing the research he had compiled. After a month on his new schedule, he organized and printed out the hundred pages of notes for each case, arranging them in brand-new, three ring binders, adding plastic tab dividers to organize the material into encyclopedic sections. It was his first book, he'd laugh over coffee, then carefully go through the document, impressing himself with the result. It *was* a book, a manual on the use of this or that medication, a compendium that stood to hermetically seal the defendant pharmaceutical house from further litigation. Far more meticulous than package inserts, he wondered if he might peddle the research to drug manufacturers.

He began to think of himself as an intellectual and took to wearing a white shirt and tie under his white coat at work. Almost coincident with his quantum increase in self-esteem came a change at the pharmacy. He imagined it was a result of the mayor's crackdown on crime, for a better class of customers appeared at his counter. He suddenly had less tsuris, even with the odd scruffy patron; for, he was sure, his patience was not as tested as it had been when there were so many of them.

At the end of each shift, he stopped at the salad bar of his store to gather dinner, visiting Sarge's Deli only twice a week. By May, he fit more comfortably into his suit, and it hurt less to be on his feet for eight hours. He occasionally walked all the way south to work.

Not often, but sometimes, he would serve an attractive woman at the pharmacy. If she showed the slightest interest, he would slide his card across the counter and remind that he was always available to answer any question. He was, though, careful to approach only women who were picking up prescriptions for someone else, and, of course, no one wearing a wedding band. It was his strict modus operandi—at first.

He got nibbles from ten or twenty percent of his casts. One woman in particular, a thinnish, hard woman, Darci Arletta, who had come in for oral contraceptives, and who habitually wore tight, tight T-shirts to the pharmacy, signed her credit card slip and added a telephone number written at the top in tiny numerals. They met after work that night. She was in the midst of a nasty divorce, she sniffed, but thank goodness her-soon-to-be ex was a gentle man, and even better, no children were involved.

They left the bar after guzzling three beers to paw at each other on the two-block stumble to her studio apartment. Their clothes started coming off steps before tripping through the door, their bodies wriggling about seconds later on the bare mattress that took up most of the floor in the microscopic flat. And seconds after *that*, they were done, and three seconds after *that*, she reached under the mattress and pulled out a baggie of white powder and a hand mirror. She sprinkled out one line, and then a second, nodding toward Elliott.

It's funny, he thought, that the first things to cross his mind were the "books" he had prepared over the past half year, the statement of hope, and of the sweat he had invested in himself. He kissed her cheek. "You know, I don't do that stuff. Lose my job in a heartbeat if I ever got caught. But I don't ever tell anybody else what to do in life. Please, enjoy yourself. I'll just sit here and look at you. That'll keep me high for a while, maybe even longer than a while. It was great. Thanks."

She showed up the next day asking to see the pharmacist, and only the pharmacist would do, for she had a burning question about side effects of the medicine she'd picked up for her dying grandmother. Elliott emerged from the break room blank-expressioned, yet another professional inquiry through which he'd smile and answer respectfully, then go back to his salad. His heart, though, vaulted into his throat when he saw it was Darci. She whispered that she needed to see him again that night.

He struggled to count pills for the rest of the afternoon. At her studio, she wore a T-shirt without a bra. She had already set out a bottle of wine on the peeling card table in the corner. They sat in white plastic chairs, had a second drink, and she was soon standing behind him, stroking and kissing his neck, her lips as soft as feathery down. Within two minutes, he was shaking as if in a Parkinsonian spell. That was when, still standing behind him, she pulled a baggie of white powder from her jeans, dipped the tip of her pinky in it, and softly touched his left nostril. She pushed his right nostril closed and told him, "I want this to be even better than last night, if that's possible."

Accepting it was just a tiny amount, he snorted very slowly. His head lurched. It was better than anything he had ever experienced, better than sex. While he was reeling, she took another bag from her jeans and spread a full line on the table. She pushed his head forward and whispered, "Please, I want you more than I ever wanted a man. Please."

He had lost the capacity to restrain himself and inhaled the full line. The immediate rush did not come, and he remembered feeling surprised, but he was still swirling from the first hit, and it made little difference. With the passage of a few minutes, though, his body loosened, and he soon perceived he was levitating, his cares suspended. After fifteen minutes, for the first time in his life, he was free of the yoke.

Darci waited until his eyes were swimming, and she drew in a full line from the first bag. Her eyes rolled back, and she purred, "Gotdaaaaaam!"

She pulled him onto the bed, and he was soon lost in a miasma of pleasure he had never suspected was reachable on this Earth. When they were done, they lay together, the night slowly passing in a fog of warm hedonism, sleep intermingled with waking. They made inflamed love yet again in the morning. Elliott was barely able to stay upright for a shower.

When he came out drying himself, considering one more go before leaving for work, Darci was sitting at the table coldly smoking a cigarette. He asked if anything was wrong, and she stared directly into his eyes. "Time to talk business, Elliott. Nothing's for free in this world. But you know that. Do you remember when you told me that if you were caught with drugs in your system you'd be fired?" His chest clutched. "Imagine you'd lose your license, too. Lotta years down the tubes. So sad.

"Well, I would like to make you a proposition; kind of one-sided, though. Without beating around the bush, I am informing you that you will start diverting OxyContin, eighty milligram pills, thank you, to our street operatives." She stopped and let him think about that.

Elliott instantly retorted with a snap. "I know what you're doing. If I don't go along, you'll run to my boss, tell him to give me a urine screen. Sorry, doll, whatever it was we played with last night, it'll be out of my system in a few hours."

"Actually, Elliott, the first was cocaine. Yep, out of your system fast. But the line, that was heroin, and that takes two to four *days*. Now, given that you are not a frequent flier, it may only be two days, if you're lucky. But if I tell your boss you're fucking the clients *and* providing heroin to seal the deal, he'll say you need to give him a sample right now. Okay, you're smart, you think, and you'll call in sick, the flu, bad enough that it takes a week to get over it. Don't want to infect anyone else, blah, blah, blah. Sorry, it's summertime; no flu around, and you had your flu shot, didn't you? Had to, right, to be allowed to continue working? And do you think he's going to buy your excuse when in comes a sexy customer, nipples poking out, whispering close to his ear so no one can hear?" She stopped and stared at him.

Elliott moaned, "Not so easy as you think, I mean, to get the meds."

"Oh, yes, it is. You know why? Because you're experienced, and trusted, and you'll be driving a cab for the rest of your life, that is, after you get out of the joint, if you don't go with the flow. Believe me, this ain't my first rodeo. So, you'll do it, won't you?"

Elliott was quiet again then looked at her with needy eyes. "If I do as you say, what proof do I have you'll still go to bed with me after I deliver the pills?"

"What are you talking about? New stage in the relationship. We're in a business association now. And you know the old saying: don't mix business and pleasure."

Elliott relaxed and smiled. "Okay, what do I get out of it?"

"A buck a pill."

"Wait a minute. Eighty milligram tablet sells for eighty bucks. Everybody knows that." When she did not respond, he put on his game face and spurted, "Tell you what. I'll deny and deny.

Take my week off, get my ass chewed, but nothing can be proved. It's a he said, she said. Then I wait a month and get the cops to raid this place, or better, have them follow you to see how your shit is distributed."

She laughed. "Maybe you're not so smart after all. First, who the hell do you think protects us? The cops run the damn organization. They suck off twenty bucks a pill, and let me tell you, it's worth every penny. And second, if you open your mouth, you will find yourself floatin' in the East River, bobbing up and down like a turd, no one givin' a rat's ass about the headless, handless bum they pulled out of the water. Deal?"

In fact, it was not as hard as he'd feared. Elliott was presented with clearly forged prescriptions for OxyContin several times a day for weeks after the night with Darci. Each Friday night, as he turned the corner toward the subway station home, a reptilian creature, sometimes white, at times black, maybe Asian, or Hispanic, a real United Nations of the sordid, bumped him and slipped a blank envelope into his hands. Their accounting was always spot on, exactly one dollar a pill in small bills. The first week's take was four-hundred-seventy dollars. He did a quick mental calculation on the subway home, and that was something over twenty thousand a year. It was a car, or a trip to Europe, or a starter house in Westchester County.

The next week, the envelope was thicker—six hundred and twenty—a trip to Hawaii.

Though absolutely a brainless move, he was unable to control himself and set out to find Darci, beg her for sex, pay her for sex, whatever it took. He waited in a local tavern until dark then left for her flat. As he turned the corner, he spotted a couple weaving toward her front door, hands groping each other madly. He hid behind a parked panel truck as they came closer. She was with a man who looked familiar, but Elliott could not place him. As the two stumbled past, Elliott's jaw dropped. It was Bobby Exton, pharm manager from the mid-town store, one of the most vocal anti-drug rabble rousers in the corporation; so obsessive, he had had feature recognition cameras installed at the counter to memorialize who had been dispensed scheduled medications, and software that alerted the pharmacy staff city-wide to repeat consumers of opioids.

By the time Elliott pulled his cell phone out to snap a picture, they had entered the building. He followed, waiting in the lobby until the jealousy short-circuited his forebrain. He started charging up the stairs toward her apartment, ready to blow through Darci's cheap door as if a DEA agent. As he reached the second floor, he squared his shoulders as he had seen football linemen do preparing for a hit. Then a lightning bolt flashed in his frontal lobe, and he took two more steps toward her door before he was able to bring himself to a skidding stop. The vision of a decapitated white man bouncing in the wake of boats from the Morris Yacht Club sobered him. He retreated and walked all the way home.

CHAPTER FORTY-ONE

By late September, he had not heard a word from Irena and did not know if she and Aaron had come to America. He called Goldstein to ask if the boy had matriculated, but the secretary would not reveal a word about students, past or present. He could not get her to put him through to Dr. Julian. Clearly, Irena and Julian had spoken.

He traded shifts, and late the next afternoon, he was at Goldstein crouching between cars as the kids spilled into the street. Prowling with his eyes, he realized how ridiculous he had become. He was searching for a preteen about whom he knew nothing, not convinced he'd even recognize Irena—it had been that long. Throngs headed for school busses, 4x4s, and vans: students, teachers, bus drivers—Caucasian, African American, Hispanic, Asian—a vibrating plasma of sameness, monotonous backpacks, predictable haircuts, predictable cars, all marking the end of yet another droning day in the great melting pot of New York City. There was no way he was going to pick out his son.

The next afternoon, he went back to Goldstein and asked one of the moms waiting in a car if she knew where the seventh graders exited. The woman pointed to a set of doors on the side of the old brick building. Elliott queried the first kids out. Did they know Aaron, the new kid from Europe? It took but seconds before one little girl answered, "You mean the boy who plays the violin so good?" Before Elliott could answer, she pointed, "There he is. Are you his father?"

Elliott sputtered, "No, just a family friend. Thanks."

Elliott locked his eyes upon his son. The boy was beautiful, sandy hair and blue eyes, his face decidedly Eastern European. His deportment was calm and knowing, clearly an old soul resided deep within. Elliott crept away, watching as the boy bounced toward an older Subaru. He clutched a tooled wooden box in his left hand, like the one in which Elliott had kept his chess pieces as a kid. It gave Elliott a start.

The boy went to the driver's window and kissed the woman who hugged him tightly. She was not, though, Irena. From what he could see, she was blond, and there was no sign of swelling in her face.

He returned the next morning, arriving an hour early. Parents in the line of cars dropping off children squinted from the glare of the late summer sun and quickly turned away from the grand oak behind which he had hidden. At seven, the Subaru pulled up. This time Elliott got a direct look at the woman's face. She was blond, yes, but now, in the spiky light of dawn, he could see the slightest wrinkle of her left cheek. On the other hand, if he didn't know, it would have been imperceptible. The woman was beautiful.

His chest clutched so hard, he imagined that, once again, he was suffering angina. How he wanted to wait until Aaron went into the building and slowly approach the car, though he knew it would distress Irena so, she might withdraw the boy from school and leave the city. He melted back into the sun and waited until the Subaru disappeared.

He thought of renting a car and following her home after she picked Aaron up that afternoon, but again, if she got the slightest wind of his presence, he would never see either of them again. Instead, while he went back to Goldstein that afternoon, he simply watched Aaron, the carved wooden box in hand, kiss his mom and run around to the other side of the car. Elliott thought constantly of a scheme to accidently happen upon them, though nothing he could think of led to a happy ending.

CHAPTER FORTY-TWO

In mid-October, the number of bogus prescriptions crossing Elliott's counter slowed, and with that, the Friday night cash handovers ceased. By early December, word had it the tally of local drug busts for OxyContin was ticking up. He dreaded that Darci and her pals had been arrested, no doubt in his mind that they would spill their guts, one name at a time, negotiating slabs of years cut from sentences for each arrest they spawned. His innards churned with the thought of the DEA raiding the pharmacy, the ugly agent in the lead, grinning. Elliott would be marched off in cuffs, his perp walk played over and over on the evening news for weeks as had Heroff's. He, too, would wind up in prison, maybe Heroff's cellmate.

Elliott missed the money but decided that if he dodged this final bullet, he would retire from any further connection with the drug scene. Since he had heard nothing, he thought there might still be time to silence Darci before she started vomiting names. He'd pay his friend Jimmy all the ill-begotten cash secreted under the floorboards. Or, maybe, he'd do it himself. She was nothing but a druggie, a whore. She would not be missed, just an expendable piece of meaningless collateral damage that had been erased by either the drug cartel, the cops, or a frightened, small potatoes pharmacist.

In his mind he counted, yet again, the stashed money, over thirty thousand by now. He would have to remove the cash and any trace of the illicit benzodiazepines he was using again, more and more frequently. He spent hours imagining a niche existed in the walls of the basement laundry, perhaps in the storage room, maybe behind the ancient pipes curling out of the fractured cement floor. There had to be a filthy corner down there not breached in decades.

But first, before his inevitable arrest and imprisonment, he had to make it back to Goldstein one more time to see Irena and Aaron. He feigned illness yet again, left work early, and hailed a cab. With the flash of a hundred in the driver's face, there was no argument about following the Subaru from school to wherever its journey ended.

Aaron had the wooden box in his hand when he got into the Subaru. He hugged his mom and they started off slowly, making a few turns until they came to a neighborhood park. Aaron got out, blew a kiss, and walked to one of ten concrete chess tables. Irena watched as an older black man rose and shook Aaron's hand then gestured toward the opposite side of the cement board. When Aaron took his seat, Elliott saw the beam on Irena's face then a reddening of her eyes. She waved goodbye, but Aaron did not notice, too busy opening the wooden box and covering his side of the table with perfectly tooled chessmen. Elliott recognized them instantly as Staunton Grand Master pieces, fairly new, he guessed, for the figures were carved in wood, ivory widely shunned. He was not surprised. The black man deferred to Aaron, hit the clock, and so began the match.

Elliott drifted toward them, stopping to watch other players who greeted him with indifferent nods. When he got to Aaron's table, he smiled at the boy, and the return beam and gentle wave stopped his heart, much as they had a decade earlier. The man looked up and, seeing Aaron's response to the visitor, smiled back as well. Elliott couldn't contain himself and spoke to the older man. "Nice set—Staunton Grand Master?"

"Yep. You know your stuff. Ain't mine though, belongs to the boy, and well it should. He's gonna be a master, this one."

Aaron blushed, and Elliott stuck his hand out to the man. "Lester Singer."

"Abraham Baker. And this here is Aaron."

Elliott took Aaron's hand weakly, nervous with the first ever touch of his son. The boy, though, squeezed a bit, and Elliott returned the gesture with a firmness that brought an even harder squeeze of Aaron's hand.

Elliott pretended to look over at other matches but stood at the side of his son's table, not behind either player. Eventually, Abraham looked up and asked, "You play?"

"Not so good as the two of you."

"Well, would you like to take on Aaron when I'm done with him which, if he makes another move like that, ain't gonna be too long from now?" The three laughed, and Abraham nodded to Elliott, "Seriously, we be done shortly. Why don't you sit in my spot and have a game? Give young Aaron here a look at another adult player. At school, all he sees are the kids. Not allowed to play against the teachers, some more of that political correctness stuff. What are we coming to?"

Elliott looked at Aaron, waiting for a nod, but it was better. "Yes, Mr. Singer, I would like to have a go with you."

His accent was decidedly French, and Elliott smiled. "Sounds as though…" he began to comment then stopped himself, for he thought better than to unsettle the kid by being a smart guy and asking if that was a Swiss accent, possibly from Geneva. Instantaneously, he realized his presence would be discussed with Irena an hour later in the car home. "Yeah, sounds as though this is serious business for you, I mean the chess set and playing at school and then after school. I think you'll whip me good."

They laughed again, but it was Aaron's move, and he embarrassedly nudged a knight into position, looked down, and spoke softly, "Checkmate, Mr. Baker."

Aaron and Elliott played one game. It could not have lasted fifteen minutes before the majority of Elliott's army was sitting pathetically next to Aaron's left hand. He told himself the drubbing was a function of his need to lose in a hurry and excuse himself before Irena appeared. He was right. A minute after he rose and shook their hands, the Subaru pulled slowly into the parking area. Elliott was gone, behind a hedgerow, staring at Irena before she looked up from setting the parking brake.

Elliott changed his shift once again and played with Aaron several times a week. He began to bring pastries, and Aaron asked if he could bring one for his mom. Elliott froze, and Aaron, sensing the change in his new friend's demeanor, spurted, "I told her all about you. She's really pretty, you know. You could meet her if you wanted to. She'll be coming to pick me up soon."

The hue of Elliott's face drained to alabaster. Abraham looked up, "You okay, Mr. Singer?"

Elliott muttered an excuse and made his way to the bushes, his last vision of them for some weeks until there was a break in the rainy season. On a clear fall day, he hired a cab and followed Aaron and Irena home to an apartment a block from the park. He watched, barely able to control himself as they disappeared into the parking garage. He paid the cabby and made his way toward the building, but trepidation overtook him, and he turned north to walk all the way back to the Bronx.

CHAPTER FORTY-THREE

By mid-December, he had not heard further from or about Darci Arletta, or from the cops, nor laid eyes on Irena. The number of blatantly phony prescriptions had dried up. He had dodged the bullet without having to murder his dangerous enemy. Conceitedly, he went back to counting pills, rote work, the task so simple, he spent a lot of time during the day on the pharmacy computer preparing for his next expert testimony.

While that aspect of his life had also slowed, he realized these complex cases took years and years to settle. He was but a sub-atomic particle in the two-hundred-billion-dollar-a-year sweepstakes that was litigation in the U.S., fully one-third of the after taxes profits of the combined Fortune 500. Still on good terms with the lawyers, it would all pay off in the end. He relaxed and smoked a joint, congratulating himself that he was learning patience, accepting that compensation for his endless hours of research would come once each case was settled. And so be it. He would work at his side gig until it matured then leave the dark smog of his day job in the rear-view mirror.

He did notice, though, that the stock bottle of OxyContin from which all the licensed pharmacists drew pills for prescriptions was emptying at the same rate as when he was engaged full tilt in the subterfuge. He became curious and searched the computer for the source of that rapid depletion, and after he saw who had filled the bulk of the scripts, his stomach soured, and he searched the paper file for the actual, written prescriptions. There were dozens and dozens of them, all identical to the ones he had filled over the hectic six months of his immersion in the scheme. Four of the five full-time pharmacists had been co-opted. It seemed only Twuck's hand had not been stained by the conspiracy.

How, he shook his head, had Twuck resisted? The answer would have to wait.

On a quiet Sunday afternoon, the streets covered in snow, a cachectic, sallow woman hitched into the pharmacy. Her face was a jigsaw puzzle of weeping sores, and though Elliott was in the back doing paperwork, the miasma of her unwashed body and rotting teeth reached him before she made it to the counter. He quickly marched up front to attend to the woman and move her on her way before she so stained the place, they would have to close early and blame it on the snow.

Irritably, she slammed a prescription onto the counter so hard, it blew off toward Elliott's side of the desk. As it floated past, he caught the letters Oxy and did not bother bending forward to pick it up. He laughed coldly at the woman, "This is a joke, right? You're from the DEA, testing me, right?"

He had spoken so loudly, one of the pharm techs drifted over, picked the script off the ground, and began to laugh sarcastically, finally taking a breath to hoot, "You came to the wrong place, Doll. What you want is the street dispensary. Go out the door, turn left, and the guy with the hoodie'll fix you up good."

The woman's twitching went into overdrive. Her face turned to Elliott, then to the tech, and back again. Without a change in her insipid expression, she hocked a loogie into Elliott's face. The tech, Javier, a good kid from nearby Hell's Kitchen, reached across the counter with his long arms and shoved her. She fell backward and hit her head on the metal stanchion that helped form the customer waiting line. The crack was so loud, the other tech from the back rushed forward to help clean up what he assumed was the most recent of the bottles that broke by the two dozen each day.

The woman's eyes rolled back in her head. She vomited, or at least there was a string of yellow-brown grot oozing from the corner of her mouth. She coughed weakly twice and turned blue. Elliott and the tech who'd pushed her vaulted over the counter and nearly retched themselves but hooted vociferously at each other, sort of a war chant, and began CPR, using the pharmacy's barrier masks. The woman shook, a grand mal seizure, Elliott was confident. He called for the stethoscope in the back room where they did flu vaccines. Though he had not listened to a patient's chest since pharm school, he was certain she wasn't breathing and, worse, that her heart was silent.

Elliott called for the defibrillator. He ripped her shirt open. Jaws dropped; gasps echoed off the walls. It was not the bilateral mastectomies that so astonished the crowd. It was the surgical wounds, tissue that had healed in knobs of scar as crude as a lava field on Hawaii. An embarrassed, yet oppressive, silence hovered as Elliott quickly applied the paddles, but then he dithered, too terrified to pull the trigger. Finally, a customer who had drifted over snapped, "DO IT, GODDAMNIT!"

Elliott called out, "All clear!" The woman's gaunt frame jerked from the floor. While Elliott knew he had not yet activated the paddles, the patient bounced around so, Elliott was unable to listen for heart or breath sounds. It didn't matter. His patient had been resurrected, now hyperventilating, a stream of profanity widening eyes as far away as the seafood department.

Elliott called for a towel from Housewares to put pressure on the very minimal scalp laceration, a scratch, really. Javier called 911. The dispatcher hemmed and hawed that the roads were impassible. The tech screamed into the phone that there couldn't be two inches on the ground, and since it was New York City, and the slop had already been falling for half an hour, it was certainly nothing but slush. "Get off your fat ass and send the aid car."

The dispatcher howled, "Who the fuck you think you talkin' to?" There was no time to answer before the connection was lost.

Elliott called for the store's wheelchair, took the woman's vital signs, and guessing they were stable, called upon all four employees to load her aboard. He had Javier push, and they made their way through the quarter inch of slush to the hospital two blocks away.

Elliott directed them to the emergency room entrance, held the door open, and called over Javier's shoulder, "This lady just had a cardiac arrest!"

The patient turned her head toward Elliott and spat, "What the fuck are you talkin' 'bout, asshole?"

An orderly who had been standing at the counter flirting with the intake clerk turned toward Elliott. "Must notta been all that bad a cardiac arrest, huh?"

Another staff member started toward the patient, resolve etched upon her face, but she screeched to a halt the instant she recognized Beverly Williams. She rolled her eyes and snickered, "Lemme guess, she turned blue, and you couldn't hear her heart. Am I right or what?"

Elliott's mouth dropped. "She's done this before?"

"You would, too, if you were living in doorways in this weather. Okay, just leave her here. We'll have the doc examine her. I'm not taking the risk of turning her out. Believe me, the first time you think you're smart and street one of these GOMERs before you evaluate them, they find a way of coding right outside the door. Then we gotta rush out to turn the body, feet, and legs toward the door, make it look like they were on their way in."

Elliott turned his head, "GOMER?"

"Yeah, 'Get Out of My Emergency Room.' You know, a frequent flier. I think she was in twice yesterday, and…" At that moment, the door from the treatment area opened into an almost empty waiting room. The orderly looked over, "Here's the doc now. She'll know what to do. She's the best."

Elliott glanced up from his embarrassed head droop. His eyes opened a bit wider, interest building as he took in the blond hair and crystal blue eyes. Suddenly, he was standing a bit straighter, but so was Javier, who waited for Elliott to speak. When his boss couldn't form words, Javier grinned foolishly, "Hey Doc, got a case for ya."

The doctor smiled reassuredly at the woman. "Mrs. Williams, what is going on? Are you okay?"

The patient looked up and moaned, "I tried to fill that prescription I got here, but this jerk threw me on the ground." She pointed at Elliott.

The doctor squinted and stared at Elliott's face, soon shaking her head in disbelief. When that did not dampen the shock, she began blinking her eyes stutteringly, trying to reset the image. Another failure, and less than one microsecond later, her color faded to a pallor matching that of patient Beverly Williams. The doctor reached up and clasped her nurse, Debbie Matsukawa, by the shoulder to steady herself. As the already searing atmosphere intensified, Elliott's color drained as well. Nurse Matsukawa surely imagined she was not in a hospital ER, but at Kabuki theater.

Elliott squeaked, "Javier, I need to get back to the pharmacy." With that, he spun on his heels and sprinted from the ER, exhorting himself to move faster and faster through the slush. While there was absolutely no smoking allowed near the store, he ran inside the pharmacy to his locker and pulled out a pack of Marlboro lights, taking the first drag before he was through the back door. He considered buying a six-pack and guzzling it in the bathroom.

When Javier returned pushing the empty wheelchair, he approached his boss. "You okay, Elliott?"

"Yeah. I think I used to date that doctor. Long time ago. Didn't end well."

"They never do. You must be right. When you left, she had to sit down in the waiting room. More like she collapsed. Looked like she saw a ghost or something. Thought they'd need to do CPR on her. And, man, I was right there to do my part for medical science, all the respirations she might need. What a fox, huh? Maybe you should reintroduce yourself, or if it ended that bad, maybe you could introduce me." He grinned and went off to restore the wheelchair.

CHAPTER FORTY-FOUR

Elliott believed Irena had known all along that he was a Doctor of Pharmacy, where he worked, and how his life had changed. And maybe she didn't, but now she would come to the pharmacy after work. Finally, they would finally be able to talk, to act like adults.

But when quitting time came and she did not appear, he felt gripped by a need to open the vault, let the demons free. He would take the initiative. It was time. He went into the store proper and bought two dozen roses then walked to the hospital and searched for her car. If she had already left, he'd walk in the cold to her apartment and sit there until she let him in.

The Subaru was, though, still in the parking garage. He went to the ER, flashed the flowers, and asked what time the present shift ended. It was already over, the receptionist blushed, but the staff hadn't yet finished their paperwork. Did he want her to go into the back and tell someone he was out there? "Oh, no. I want this to be a surprise."

He returned to the parking garage, pulled the petals from eight flowers, and sprinkled them from the elevator door to the Subaru. The other sixteen roses were held in abeyance behind his back. When the elevator door opened a moment later, Irena emerged with a nurse, both women's mouths agape. Irena's head shook. She spoke softly to her companion, who giggled kindly and went her own way.

Irena turned a full circle looking for Elliott. When he stepped from behind a concrete column, she stood motionless. Instead of pacing toward her, he walked blandly in the direction of the Subaru, careful not to get too close. As she approached the car, he took steps in an arch, keeping a ten-foot radius.

Elliott pulled the roses from behind his back. As she peered at them, her eyes clouded. It was the first time anyone had ever brought her flowers. "Irena, please, just listen for one minute, and then I'll be on my way. I mean you no harm. I will not block your sunshine. I did something terrible to you. I swear, to this day, I do not know what it was; but I will admit I did not treat you like a lady.

"I thought, Irena, that we were friends with benefits. I mean we weren't like steady dating when you asked me to come to the USSR. And what the hell was that about? Never been outta New York since I got here as a little kid. Next thing you know, I'm off to the moon—no, fuckin' Mars. Then I'm smuggling a hundred thousand dollars' worth of diamonds out of a communist country into the US. What the hell is that about?"

As he went on, his passion grew. "And you have to be honest, I never tried to fool you. I adored making love to you, you…"

She shooshed him. "Not so loud. Around here, I am respectable woman. Not what you see in me." Now *her* voice rose. "Object. That's all I was to you. No woman wants to be piece of meat. You found me deformed fucking freak," her tone mounting, "easy prey, low hanging fruit, didn't you? *Didn't you*?"

At that moment, the elevator doors slid open, and her two orderlies emerged. They stared at Irena's face, then at Elliott. In two seconds, they started walking toward him, daggers in their eyes. "Hey Doc, you okay? Need this guy tuned up?"

The other one huffed, "Hey, ain't this the dude brought in Beverly?"

She laughed. "Don't worry, he is so defective, tune up isn't going to fix anything, but thanks." She paused, gazed at the flickering florescent lights, then continued softly. "Yeah, he is that dude. You have to admit it was good of him to go through streets to bring her to ER. She is handful."

"Yeah, okay, Doc. See ya in a couple a days. Good workin' with ya. You're our fav, ya know?"

Elliott could not help himself. “Mine, too.”

They walked to their cars. Irena waited until they had driven off. “Elliott Sass, I have been carrying that hurt in my heart for many years. You had to remember only man who ever put hand on my body before you was pig who raped in my village. Even my father never, not even to change diaper. It was only women, and then so rare, I have no memory of human touch before village maggot. You, but you had my heart in your hands. Don’t you understand that for woman it is not just roll in sack, at least not for me. Yes, I loved what you did to me in bed, but you had to know I had such strong feelings for you. I could not keep separate, even if I tried.”

“Irena, I swear I did not do anything purposely to hurt you. I thought it was just me who was growing close. You have to admit, you yelled at me a lot. Yeah, I screwed up a bunch of things in Russia, but I had no idea what the hell was happening. I was a goddam teenager. Wasn’t even twenty yet, not even nineteen. You sure didn’t seem to respect me all that much, putting me down all the time.”

“It is way we are raised. Way I am raised. Outcast, not to be spoken to, but commanded to, every adult squeezing every drop of labor out before I die from my curse.”

He stretched the bouquet toward her. She stared at it for a moment then reached forward and took it softly, almost tenderly. She lifted the roses a few inches and breathed in the scent. Her eyes reddened, and Elliott thought a tear fell.

Elliott turned but called over his shoulder, “You know where you can find me.”

CHAPTER FORTY-FIVE

With Christmas approaching, customer flow in the pharmacy slowed as it did yearly. The chronically ill, mostly lonely elderly, were too depressed to leave the house. In the good old days, during the Seventies and early Eighties, the desolate were allowed to spend the holidays in the hospital, “social admissions” listed on the intake documents by the residents. As the business of medicine ripened, that practice was not only abandoned, but every second in the hospital had to be defended with proof that the insurance company was on board to cover the charges. Specially trained nurses trolled the hospital halls digging and scratching to unearth and blot out even a single hour of overstay, the cost of which came directly out of the corporation’s bottom line, and eventually out of the doctors’ pockets. The atmosphere in the hospitals slowly decayed into tribes, those committed to the bottom line, and those sentimental physicians who were better served by finding workplaces elsewhere.

The younger patients also stayed away from clinics and pharmacies, too busy with shopping and partying to worry about silent bodily dysfunction. Afterwards, there would be a frantic rush to lower blood pressures that had skyrocketed with weight gain and salt overload, and to address cholesterols that had zoomed far above two hundred; but for now, it was quiet.

Elliott was bored to tears. He spent a portion of his days wondering pensively if Irena would call. He was never peaceful, not for a single moment, though he tried to smooth the unease by reminding himself that she had, at least, listened to his version of history and seemed moved. But this did not blunt his needs, and he was casually seeing a sprinkle of local ladies, not one of whom piqued his interest for more than forty-five minutes. That changed when he met an anesthesiologist at a party thrown by a colleague from the pharmacy. He was smitten the instant she spoke her name, Antoinette Chugunkin. The heavy Russian accent stole his breath. He managed to get out of her that she was from a wealthy, refugee, Russian Jewish family. He tried to impress her with a few of the Russian words he remembered from so long before. She was, though, not terribly receptive, rolling her eyes several times at his battered pronunciation, and more at the content of his vocabulary, which was essentially profanity.

She finally asked, "Do you know a single intelligent word in my language…or yours?"

"No."

A cold Russian shoulder was tipped at him for the rest of the night. That made him even more crazy. While he finally wheedled her cell number, the phone usually went to voice mail, and when he borrowed a phone to call her, she always had a work excuse to avoid seeing him. Elliott, though, would not suspend his efforts. He would have this Irena or the other one. He had nothing to lose.

He wondered if he had anything to fear, that maybe the two would cross paths. Yes, both were Russian women, Russian physicians, but they practiced miles apart. New York was a city of six-hundred-thousand Russian emigrees, and there were tens of thousands of doctors sprinkled throughout the five boroughs. The chances the two hopelessly busy women would ever meet was diminishingly small. And so, he kept up the barrage of calls until she screamed, "Go away, asshole!"

Anyway, he became suddenly quite busy preparing for a malpractice case in late January. He had already put quite a bit of time into research despite the whole project being worth only a couple thousand. When he divided his hours into the payoff, it came to a few pennies less than he was making per hour at the pharmacy. Also, the lawyer he was assisting was small change. The future there was pointless. He would do this case, then concentrate on finding opportunities that would lead to real wealth.

It came to him during a commercial enticing the family members of those who suffered from mesothelioma to choose its law firm to represent them. The ad invited sufferers of this rare form of lung cancer to join their class action lawsuit against the manufacturers and users of asbestos. He had heard of this sort of litigation but had little idea what it meant. He Googled the term "class action" and found it referred to trials in which thousands of victims, all harmed by the same corporation or product, could file suit as one person and split the jury award. These lawsuits sometimes settled for billions; the attorneys became obscenely rich while the victims rarely got more than a pittance, a slap on the back, and the satisfaction that they had obtained justice. It was enough to shut them up. Yes, he would find a law firm engaged in the big time and offer his services as an expert witness.

Two days later, a customer came to his counter asking to fill a prescription for Accutane, tretinoin, probably the most effective treatment for acne ever formulated. The drug, though, had been under attack over several decades for a host of side effects, the worst, birth defects in the children of women who had taken the medication within a month before, or during, pregnancy. There were also accusations of depression, psychosis, Crohn's disease, and metabolic abnormalities that covered essentially every bodily function. As with most products, or human endeavors, if one read the list of side effects, the product would die on the vine of its own weight. Accutane, though, had not perished. It was that effective.

A lot of money was on the line with Accutane, for the manufacturer was still reaping huge profits, and at the same time bleeding preposterous amounts to patients who could prove they had been harmed. As a pharmacist, Elliott was quite familiar with the medication in terms of dosage, time frame for treatment, and side effects. He was also aware that any woman contemplating taking it had to sign a contract of sorts swearing she would follow strict pregnancy limitations. But working in retail, he wasn't terribly acquainted with the drug's mechanism of action and wanted to look into that more carefully, he imagined, than would most doctors.

He found it a complex molecule, one similar to Vitamin A, but different enough to give the drug its power to do several things: reduce the number of oil glands in the skin, limit the size of those that remained, and most important, severely limit the amount of oil they produced. It was the oil that created a favorable environment for the special skin bacteria that gave rise to horrible acne, and which grew especially well when locked into the skin by a blackhead. Accutane basically limited clogging of skin pores, allowing the body to expel the bacteria before they could set up shop.

He studied the molecule and the process for several days until he had figured out a way to synthesize it in the laboratory. He called the pharmaceutical company in Chicago over and over until they put him through to an administrator. He floated a proposal. As he was both a graduate chemist, a pharmacist, and had developed good knowledge of the medical malpractice scene, he wanted to join their team to fight the frivolous lawsuits filed against the company.

Two days later, he got a call back from Ellsworth and Ellsworth, the law firm representing Accutane's manufacturer. They were interested. He would be sent a ticket to fly to Chicago. He was to bring the corpus of his research. A date would be chosen in short order.

That evening, Elliott received an email from Irena.

Elliott Sass,

You are invited to celebrate Hanukah with us. The date is 20th December. RSVP.

Irena

He wrote back in a heartbeat.

I will be there. Can I bring anything?

The next evening, there was an email from Ellsworth and Ellsworth. He was to present himself on the 19th of December. The interview would be in two parts over two days, finishing late on the 20th.

Elliott sat in his mother's chair and smoked a joint. Then a second. After a swig of bourbon, he pulled the laptop in front of him. In an hour he had written drafts of twelve letters, six to Irena begging she forgive him for cancelling Hanukah and six to Ellsworth and Ellsworth begging the interviews be rescheduled. He twisted in the wind pondering both sides. With the Accutane project, he'd be vaulting several stories over the rest of the pharmacists who had branched into the sphere of litigation. Accutane promised a steady income for several years; there were that many pending suits. He could not think of another way of amassing enough capital to reach his dream of escaping retail, starting his own company, and milking his computer skills to milk the online pharmaceutical industry. This time he would be smart, staying an inch from the line, never again crossing it. He was done looking over his shoulder. Those days were gone forever.

It wasn't, he finally decided, an either or. The more rationally he considered his problem, he understood he could do both: see Irena *and* present himself for an interview. Certainly, Ellsworth and Ellsworth would understand, what with the holidays and the months before the next lawsuit scheduled for trial, which he discovered wasn't until late March. Calmly, he opened a new document and wrote apologies to the law firm, suggesting he was, other than the 19th and 20th, totally free to appear at their convenience. The reply was there in minutes. He was to return the airline ticket forthwith. They would call him if the need arose.

CHAPTER FORTY-SIX

On December 20th, Elliott wore his just-dry-cleaned suit and his just-shined shoes, stopping first at an upscale Jewish bakery in Washington Square. He brought a bottle of first-rate kosher wine and a challah. As Elliott was the last customer before they closed to celebrate the first night of the holiday, the woman at the counter smiled warmly and pushed back his credit card. "This is a Hanukah gift from my family to yours, sir."

He was rendered silent for a moment but took ten dollars from his wallet and placed it on the counter. "From *my* family to yours, ma'am." They touched hands.

Elliott was so nervous when he pushed the front buzzer, the bread slipped out of the bag onto the concrete steps. He looked about furtively, and with the coast clear, brushed off the dirt with his sleeve. That left a patch of schmutz on his suit that he did not see in the dark. Irena buzzed him in, and at her apartment, he lost the bread again and was picking it up when Irena opened the door.

She shook her head. "Come in, Elliott Sass. Let me dust that off." She took the wine and bread then stretched her arm out to invite him in. "There's someone I want you to meet." Elliott's heart pounded so hard he imagined Irena could see it through his jacket.

In the living room sat a woman facing slightly away. From what he could see of her profile, she was decidedly Eastern European, probably Russian. "This is friend, Antoinette Chugunkin. That means cast iron in Russian. And she is, so you better mind yourself."

He did not appreciate the name for a moment and froze, thinking that Irena had brought over her lesbian lover from Geneva. He had, yet again, been made a fool of publicly.

Irena started to speak, but the woman gasped and let go a string of foreign sounds that had the warp and woof of obscenities. Irena stared at her friend. She asked in Russian, "Are you okay, Antoinette?"

Antoinette sighed, "We've already met." Then she sat back and guzzled her wine.

Irena's jaw dropped. "Oh, my God, this is one you told me about?"

She hooted, "It's the one," then turned away.

Irena shrugged. "Why I am not shocked? Anyway, Elliott Sass, there are others to meet. I trust these two are strangers." She called in Russian and two young boys came out of the bedroom clutching handheld computer game consoles. They barely looked up until Antoinette snapped at her son, "Gregor, say hello." He did in a mumble, though his eyes had already dropped back to the computer toy. The other child, though, gasped so forcefully, Irena flinched.

The boy blurted, "Mr. Singer. Is it really you?"

Irena took a step toward Aaron and asked in Russian. "Oh, my God, what did you say?"

He repeated himself in English then spoke almost breathlessly, "Mama, this is Mr. Singer, the man I told you about who plays chess. He's really good. He was really nice to me and Mr. Baker."

Irena made a comment to Antoinette in Russian then shooed the boys back to the bedroom. Her face was as pale as the day Elliott had shown up in the ER wheeling Beverly Williams.

Antoinette asked gently, "Irena, do you want us to leave?"

"No, I want us both to see how he gets himself out of *govno* pool he is swimming in."

Antoinette laughed, "Yeah, he floats face down."

They stared until Elliott took a prolonged breath buying time. "Okay. So, I play chess…"

Irena snickered, "If you can call it that. Go on."

"I was walking through the park, and I saw you. Didn't recognize you at first, but the line of your face, it was so beautiful…"

"Stop *govno*, go on."

"So, finally, I recognized you, and I realized that Aaron was Aaron."

"So, who is Mr. Singer?"

"Hey, I'm a local pharmacist. Anybody could follow me home, hit me in the head, and search my place for opioids. You know that. Do you use your real name on the street?"

"Yes."

"Well, I don't. And I never even had a conversation with Aaron. He was a polite kid, and I was, to be honest, happy to see he's turned out so well."

"Oh, that is such surprise?"

"Irena, stop."

"No, you stop. You have stalked me. That is how you knew which was my car in hospital parking garage. True, yes?"

Antoinette inserted herself, "And stalking *me*, too."

"I have not been stalking either of you. Did I ever show up at the hospital again? No. Who wrote to me? Was that you, Antoinette?"

Antoinette twisted her lips, "You Americans say, 'yeah, right.'"

"Look Irena, I couldn't get you out of my head. I met Antoinette at a party. She reminded me of you. Is that so hard to understand?" Irena stared at him silently. He went on, "I asked her for a date. Is that stalking? When she told me no, I never called her again. Did I ever call you again?"

Antoinette grunted, "No."

"So, I met Arron. Big deal. I didn't ask him about his mother. I didn't ask him where he lived. I am innocent of all wrongdoing."

"Elliott Sass, you are never innocent." She turned to Antoinette. "Shall we let him stay?"

Antoinette rolled her head left and right skeptically. "He is man. You will never get straight story out of him."

Irena thought for a moment. "Elliott Sass, you may stay." She lifted her head toward the bedroom door. "You two, come out, and leave games in there."

When Aaron appeared, he walked straight to Elliott, who stood and shook his hand. "Aaron, I'm sorry, I don't use my real name on the street because I am a pharmacist, and we carry a lot of controlled drugs in the store, and I don't want people to know who I am. I'm sorry I misled you."

Aaron smiled. "That's okay, sir. Mama says your real name is Mr. Elliott Sass. May I call you Mr. Elliott?"

Elliott suddenly blurted, "How 'bout you call me Uncle Elliott?" Both he and Aaron turned sheepishly toward Irena.

With a not-so-veiled twist of the lips, she added, "Well, *Uncle Elliott*, maybe you should tell Aaron work you do in pharmacy."

"What's there to tell? I count twenty pills and put them in a child-proof bottle. My hands get tired at the end of the day and burn by the weekend. So that's what I do. Your mother, on the other hand, she does something for humanity. Be like her, not like me."

"Yeah, Aaron, I give drunk man emesis basin and call nurse to hold head over bowl so they do not get it all on me."

Aaron's friend asked, "Irena Ledderova, what is that thing you just said, an emma…?"

"Emesis basin, Gregor. Little bowl to, what is word? Antoinette! You know, *izvergot*."

"Puke."

"Thank you. Yeah, my job is great, Gregor, like your mama's. But she has it better than me. She does not have to talk to patients. In operating room, she checks name, hospital number; she says, 'You go to sleep now.' Put mask on face, boom, done. Anesthesia nurse comes in, take over for mama, then mama goes to next victim, same thing. Five patients at one time, all sleeping peacefully. Pay is more than surgeon."

As Irena was speaking, Antoinette grasped the bottle of wine Elliott had brought, inspected the label, shook her head *comme ci comme ça*, poured herself a nearly full glass, then filled

Irena's. She blurted, "Your mama knows all about surgeon income, don't you, Irinska?"

Both women laughed and took healthy gulps of wine, turning away from Elliott to chatter in Russian. Elliott leaned back, slowly letting his head slump. He wondered if Irena would allow him to stay after her friend left, if he would ever have a single instant to talk with her privately. As the conversation waned, he looked up a couple of times to see Antoinette glancing at him. Both times, their eyes locked, but Antoinette quickly turned back to Irena, and Elliott dropped back into his stupor.

Elliott finally leaned forward stiffly and poured half an inch of wine into a used water glass sitting on the coffee table. He sipped for a moment, smiling inside as Aaron and Gregor twitched, waiting to get back to their computers. He was about to ask Irena to let the boys go off to the bedroom when she stopped chatting and sent them off.

Elliott finished his splash of wine. It was enough to temper his self-imposed need to remain sober, to exercise complete control of his emotions. He refilled his glass, lifted it toward the women in a silent toast, and took a deep swallow. It was not long before his face reddened, and Irena mocked, "You look like borscht I have boiling for dinner." His blush drained. "Antoinette, you see, he hates borscht. Only reason to invite him is to make him eat it. He must, to be polite." After a pause, she laughed, "No, Elliott Sass, I did not cook borscht."

The color began to return, and he smiled weakly. "Thank God…"

She watched him searching for something else to say then let her jaw drop. "Elliott Sass, this is first. Your tongue is tied!"

And so he remained for the next two hours, during the brisket of beef, latkes, potato pancakes, and *sufganiyot*, round jelly doughnuts, the same meal his mother had prepared every Hanukah. During the second bottle of wine, he wondered why she had invited him. The third bottle rendered him maudlin, twisting inside. Irena had humiliated him publicly, final retribution, he guessed. The only way to stop the bleeding was to leave. He would never see her again, and the way he had been demeaned, never would be too soon. Conceivably, this was her Hanukah gift.

Antoinette watched Elliott staring into the blank TV and murmured to Irena, “I think we should be going.” Irena did not protest.

After they left, Irena told Aaron to get ready for bed, which he did without a fight. Irena checked on him minutes later. He was asleep. She came back into the living room and sat on the couch. “Elliott Sass, I am glad you came tonight. I thought we would see old Elliott Sass. I wanted to see for sure. I am probably wrong, but maybe you have changed. You are good with boys. You are honest about Antoinette. It made me sad that you are lonely for Russian girl. The best is, you make honest living. A professional!”

Elliott was shocked. It took a few seconds to come up with a response. “Well, by itself the pharmacy pays shit, but I have a gig on the side.”

“Oh, my God. It is legal?”

“Ha ha.”

“No, I am very serious.”

“I testify as an expert on pharmaceuticals in malpractice cases. Don’t worry, I’m on the doctor’s side.”

“That is nice, but you get paid by insurance company?”

“And?”

“In your work, it does not matter the side you are on. It is always wrong one because patient always loses, always. You are paid to hurt patient who came to you for help. That is going over to dark side, if you did not realize. Be careful who you associate with. Ever heard that?”

“What are you talking about? They pay me about five hundred an hour to say, ‘Don’t blame the doctor or the drug manufacturer. The warnings were all in the package insert.’ How is that immoral?”

“You know well. And, big deal, five hundred every three months?”

“Not quite. I testify very, very slowly,” his voice decelerating into a protracted pronunciation of syllable after syllable.

"Quite moral. So, you are stealing from stealers, huh?"

"Look, Irena, I'm not some fancy doctor. Put in the same amount of time in school as you, and, still, I'm a second-class citizen. I make babkas for the years I put in."

"Who made decision?"

"Okay, you're right. Stupid me. Maybe better if we talk about you. Did you get married in Geneva?"

"No way."

"Boyfriend?"

"None of your business." She stopped for a moment. "I will be honest. I am seeing doctor from hospital." She watched Elliott's eyes. They merely blinked. "He is orthopedic surgeon."

"He's Russian, Jewish?"

"Oh, God, no. He is WASP. Wealthy, wealthy home. Sometimes, that is problem with parents."

"Are you planning to get married?"

"Probably."

"Are you in love with him?"

"It matters? Wealthy home, good salary, money on top of money."

"Okay, but you're a doctor. You're rich on your own, or you will be in a year or so. Why marry someone just for money? You, of all people."

"You know, Elliott Sass. You remember how I lived as child, if you can call it living. When I was here first, my English is so bad, even more than now. Nobody will look at me, nobody speak to me. Never one lesson in English. In Moscow college, some students come together and play games to speak English. We make up new language. Worthless here.

"In U.S., I never leave apartment. How could I? Even if not such monster, still no one understand me, nothing in my pocket. I live two years with no idea of life here.

"When I go back to Russia to see father, from what I know of America, not much different. In Russia, I understand whispering behind back. Nobody in Russia have penny more than me. Here I am freak with no money. Still freak with little money."

"You are not a freak, never were."

"Elliott Sass, thank you very much, but you are full of *govno…*"

He interrupted, "And that's another thing. Your pal, Antoinette. Why is she so mean? All I did was ask her out on a date, tea or coffee, that's all. I was dying to see Irena Ledderova. She wasn't you, so I tried to pretend. Even said a few words in Russian. She yelled at me that I was a moron *and* had a foul mouth. All I did was use the language you taught me. What the hell did I do to her? Bitch!

"Maybe not everything on Earth is about Elliott Sass. Maybe she has own problems." Irena stopped, filled her wine glass, and chugged half of it. "I should not tell you, but she suffers with breast cancer. She is young; it is certain to be aggressive. What can she do to protect son when she is gone? Her life is shit; it is almost over, and nothing she can do. Decades of work to get M.D. wasted. You still want to call her bitch?"

Elliott gasped. "How was I supposed to know?"

"You were not. It does not matter if you know or do not know. We Russians do not 'share our feelings' like American snowflakes. Hello, bright morning sunshine; ach, *gov…*" She stopped abruptly, "I teach you to be polite. *Yurunda*—nonsense. Russians see only dark future because we know there is only dark future. You *Amerikanskiy*, we laugh." Her eyes reddened. "You are weak, lazy; in school, in work, in life. I despise Communist Party. America is only hope to control Russian Federation. If you *Amerikanskiy* do not start to work, you will learn more than Russian cursing. Borsht shop on every corner. Those *ublyudok* are hard like steel. You remember *ublyudok*?"

"Bastard."

"If only you know p. chem like cursing." She took another swig. "So, I do not care if I 'love' my surgeon. I want this man not to beat me or son. I want to eat like I want—borsht, borsht, borsht. I do not want to be cold, ever again. If I have all that, I will roll up inside Mexican jumping bean and be quiet. That will make satisfied Russian."

Elliott had nothing to say for a while. He poured half of the last of the wine and mumbled, "Well, that sure brightens my holiday night." He paused again. "Let's not talk about you getting married for a while. I got an idea. Why don't you tell me where you've been for the last decade, not that it's any of my beeswax."

"It is not. But I will tell anyway. After we are back from Russia, first time in my life there is second person. Maybe someone loved me. That was gone very fast. I was locked in apartment hiding my face again. NYU students, ach, pitiable. You last one week, maybe three days in Russia if you are so lazy as that, but I already said so to you.

"So, I decide I will run away. I am weak from living here. Sorry for myself. Looking in mirror is harder every day. I know I understand people in Europe better. Not so many cowboys. Civilized."

Elliott raised his hand as if in class. "How did you pay for it all, I mean losing your stipend and free apartment?"

"So nosey." She poured the rest of the wine into her glass and finished it in one gulp. "I sold some diamonds here in New York. Went through Eastern European mafia—scum—but they gave me something, enough to leave precious U.S.A. You know, I am not in love with Germanic culture either, but there is quick fellowship in Geneva. Free rooms for fellows. First thing to do, I paste up mezuzah. Did not nail. Maybe have to take down fast when they figure out Ledderov can be Jewish name. Next morning, I get note dean is to see me at end of day. Should I go? Antisemitic *ublyudok*, I am guessing. Be out on rear by sunset."

Elliott interrupted. "And a nice rear it is."

"Could you be serious for one minute?"

"Excuse meeeee."

A weak smile curved her lips. "Never mind. This guy, dean, he pulls out two wine glasses. I am thinking, here it comes. So, he will allow me to stay if he gets what he wants, or he would relax me so I wouldn't make scene when he tells me fellowship is all big mistake, sorry. You know what, Elliott Sass, I did not care. Door One is way to get ahead in world, so I will go along with what he wants.

"One minute after sitting down, knock on door. Wife and kids have come to welcome Irena Ledderova. Such beautiful people. Daughter is babysitter. They pay her behind my back. In Europe, they say, responsibility of university to make sure student body is safe and cared for.

"He calls me back to office one month later. No wine. I only could think of ogre in village. But fooled again. He says facial surgeon is friend, plastics in Third World, much experience in revising my problem. Doctor has private practice in downtown Geneva. Elliott, that is high, high, rent. Patients come from all over world to this guy.

"Dean admits he already pointed me out. Doctor thinks he has chance to help. I ask in Geneva about fees—tens and tens thousands of dollars. He said several surgeries. It could not be done with salary of graduate fellow.

"I thank dean very much, but I must go back and work on degree. Maybe someday. Then, I think what did I learn in U.S. What is one good thing? Always alternatives, always." She slapped her forehead. "Next weekend, took train to Antwerp to sell diamonds left over. Did not know how much they sell for, but on train back to Geneva, thirteen hours, plenty of time to count money. I am richer than in dreams. No little mouse working in chem lab ever have such money in pocket, ever in world history. Dean is ecstatic, offers leave of absence. As much time as needed. Then he stops. 'You have considered medical school, yes? Use God-given talents to make people feel good?'

"I asked to stay in program; maybe become doctor after I finish research. That was fine. Could I have first surgery, then two weeks rest, then back to work? No problem.

"When you have come to Geneva, I was maybe halfway finished, still freak, but not so much." Her voice cracked. "First time in life to walk into room and people stare, yes, but only for seconds. Then boys drop eyes onto chest.

"Do you know what that..." She began to cry, then sob, and soon so hard, she could not speak. Gruffly, she opened her laptop and typed, "Do you know what it means not to be disruptive because..." She picked up an English phrase book, searched, and typed, "*Through no fucking fault of your own*? Do you?"

Elliott had never seen her that vulnerable. She remained wordless for a minute then heaved a deep breath. "And here we are."

Elliott could not speak and raised his wine glass, tipping it toward her as an offering. She shook her head, and he put the glass down. "Irena, you are free to do anything in your life now. You do not need to explain a damn thing to me, of all people. I'll tell you the truth. You may have had a superficial problem that seemed beyond repair, but it was not. My lesion is so bottomless it cannot be reached with a hundred scalpels, or a thousand pills, or five thousand hours of counselling.

"And I'm not asking for your pity. Don't deserve it. I just wonder why you invited me here tonight. I know it wasn't to torture me by letting me see my son. As much as you hate me, that isn't you. You deserve a surgeon, not a druggist. Even he probably isn't good enough for you…sorry, that was dumb."

"Elliott, you will stay with me the night? I do not want sex. I only want you to hold me. I want to bring back my most remembered moment."

"What?!"

"Things are easy now for me. Big doctor, not dog anymore. Patients always hitting on me; females, also. It is too easy. I begin to forget struggle to get here. You were vivid color in my life—for the few days. Hope. The only color I have ever seen. Hope. First time I saw you—you remember interview?"

"What man could ever forget?"

"I am more nervous than you. You are first one I am to interview. Dean was thinking to be in admissions process maybe helps student shyness. He knows I am hammer in p. chem, but not so much in life. He is good man, still important friend.

"When I saw Elliott Sass first time, I forgot to be professional. I am thinking only to make love with you."

"Really?"

"Really. How can I tell you this?" A smile crossed her lips. "That day, outside in garden, I look down there, you know, you know where I mean. I wonder what it looks like. Next thing, I am doing everything to get you to apartment. *Amerikanskiy* will say, 'I fell for you.'

"Sometimes, I was not nice to you. I am sorry. It is my defense. I could think only that what we did was dirty, soon you will be tired of me, of my body. Then, off you go. How many days we are home before I will never see you again?"

Elliott sighed. "What a mess, Irena. But I will no longer hurt you by confusing your life. I think I'll go home. I do not want to be here when Aaron gets up. It isn't right." He was about to say, "I will think about you for the rest of my life." Instead, he touched her cheek, grabbed his coat, and let himself out.

CHAPTER FORTY-SEVEN

In the week after seeing Irena, it was not until Friday that she returned his emails. She wrote back only, "Not to worry, I am sobered. Russian sensibilities return."

He was unable to sleep without Xanax. They helped for only a few nights, and when he doubled up, he was unable to think clearly for the next day and a half. Alcohol made it worse, throwing him into fits of despair that had him crying in bed.

Then an offering emerged from the ether. A customer returned a prescription of Vicodin, hydrocodone, an opioid not as potent as OxyContin, though only by a whisper. Elliott slid the bottle in his pocket, once again nodding to himself that he'd do the paperwork at the end of his shift. And once again, he did not. After a Xanax and an hour of tossing in bed, he went to his pants, stared at the bottle of Vicodin, and with less than a single additional second of further rumination, swallowed one. In fifteen minutes, it was pleasant enough, but more crucially, he slept. He did the same thing the next evening, and the next. By the fourth night, he waited impatiently for the warmth to encase him. It came but was decidedly muted. The Xanax did nothing. He added half an additional hydrocodone. That sufficed for a couple of days; a second full tablet helped after that, but it also quickly depleted his stock.

At work, he noted a concurrent uptick in the garrulousness of the clientele. It angered him to the point he became short with the staff, and soon there was a visit from Twuck. Elliott apologized and agreed he had been in a bad mood, a personal problem, and that he'd correct his attitude.

He did that by replenishing his opioid supply, this time accepting back a bottle of thirty oxycodone. He knew he was pushing his luck, but into his pocket went the pills. Finally, on a particularly restless night full of awful, threatening dreams, he startled awake as a police car sped by on Jerome Avenue, passing right under his window, siren blasting, the cop no doubt pissed he had been sent on a call at 2 A.M. Elliott jumped from bed and stood at the window screeching profanity and threats at the long-gone patrol car until, fully awake and trembling with anger, he dropped into his mother's chair.

Still unable to keep his eyes closed, he got a bourbon and sat back down to count the number of oxycodone left. That fueled a sense of dread, for no matter how hard he shook the bottle, no matter how many times he counted, there were only five tabs. He spent the next minutes scheming, seeking a new source of dope, no matter the lawfulness, morality, or consequences of the scheme. Finally, his body went limp, acknowledging he had become nothing more than a dyed-in-the-wool junky.

He was the precise creature, a pathetic addict, that course after course in pharm school had warned about being the greatest jeopardy to their careers. They taught addiction was a medical disorder, a disease, the patient to be solaced, even pitied, for it was a syndrome in which the brain has been restructured. Therefore, the patient was no more responsible for the disease, they harangued, than the poor soul who'd suffered a stroke. Elliott knew damn well this was but lip service paid to the tsunami of liberalism washing over American medicine. That might be fine to believe if you were a professor in your ivory university tower, or an internist on Park Avenue, but not so much on Jerome Avenue, where, if you were a cop, a medic, or doctor in a storefront immediate care clinic, that pat on a patient's back after revival with Narcan was more a veiled lashing out, a figurative stab, than an act of warm human caring.

Back in bed, still unable to sleep for the sweats and cramps, he lay awake trying to conceive of a new source of pills. Waiting for return prescriptions from senior citizens was unreliable, but focusing on the elderly had to be the solution. As he tossed, he remembered his old soliloquy warning frail, senior customers, "You know, Mrs. Jones, even one full pill is far too much to take at a time. You might get dizzy, fall, break a hip. Then we'll have real problems. We care about you. Why don't you let me split the tablets into quarters and eighths? No charge." Then he would skim two whole pills off the top like Jimmy had instructed, chop up the remaining thirty-eight tabs into pieces so small—and considering the dust and tiny slivers—no one short of the FBI could determine how many total pills were present. With this scheme, by writing the original, doctor-ordered number on the label, all accounts within the pharmacy would remain pristine. But he also reflected upon Jimmy's warning that there had been arrests for such duplicity. Those, though, were stupid pharmacists who had not planned well. His scheme was foolproof.

The next morning, he decided to try a few dry runs before actually pruning product. The first customer with a prescription for OxyContin was an aged man who looked to be eighty, one foot in the grave, the other on a banana peel. He could not believe that the man had been sent home with a script for ninety tabs. While it was enough to sedate the entire Bronx Zoo, the patient standing before him was so ancient a soul, he would have been well advised to avoid taking anything more than a breath of the medication powder as he opened the bottle.

Elliott shook his head at the low-hanging fruit dangling before him. He made a quick reassessment and decided to make this more than a dress rehearsal. He launched into his speech. The customer listened quietly for a few seconds, staring as if Elliott was one the legions of psychopaths he'd dodged on the subway to get there. To Elliott's surprise, the man's face suddenly flashed a ruddiness that matched the diatribe into which he launched, one that raised the temperature of the pharmacy a good seven degrees. "What the fuck are you talking about? You little prick, don't tell me how much pain I need to feel before I take my fuckin' goddamn medicine. I know about you little shits skimming pills. Everybody knows! I'm callin' the cops."

The word "cops" should have shut Elliott up, but he could not help himself. As words flew, it would have been hard for an observer to tell who was more desperate for the meds. When the customer howled, "You fuckin', big-nosed Jews, always ripping off the little guy…" Elliott dashed around the counter, fists clenched. A tech wedged himself between the two, another ran to fetch the store manager.

Elliott vociferously accused the patient of drug seeking, calling him a well-known opioid abuser. The manager ordered one of the techs to call the doctor in question and find out if the script was real. In retrospect, it might have been wise for Elliott to have taken a couple of seconds to inspect the paper prescription, not just the first two lines of computer input. It was from Irena's hospital, specifically the ER, and the doctor on the phone confirmed the poor man's script had been issued only after she had spoken with the patient's oncologist. The voice then accused that the delay at the pharmacy, forcing the dying man to wait, "…even a half-hour longer than necessary, is cruel and unprofessional."

The doctor went on to explain that, in fact, the customer was only in his 50s, suffering from end-stage lung cancer, the result of exposure to shipboard asbestos during naval service in Viet Nam. He wasn't even a smoker. The doctor related that two, and even three, OxyContins per day were no longer controlling his abject pain.

The tech answered, "Yes, Dr. Ledderova. We'll let the pharmacist know."

"And who is that, if I might ask?"

The tech hesitated but realized there were no grounds to refuse that information and piss off a local doctor. "That's our Dr. Sass."

That evening, he began a self-detox. Within a few days, he'd weaned to a quarter tab every other night. He believed he hadn't needed the taper, hadn't really needed to stop the dope in the first place, though he had to admit that only ten days later there was another grand shift in the mood at the pharmacy. Even the clientele had become far more cooperative.

He had also met a new girl, a doctor from somewhere in Central Asia, a country Elliott could not pronounce. She wasn't terribly pretty, wasn't terribly nice, but her accent was not that unlike Irena's. Her father was an aerospace contractor who had spent decades buying commodes built in the slums of his city for thirteen dollars and selling them for over three thousand to Western aircraft manufacturers, Boeing in Seattle, and Airbus in France. The daughter was filthy rich, so rich, she had her twelve-cylinder Jag XK serviced twice as often as recommended. At four thousand bucks a clip, one tune-up would have paid his groceries, electric, gas, water, and carfare for over a year.

There were other red flags. Most concerning was her foot fetish, a mania that worsened with each visit to her condo in the Dakota Apartments. The first time he'd gone there, she met him at the heavily gated front entrance and dragged him past #72, John Lennon's old apartment. He turned away and dropped his eyes. She laughed mockingly. "Oh, so sorry, Mr. Sensitive Plant."

It wasn't long before they were in her bedroom. He was ready, but she made him show her how he took off his socks and put them back on. Once, okay, maybe she wanted to look at his feet to make sure they were not deformed, that he was well groomed. But it was over and over, maybe twenty-five times, until a toenail caught and ripped a hole in the cheap material.

Then there were the late afternoon assignations in the Jag parked behind the pharmacy, and in the staff bathroom at the back of the store. It was exciting, but the prelims, taking off and putting on socks, ate so much time, the trysts went beyond his allotted break. He got a call from Twuck asking him not to leave the pharmacy unattended for so long. Finally, he came up with a plan. He would not wear socks. It was at the next rendezvous, after a full day in just loafers, that she shoved him out of the bathroom, hurled a loose roll of toilet paper at his head, then ran from the store to peel away blindly in her Jag.

He was relieved. For a few days after the breakup, he was surprised that access to unlimited piles of dough was not what it was cracked up to be. Subtracting her cash from his life's equation was actually comforting, and he refused to take her calls on his cell or the pharmacy line.

She returned three days later. Confronting him in the pharmacy proper, he demanded she leave, or the cops would be called. She gave him the old two-finger, the backward peace symbol used in England and her colonies, an equivalent of the American lone middle finger. She spat at his feet, raked her left hand over his face, and started tossing bottles of decongestants at him, again using her left hand. One of the techs, an East Indian guy, was shocked but managed to explain that in Central Asia one never touched other people with the left hand, particularly on the head, and never, ever, on the face. That was the hand used for personal hygiene in a country where toilet paper was a luxury.

The next morning, during a visit from the district manager, Elliott was presented with a bill for hundreds of dollars of stock to be replaced at retail. Corporate administration also concluded that the ire he'd raised in a local medical doctor could not possibly serve their business interests. He was to apologize to the woman. While Elliott crawled back, it was only long enough to solicit funds to pay the bill and beg her to withdraw the formal complaint.

For that Saturday night, he bought a pair of good socks, and when they were done with the carnality, if you could call the one-sided engagement with a motionless, near-corpse, making love, she took him to Jean-Georges in the Trump International Hotel and Tower. On a sheet of her office letterhead, she wrote a note stating that Elliott Sass was not responsible for what had happened and enclosed a signed blank check for the damages. After the *Ten Course Omnivore* tasting, she went off to powder her nose, asking him to order dessert. He could not help himself. Recalling that she had once puked at the sight of Munster, he ordered the cheese plate featuring Stilton, Blue, Roquefort, and the *pièce de résistance*, Limburger. He also ordered the Berry Garden, her favorite. As the waiter placed both orders on the table, she cursed in a foreign tongue, swept the Berry Garden off with the back of her hand, and threw three one-hundred-dollar bills on the table as she marched out gagging.

He quickly wrapped the wedge of limburger in a napkin and slipped it into his pocket. At the driver's window of the Jag, he apologized that he had not been aware of her aversion to cheese. She frustratedly reminded him of the Munster incident, but he swore, "That musta been with a different guy." She gave up with a huff, forgiving his male insensitivity with an outstretched hand stroking his privates.

At her place, he waited until she went into the bathroom to recharge her diaphragm, laughing to himself how unlikely Round Two of the sleepathon would ripen to fruition. With his smile decaying into a malevolent twisting of features, he reached down and very deliberatively peeled off his socks and slipped them under one of the pillowcases. He jammed globules of the Limburger between his toes, then reclined and waited. It wasn't two minutes before he was running sockless, feet squishing in untied wing tips, from the Dakota. He never heard from her again.

Elliott sent Irena email after email forging excuses for denying the patient with cancer his OxyContin. He told her of the man's aggressive antisemitism, but there was no reply. At the end of February, there was a note from her; but she did not mention his bedside manner, nor their relationship, just that Aaron had earned all A's despite his limited English and the demands of an unfamiliar school. She had been bursting to tell someone, but there was only her surgeon friend, "And he has kids of his own…enough said."

Elliott wasn't sure why she had confided in him. And where had she been for the last eight weeks? She knew well her email would torment him, reringing the bell that she was having the time of her life, back again with the rich, successful doctor who demanded little of her. She was patting herself on the back for having reared a good son from whom he was, callously, by her hand, estranged. He replied that he was proud of them; she had done a great job raising a child in so dangerous a world. He asked to see them. She did not write back.

CHAPTER FORTY-EIGHT

There were a few scraps of OxyContin left. He took the pills over two nights. Just that quickly, three blowups at the pharmacy culled a talk with Twuck. There would be no weaning from the opioids this time. There were none left. What he did was take a half Xanax during the workday, enough to mute his bitterness but not enough to blunt his professional skills. By the end of the week, the turmoil in his chest had faded sufficiently for him to take stock, once again, of his life.

He knew what mattered: first, Aaron's smile and the remote hope he would regain Irena's affection. Next came research for the attorneys, particularly working alone and netting three hundred fifty an hour for testifying in depositions and five hundred in court. He decided to go looking again for a sugar daddy law firm to keep him busy over the next three or four years.

He called Sanford Barron, the pharmacist-cum-professor-cum-attorney-cum-expert witness at NYU. "There may be some action," the man spoke collusively. "Just read in the *Times* this morning that Marlancor Inc.'s Ampfloban's already in trouble. What, been out for six, eight months? I'm sure you know all about it."

Elliott blustered he was quite familiar with the new non-opioid created specifically to block pain signals from herniated and damaged spinal discs. In truth, Elliott's cliental subsisted far from the level of affluence needed to purchase the drug. In fact, he had dispensed it just once, to a baseball player from the Yankees who'd paid cash so the team would not find out his back was a shipwreck. Elliott had told himself to look it up at home that night, but he had forgotten.

Barron nodded, "Good. Tell ya, you don't need a crystal ball to figure out there's gonna be a lot of litigation. I'm thinking, maybe we should position ourselves to be their go-to guys, available the day the shit hits the fan. When the court cases begin, there'll be plenty for those who get in early. Why don't you put together one of those binders of yours; I'll give Marlancor a call and tell them we're already working on it. If they bite, you and I'll get together soon."

Elliott spent the next evenings reviewing Ampfloban. Marlancor Inc. claimed it to be safe and effective, bragging it was a Nobel Prize-worthy breakthrough in pain management. Its efficacy and safety, however, had nothing to do with whether it survived the gauntlet of coming litigation. What it had on its side was that hydrocodone, standard release oxycodone, and OxyContin were presently the mainstay treatments for chronic low back agony. The side effects and the potential for addiction of all three were well known and deadly. But that did not matter. What did was that this new drug was a direct challenge to the opioid industry, and there was no question it would be attacked viciously, litigation fees reaching the moon before all was said and done. On the other hand, in terms of ROI, return on investment, it was worth the hundred million the legal narcotic cartels had put aside for a rainy day.

The problem facing Marlancor, one of the true pharmaceutical giants, was that the FDA had already begun evaluating Ampfloban's side effects, particularly a dangerous elevation in liver function tests that could presage eventual liver failure. How a medication affected the liver was always the laser focus of FDA approval for a new drug. That was not unreasonable. The liver is a chemical jack-of-all-trades, said to conduct five hundred separate chemical processes over the day, many of which are to manipulate and detoxify the constant barrage of contaminants that find their way into the blood. All drugs are toxins, for they artificially alter bodily functions, and all drugs have to pass eventually through the liver, most reworked there to render them less malicious. During that process, if a medicine is sufficiently noxious, some of the liver cells that try to tame it will become inflamed and perish. When the cells die, they rupture and leak their contents into the blood. Measuring the level of those escaped chemicals is done by taking liver function tests. If they are elevated, that indicates more than normal death of liver cells, and thus damage to the organ. While the liver can repair itself at a good rate, if it is dying faster than it can be replaced, healing falls behind, leaving a net destruction. Eventually, there will be insufficient liver left to carry on, and that is called liver failure. It is fatal without a liver transplant.

The FDA got wind of three patients who, during Phase II trials, were found to have a rise in liver enzymes. Phase II is composed of hundreds of patients, and while that raised eyebrows, the elevation was mild. The affected patients simply discontinued the medication, healing caught up within a month, and all liver function tests quickly returned to normal. The bump in the road was so small, Marlancor issued a statement that the original data was likely erroneous, simply an aberrant signal.

In Phase III trials, testing the drug in thousands of people, the same seemingly insignificant percent of subjects suffered mild elevation. Some of the affected even continued on the medication, and the liver tests stabilized a bit over normal. At that slow rate of destruction, the liver's corpus would last a hundred years before running out of tissue to perform its cleansing duties. There were also six subjects who had accelerated rises in liver tests. When Ampfloban was discontinued, they, too, saw their numbers return to normal, though more slowly than those with only mild elevations. Marlancor was satisfied that if doctors checked liver tests on a frequent basis for the first few months, they could winnow out the rare strong reactors and take them off Ampfloban for good. Those with mild elevations might even continue, as long as they were tested every three months or so. If levels never got too high, who cared? The body could easily tolerate the mild problem. There was even data indicating that the percentage of those who developed any liver involvement was lower than the percentage taking the comparison sugar pill. There was no need to stir the beehive over a triviality. It was certainly preferable to taking narcotics for the rest of your life.

Conversely, if you were the fabricators of the very narcotics that Ampfloban was designed to replace, it did not matter that the major side effect of *your* product was death, a lot of it, a full NFL stadium's worth every year. And that was just in the U.S. But what counted in the drug wars was if a new rival product exhaled the slightest breath of a side effect, no matter how benign, it was grounds for a fight to the death in the courts to have the medication banned, hang the fortune in legal and lobbyist fees.

Eventually, Ampfloban's liver abnormalities came under the FDA's purview at the hands of a whistleblower at Marlancor. She had sold reams of computer files to several makers of hydro and oxycodone, but the volume of data was so immense, it was impossible to tease out that the dangerous elevations of liver enzymes had been found in but a handful of Phase II and III patients.

But mathematics had no bearing for the opioid industry, which manipulated the data on the toxicity of Ampfloban then cajoled a U.S. senator into hand-carrying the results to the Commissioner of the Food and Drug Administration at their headquarters in White Oak, Maryland.

It was, though, too late. The FDA had just, hours before, cleared retail sale of the drug. Marlancor, aware of the leak of their data, had already dispatched the first shipments, tractor trailers of the stuff waiting in parking lots, surrounded by legions of taxis co-opted to drop off individual boxes at local drugstores the instant the medicine was declared legal.

As with most drug releases, doctors were quickly descended upon, enticed into, and richly rewarded for prescribing the medication as fast as they could scribble illegible prescriptions. That generated an early momentum of sales, obviating a quick recall.

Oh, to be a fly on the wall of the CEO's office the day, three weeks later, even more reports of cracks in Marlancor's golden egg were passed to the FDA. And what about the day the lay press got their hands on death certificates memorializing liver failure in two patients taking Ampfloban? While it appeared the bottom line was about to be strangled, it really wasn't the end of the world. Even when two more deaths made it into the papers, the CEO soothed the board, reminding that any publicity was good publicity—name recognition. The corporation simply increased their TV and medical journal ad blitz, to say nothing of authorizing inflated funds for hospital administrator junkets to Paris and Madrid. And then there were the endless steak dinners at Ruth's Chris for local providers to persuade them over good wine that rumors of liver disease with Ampfloban were vastly inflated by the purveyors of the narcotics that were killing their patients willy-nilly. Even if believed, the mortality rate was diminishingly small, less than for Motrin.

In the trenches, local practitioners listened to hurting patients plead, "Doc, I want some of that Ammoban. Heard about it on the news. Gets rid of pain. No addiction."

"But, Mr. Jones, there may be some side effects."

"I don't care. You gotta get rid of this pain for me. I wanna try it."

Marlancor was soon making such a killing, they invested further gobs of money in disguising the not-so-sparkling, real world data that began flowing in as fast as the profits. Their bet was that the FDA's response would be sluggish. It was. For the feds to allow there was a problem meant they had failed in their sacred duty to guard the public, no matter that their real mission was to shield big pharma. Marlancor's strategy was to pose their defense in the form of a question, flippantly asking at press conferences if it was such a great surprise that the legal narcotic drug cartels were out to get them.

A high federal court ruled that a lower court's order to delete Ampfloban from the drugstore shelves was premature, especially since the FDA experts had approved the medicine in the first place after years of testing. A *writ of certiorari* was denied by the Supreme Court, at least until the FDA was finished with its probe. While the endless investigations chugged on, so did sales and an accumulation of interest on the nest egg Marlancor had created with the first wave of profits.

While it was common lore that it cost two billion to develop a drug and deliver it to the worldwide market, a powerful study by the AMA claimed it was really more like five hundred million, plus or minus a hundred million here and there. Since serious medication adverse effects were commonly not exposed until after the potion had made a name for itself, the pharmaceutical houses devised preemptory schemes to make the eventual demise of a bad drug nothing more than a blip on the radar scope. They kept their lawyers busy exploiting cutthroat legal, and not so legal, tactics to delay the retirement of their product. When the cat was finally out of the bag, there came negotiations with the FDA to delay withdrawal of the medication from the U.S. market. Marlancor agreed to print black box warnings on each bottle to remind vulnerable patients and ignorant doctors of the risks. When the meaningless alerts failed, and enough patients had died, and the drug company was forced to "voluntarily" pull it, there was still a decade before the foreign market imploded, and never in the Third World.

When it was clear to the corporate principals that a rocket had been aimed at their profits, they squirreled away vast sums before the years of class action lawsuits were even filed, to say nothing of settled. At seven percent interest, it took about ten years to double an initial investment, so if they could cut a corner here, one there, and come up with a billion in profits early on, then invest it soundly, there would be no need for long term efforts to protect a medication that was eventually going to be removed from the market no matter what they did. While they'd pay the piper one day, in the meantime, all efforts would be devoted to slowing the wheels of justice even more than usual and allow the money to earn interest while they impeded litigation.

To Marlancor Pharmaceuticals, if that meant paying a piss ant pharmacist five hundred bucks an hour and covering a musty room at a Holiday Inn Express, so be it. It was a submicroscopic irritation, zero cost in the grand scheme of things when said druggist was able to fritter away a couple of days of court time. If, through mountains of motions among other nefarious but legal tactics, Marlancor could suspend the penalty phase for a decade, they could earn that extra billion in investment interest. If there were two hundred and fifty court days a year, over ten years, that came to $67,000 profit for each wasted hour before a judge—$400,000 a day.

Sanford Barron ordered Elliott to report to him with his binder of research in a week. That meant basically no sleep. There was little choice but to raid the Concerta supply at the pharmacy. He pocketed two weeks of this legal form of recreational methamphetamine that was prescribed for attention deficit disorder. More and more commonly, though, it was bought on the street by students and professionals wanting to improve concentration, decrease the need for sleep, and to lose weight. He would figure out a way to replace the tabs as soon as the present dilemma was over—first things first.

Barron was impressed and had Elliott meet with Marlancor's chemists and pharmacists at their plant in White Plains, thirty miles north of the City. He would be paid one hundred dollars an hour for travel, two fifty an hour for deposition testimony, and five hundred in court.

What he learned from the day off work he'd taken to meet the Marlancor chemists and lawyers was that he was not to answer questions about what the company did or did not know during the testing and approval process. No matter what he had read in the professional or lay press, he was to testify only that he had not been involved in the development of the drug and had been consulted only as an independent pharmaceutical professional. He was allowed to offer that he had dispensed the medication and understood its mechanism of action. He was to state that he could find no connection between what the drug was accused of causing and the actual molecule.

Essentially, he would be paid only if he answered each question, "I don't know." How he delivered that phrase was up to him, but it better be good because the attorneys, four of them, would be in court to scrutinize every second of his testimony. As the lawyers coached over and over, his value to the corporation was based solely on the nebulous answers he was able to cloak in obscure scientific jargon. "Let's force the plaintiff's attorneys to spend a shitload of time untangling all the garbage you can generate. And I'll tell ya, one of the best props is how thick your three-ring binder is; maybe bring two—I don't care, fill 'em with shit paper—and let's not forget, a crisp white shirt, a good silk tie, and those wingtips, Christ, they smell like bad cheese."

When the lawyers were done, they could see in Elliott's eyes that he was not convinced of the propriety of the case. In fact, he wasn't. He had spent much of the time thinking about Irena, his attention unfocused. He asked himself if there was still a way to make her respect him professionally. The question left a morose pressure in the middle of his chest.

He was, a moment later, shaken out of his reverie by an impatient, "Look," the greyest of the attorneys huffed, "I assure you the plaintiffs in this action are nothing but greedy frauds. It's your typical money grab. You're on the right side. You'll get a good look at these people during trial—trash, willing to tell any lie to suck a few dollars from a legitimate corporation, from people who actually work for a living. They hurt you and your customers. *They* are the ones sending up drug prices, not us. Well, that is not going to happen here. We are fighting back this time—finally."

Elliott's sentience snapped back into the posh office, his attention a function of the vituperative tone taken by the lead lawyer, not as much as by his words. A lesser attorney took up the harangue. "Here's our theory of the case: the plaintiff, an old man, is deceased. Died some time ago of liver failure. Yeah, he'd taken Ampfloban for several months to treat chronic low back pain, but what they don't want you to know is that he was a low-level grunt in Viet Nam. Guy was stuck out in the rice paddies, exposed to Agent Orange for a full year. That by itself is enough of a medical history to rot a liver, but what they're really trying to hide is that he was also a drunk for his entire adult life.

"Let's look at his reasoning for taking Ampfloban. The family claims his back hurt so badly, he couldn't go to work anymore. Yeah, right. That's, in and of itself, sufficient to raise red flags about the man's moral character. Everybody knows so-called debilitating back pain is simply another excuse for malingerers.

These are deceitful patients, specialists at ripping off the state worker compensation program. Bet you dollars to doughnuts the guy was a laborer, hated his boss, chip on his shoulder, drug addled, typical injured worker syndrome."

CHAPTER FORTY-NINE

Elliot was on afternoon break when he was summoned to the front of the pharmacy by a tech who looked as though she'd swallowed a crow. Elliott smelled stale booze thirty feet before he focused on a greasy man who, upon seeing Elliott nearing, swung his arm forward and down as if slamming a hatchet into a round of firewood. Elliott took a step back until he realized the man was only whacking a thick envelope onto the counter. "Sign here," he slurred, shoving a clip board in Elliott's face.

Elliott scribbled a signature and in the same breath opened the envelope. The words SUBPOENA and NOTICE OF APPEARANCE stole his breath. He was finally being sued for one transgression or the other. He went into the back bathroom and sat on the commode to read the document. Actually, it was Marlancor's lawyers ordering him to materialize early the next morning for court testimony regarding Ampfloban. When his heart rate dropped to one twenty, he read further only to choke again as he discovered the venue was the Supreme Court of the State of New York. Since when had this become the trial of the century? He got on the computer and looked up the Court's description. His heart rate dropped back to one twenty again when he figured out this was what the local civil court had been puffed up to call itself in New York City.

He planned to leave work immediately to prepare, but an emergency meeting of all pharmacy staff was summarily ordered by the home office in Toledo. It was to commence at 4:00 P.M.; however, it did not get started until the district manager darted in at 6:00. In front of the overfull break room, the man charged that a pill count discrepancy had been uncovered in a surprise audit. Elliott held his breath.

A recent inventory of the Schedule II medications in the store showed the tally of Concerta, the pills Elliott had borrowed to stay awake and do his research on Ampfloban, had come up short. It was a drug regulated by the DEA with the same fist as OxyContin and the other opioids. “This is a major crime,” scolded the district manager. When that brought only a grating chorus of mocking snorts, his jaw gnashed. “People, this is a felony, a *federal* crime, in fact. Lots of prison time.” When a few backs straightened, his pique tempered a tad, but intimidating only a handful of his hostages, his voice raised once more. “Well, maybe this will get your attention. Top management has ordered *all* pharmacy staff to submit to a polygraph.”

A few, “Whoas,” meandered through the congregation, but most of the staff looked at watches or stared into space.

“Not impressed, huh? Well, guess what, those who refuse or fail the test will forfeit their jobs, and we will make sure their licenses, too.”

As the gravity of the threat drifted about the room, anyone standing at the front of the meeting would appreciate the curtain of white descending over myriad faces. Elliott, however, sitting at the very back so he could escape first, was not able to see the guilty consciences playing out. Unaware he was but one of the heap to suffer such shamefaced hypotension, Elliott clenched his chest as if holding his last breath in the gas chamber. This forced his blood pressure north sufficient points to regain a bit of color. It was a trick of the trade he’d developed after years of standing in front of probing teachers and vice-principals. He, nonetheless, left the meeting shaking, accepting he was going to pay for this one.

The threat from management was his second shock of the day. As all things in medicine come in threes, or so he had been told by his professors, he came close to passing out on the subway home waiting for the third shoe to fall.

He called Barron in a dither, hoping for a continuance, or whatever it was called. The old man laughed. “Look, Elliott, lawyers and judges call you when they want, not when you want.

Half the time, they subpoena you for testimony the next morning, you take a sick day, and when you get there, you find the case was settled at the last moment on the courthouse steps. Never heard of a lawyer phoning one of their witnesses and letting them know. Just the way it is. To them, you are nothing more than a lifeless nail, one of a box of five hundred. Bend one, toss it away, pick out the next, and hammer it until it's gone. You like the few hundred dollars an hour they dangle in front of your nose, you do as they say."

Barron went on to explain why Elliott had been mustered so abruptly. "Apparently, the judge in this case is notoriously parsimonious in his allowance of expert witnesses. In fact, he has allowed only one per side. It isn't right, but a judge is king of the court. Elliott, let me be frank. You were not their top choice, but the drug company's expert fell from grace with a thud, actually more like a cow dung bomb. It was so bad they struck his testimony from the record. Marlancor had to get on its knees and petition the judge to allow one more voice for their side. Again, being honest, you weren't second either, or the third, but you were the only one they could make available on short notice. Sorry to tell you."

"You sure hate to be the last guy in the playground picked for the team. Maybe I should have some pride and tell 'em to go to hell."

"You can, and I wouldn't blame you, but if you do a good job, your stock will rise. Again, it's just the way it is, Elliott. Look, let me tell you what happened. First guy really screwed 'em. You might want to cut 'em a break."

He described the initial authority as a retired pathologist flown in by Marlancor from Allentown, PA. His testimony had been quite terse: the plaintiff died as a result of garden variety alcoholic hepatitis, not from Ampfloban toxicity. The doctor presented a series of tissue slides via computer projection, the first from the normal liver of an old man of the same age. Then he showed the slide of a booze-marinated gland from an autopsy at a VA hospital. Next was an Agent Orange-poisoned liver. Then he flashed the plaintiff's liver. Final screen, he compared all the slides. There were signs of both problems in the plaintiff's liver. So, the conclusion was that the plaintiff died of cirrhosis caused by alcohol *and* Agent Orange, in which he had been pickled as a grunt in Vietnam in the Sixties. He even went over pathology slides of other causes of liver disease: cancer, typical medication-induced hepatitis, infectious hepatitis, exposure to chemicals, and radiation. The only conclusion the jury could come to in the face of such scientific proof was that alcohol and Agent Orange killed the poor man, not Ampfloban.

The moment the doctor's testimony finished, the drug company asked the judge to summarily dismiss the case against the corporation; there was obviously no point in further wasting the jury's time. Before, however, the judge could take a breath to ask the plaintiff's attorney for a counterargument, the latter flew out of his seat and objected so vociferously, the soot-covered Centre Street Courthouse windows shook.

"First of all," he heaved, "I have never seen this tissue sample. I demand I be given the opportunity to call my own pathologist to verify what this long-retired doctor has tossed in front of the jury."

A two-day recess was granted, not cheerfully. A neutral pathologist was recruited. The judge phoned him from chambers in front of the attorneys for both sides. Over speaker phone, the doctor explained that although the patient's slide had what appeared to be a label of his name and date of birth, said label was impossible to read, having been mysteriously obliterated by a splash of purple staining material. "You must have seen that, Judge."

"Yes, of course. Go on."

"Well sir, I, personally, can't make out a single letter of the name. That is inconceivable. Labels should never be applied until after slides are stained, washed, and dried. Pathology 101," he scorned. "But you know what's worse?"

"I'm afraid to ask."

"You should be. I checked records for the autopsy done on the plaintiff. Already been lost. Faster than usual when a lawsuit's involved. And you know what, Your Honor?" The judge grunted;

the pathologist went on. "I found an image on the internet that matches the slide, cell for cell, the defense told you was from the deceased."

The first expert's evidence was stricken from the record. Marlancor's attorneys stood before the judge and swore to God they had no idea the initial pathologist had perjured himself. They were handed a first and last warning. The judge gave Marlancor twelve hours to find a new, and final, expert. Hence Elliott's late afternoon call.

As Elliott put the phone down, it rang within a millisecond. It was Marlancor's attorneys on a conference call. "Sorry we gave you so little notice, but we had a pathologist on tap. That seemed the smartest way to go, don't you agree? But one of us looked up and said, 'Hey, you remember that really sharp pharmacist…' and here you are."

Against all court rules, Elliott was briefed on the testimony ralphed up by both sides then bluntly ordered to study a fax they had just sent, one with the word-for-word testimony they expected him to include in his appearance.

Over a scotch, Elliott perused the transcript, including the marginalia added by Marlancor's CEO. As he started to memorize the suggested testimony, he realized their case had been created from whole cloth, a fairy tale woven to exonerate the corporation. Basically, he was to declare that the Ampfloban molecule was, at its heart, a common non-steroidal, non-narcotic medication that had been taken in billions of doses over the past fifty years, and within the bounds of acceptable safety. He was to turn to the jury at that moment, smile subtly, nod, and speak evenly: "I imagine everyone on the jury has used it, even given it to your kids, and many times. There's no more evidence that it harms the liver than does a diet ginger ale."

He was to convince the jury that all Marlancor had done was connect it to another harmless moiety, one used universally for its ability to relax spasming muscles. And that was it. That's all Ampfloban was. It was the process to connect the two molecules into one that became a testament to the genius of Marlancor's futuristic corporate leadership and its top rate chemists. That was what the flurry of excitement and talk of a Nobel Prize was about. It was like mixing oil and water into a pure, third, miracle substance that was neither greasy nor watery.

He was to end with the final words, scripted by the lawyers. "It was our hope, we health care professionals, doctors and pharmacists working so hard on the front lines, that Ampfloban would change medicine forever. Finally, there was a safe pharmaceutical for patients suffering from debilitating pain, a safe medicine that did not cause addiction three days after you start it. Something to give patients hope. Please don't take this important tool away from us."

CHAPTER FIFTY

While Elliott had fully intended to deliver his lines as ordered, by midnight, he feared there was simply too much to absorb in a brain that had had so much wrung out of it in the past twelve hours. He searched for a single Concerta, but he knew well the cupboard was bare. He substituted two glasses of scotch. While the foreboding faded, so did his consciousness, and he fell asleep at his desk, only to wake with barely an hour to shower, dress, shine his shoes, and hail a cab.

He stumbled unsteadily into the witness chair. Cotton mouthed, he swore to tell the truth then spent an hour stammering over answers to questions posed by his own attorney. As his performance deteriorated, he began to tremble, thinking about the coming cross-examination. His infirmity intensified the static jetting from his employers, their butts lifting centimeters from seats with each of his anemic responses. He finally looked up from his notes to take stock of the lawyers whose wrath was now etched on their twisted faces. He was so frightened, he turned away, his eyes darting past the plaintiff's table, finally taking refuge in the smoggy sky outside the courtroom window. Something, though, drew him back to an African American man, his affable visage belying the spit-shined army uniform and gold leaves on his epaulettes. Elliott thought for a moment the man was a military attorney sent by the Veterans Administration to deny Agent Orange in Viet Nam had a single thing to do with the deceased's liver failure. He was, of course, there to insulate the government from yet another lawsuit growing out of that bedeviled conflict. The man, however, smiled respectfully at Elliott, who smiled back.

During a break in testimony, Elliott went to the men's room. The soldier was washing his hands but turned to Elliott and greeted him with that calm smile. "Dr. Sass, that is some sophisticated chemistry you outlined. Now *that's* what you call rocket science."

Elliott snickered, "You do it all day long, it ain't so special. I imagine what you do for a living isn't child's play."

"Yeah, pretty dangerous. Gotta keep your head up all the time."

"I thought you guys had to keep your heads down."

The man laughed. "You got a point there. Just got in from Iraq for the trial. Don't know if my head's supposed to be up or down. Takes a couple of months each time I get back, you know, to appreciate a world where every soul isn't plotting to behead you."

Elliott frowned. "You sure you're in the right place?"

"You got another point." He laughed again. "Hey, sounds like you're from the City, like me. Go to junior high school here?"

"Yep."

"Where?"

"P.S. 86."

"I'll be darned. My dad, he taught up at 86 for a lotta years, then he became principal over at Stuyvesant."

"What's his name."

The man looked curiously at Elliott. "*Was*…same as mine." He pointed at his name tag. For a moment, Elliott was confused, for it was, indeed, the same as that of the late plaintiff—Cromartie.

"I didn't realize."

"Yeah, and he was a great guy. Don't believe these lawyers when they say my father was a drunk. Some old schoolmarm said she saw him take a single glass of wine at his retirement party. She didn't remember what year it had been. Couldn't even remember the decade. Not even the dates *she'd* taught there. Then my mom testified he did indeed have a single glass of wine at that party. She remembered it so well because he made her drive home, and her driving, according to him, was more dangerous than riding in a jeep in combat. And *I, personally*, never saw him take one drop—

ever. He had all these programs at his school trying to keep kids off alcohol and drugs. And now these charlatans make him out to be the opposite of what he lived his life trying to address."

"That doesn't surprise me. These guys are pretty slimy."

The man's face tightened. "Then why do you work for them? You're a pharmacist. A health professional. You have to know Big Pharma is screwing your clients. You gotta be seeing it all the time. These are innocent people. Can't afford even basic medicine, yet the drug companies are hiring the most expensive lawyers on the planet to protect their obscene profits. Seems you're a smart guy. Can't you see it?"

As Elliott scratched for an answer, he was distracted by a flush from the far stall. He looked up to see one of the defense attorneys walking toward the sinks. Unsure if the man had overheard the conversation, Elliott froze, nodded at the soldier distractedly, and scurried from the room.

As the players drifted back into the courtroom, Elliott could not ignore the wired glowers from the defense table. The moment court resumed, the chief drug company attorney rose and asked the judge for a five-minute recess to confer with the witness. His three assistants followed obediently into an empty courtroom, where they took turns reminding Elliott, "We know you are not a lawyer, so we are guessing that you were not aware that it is verboten to, shall we say, fraternize with the enemy. That can be forgiven, but you are going to tell us what was discussed."

Elliott fumbled for a couple of seconds, unsettled by the phalanx of menacing faces, and quickly blurted, "He told me that his father was not a drinker, that's all."

"And did you believe him?"

"I don't know."

"Well, you're not to. We already told you who these people are, and now you can see for yourself." There was an angry pause. "This has nothing to do with the family patriarch. It has to do with stealing money from Whitey to buy booze and drugs. Surely, you understand that.

"You are to follow our plan to the letter. Your future depends upon it."

When direct examination began again, Elliott could not miss the quivers of poison-tipped arrows primed to tear from the defense table. He answered the first few minutes of questions by the defense attorney per script, until his eyes were drawn to the plaintiff's son, whose face had grown, not cold, but accepting of the coming smack in the lips. The outcome of Elliott's testimony, of the trial, of the man's future, and that of his family had never been in doubt.

Elliot thought of his father, of the one time he had taken Elliott aside not to whack him for some imagined or real felony, but to remind him, warn him, that he was a Hebrew and would never wash that stain from his being. He would always be a filthy Jew, as it had been since antiquity. There was nothing he could do. "They're jealous, the momzers, because we're smart, smarter than all the rest. And we work hard, like dogs. It's in the blood. And when you stick your head above the crowd there's always going to be someone looking to lop it off."

Major Cromartie turned away, eyes far from the courtroom, as if reliving the day his own father, the school principal, had taken him aside and given him *The Talk*. The Cromarties were as likely to be awarded justice as the Jews of the Holocaust.

Elliott was moved and fought back, throwing up a barrage of pharmaceutical flack laced with the jargon of physical chemistry that not even Barron, who had slipped into the courtroom during break, could follow. On cross-examination, he was so obtuse, the plaintiff's attorney asked the judge to declare Elliott a hostile witness. He did, and Elliott was soon dismissed. Barron turned away as Elliott slunk from the courtroom.

Elliott chose to walk the eleven miles home to the Bronx. As he crossed the bridge over the Harlem River, he was blanketed by a sense he had finally done something for someone other than himself. There was no way Marlancor could prevail. They had not mounted a cogent defense. The entire case against Principal Cromartie was that he had been a drinker and burned out his liver on alcohol—a single glass of wine. His back straightened, and his stride lengthened. He wondered if Marlancor would pay him for his tepid performance. He smiled to himself that even if they didn't, he would reap the reward: a dose of good karma, probably his first.

He stopped for a cup of coffee at Starbucks and emailed the pharmacy, moping that he had contracted an awful flu and would be absent for several days. The next morning, he withdrew from his checking account the expected recompense from Marlancor and bought return, first-class Amtrac tickets for the Jersey Shore. In Atlantic City, he lost hundreds on the slots, far more than he'd calculated his testimony would fetch. So much for karma.

On Monday morning, he settled into his first-class dining car seat back to New York. He looked about, twisted his lips superciliously, plopped two sugar cubes into the porcelain cup, and wrangled with the silver carafe trying to open it. The waitress sidled up beside him and surreptitiously pressed the button above the handle.

Next to the saucer on his white tableclothed breakfast tray sat a neatly folded copy of the *Wall Street Journal*. He leaned back, sipped the coffee, and glanced at the headlines. He took another satisfied sip before turning the paper over to peruse what lay below the fold, eyes instantly opening as wide as his saucer. His chest clutched so brutally, he coughed up spurts of coffee to the stares of his genteel fellow travelers.

Marlancor had won the lawsuit. The drug, itself, the jury found, was a miracle, so complex, so elegantly fashioned, the plaintiff's expert witness did not hold a candle to the chemist/pharmacist Marlancor had put on the stand. They were angry at the judge for dismissing Elliott.

That was good, he imagined, for his ego, and further Ampfloban litigation into which he might be drawn. He ought to be able to squeeze them for six hundred an hour next time. On the other hand, the outcome did not seem promising in the realm of karmic destiny. He wondered if he should contact the Cromarties, express his sadness, and ask if he could do anything. Yes, he would do that, in a few days.

CHAPTER FIFTY-ONE

When he returned to work, his first act was to stop by his pharmacy mailbox for the check from Marlancor. The cupboard was bare. He called the law office and asked prickly if there was a problem, but the secretary said she knew nothing of the matter. When Elliott insisted he be connected to one of the attorneys, the next words were a legal assistant's voice mail.

There was also nothing in his cubbyhole regarding the date he was scheduled to sit for the polygraph. As the tension built in his chest, he ripped the cell phone from his white coat pocket and dialed the district manager's emergency number. Before he had bristled halfway to the back door to take the call from the old employee smoking area, the manager answered. Elliott snapped, "Look, when am I scheduled to take the lie detector test? I want to know."

The man was circumspect at first, blabbering corporate speak before tightening his tone. "And tell me again why you're so interested. You have something you need to tell me?"

Elliott gulped but recovered quickly to growl, "Tell ya why. I'm uncomfortable not knowing if a rogue employee's on the loose."

"Yeah, why don't you just leave human resources to me? You do your job, I'll do mine. We'll let you know when it's your turn." And that was the end of the conversation.

Elliott asked around surreptitiously, he thought, if anyone had been canned; but the scuttlebutt was that the pills had magically reappeared, in fact an extra two were counted, and the incident was written off as a clerical error. The store manager suggested he forget the whole thing and never again mention it.

With that anxiety lifted, his chest relaxed. In fact, it was the first time he could breathe in days. With a future not interrupted by a good seven years in Sing Sing, it was time to start cleaning up his life. He also stopped ordering marijuana from the local grease ball, the man having been busted during Elliott's lost weekend in Atlantic City. It had been a sting operation, a slew of customers swept up in the raid. Had Elliott been home that Saturday afternoon, he too would be facing felony drug charges, the automatic revocation of his pharmacist's license the least of his problems. Perhaps it was trace evidence of his new-found good fortune. While the dealer was already back on the street, Elliott decided to do without dope for a while.

That lasted a week, until he and Jimmy Prince found themselves on the same shift. Jimmy suggested a new dealer, Rhianna Gene, a six-foot-three, two hundred seventy-five pound drag queen; though, Jimmy smirked, that was in heels. She typically sold exclusively to Wall Street executives, but when she discovered Elliott was a fully-employed retail pharmacist, she proposed the latest iteration of the never-ending pain pill conspiracies. They met in a Starbucks not far from the pharmacy. She nudged Elliott into a seat, abandoned the falsetto, and spoke guardedly. "You know, you're about to become a very rich man. Oxy, Vicodin, and we've also got the market on steroids. All the local gym rats use us. Guy comes in with a script for the usual thirty tubes of monthly testosterone gel, you fill that one, then make a copy of the script, change the name to one of your old, retired patient farts, and push that script through Medicare. First guy's happy with double the usual dose of anabolic steroids; stupid old man whose name you borrowed has no idea because you cover the co-pay."

"*I* pay the co-pay? That's like seventy-five bucks."

"Hey, you gotta spend money to make money. Ever heard that? Listen to me, Cupcake." She put a hairy hand lightly on Elliott's forearm. As he started to draw free, she tightened her grip and blared, "Just listen!" He paid attention to the first few lines of the sales pitch. "Oxy ten brings a buck for each tab, two bucks for twenties, and eight for eighties. The testosterone's five bucks a tube."

"Does that go for the second, phony steroid script, five bucks a pop?"

"Oh, my God. This isn't Christmas, Sweetheart." She relaxed her grip and fondled his arm with calloused fingers. "But you do get a hundred fifty bucks for the second script; that's seventy-five bucks—clear, plus the one fifty for the first prescription. Two transactions a day, that's a hundred and fifty for three minutes at the Xerox machine. Let's say you can do this forty weeks a year, and that's a bad year. You're looking at thirty K. New ride every January, and that's not countin' the Oxy. And that's where the real money is."

She lowered her eyes and voice. "By the way, some of our more active pharmacists collect a premium for their efforts." Elliott looked at her questioningly. She rolled her eyes. "Get your pipes cleaned, on the house. We can talk about that, yes?"

He hadn't heard the last sentence, his concentration so locked on the spoils that sat before him. He calculated the conspiracy would last, at best, a year, long enough to make many tens of thousands before it imploded. Mumbling to himself a justification that everyone and their uncle in the health care industry was doing *something* felonious, he agreed to the terms.

Yet there was a nagging in his solar plexus, and he stalled calling Rhianna Gene for several days. He was not quite sure where the disquiet was coming from, for there was no illegality in filling prescriptions. "We've been through this before, schmuck," he scolded himself aloud as he sat down to call the pusher. "It's not my job to check signatures. And even if it was, I can always call the doctor's office and verify they ordered that drug. I don't have to ask if the script was for a double dose."

He started to punch Rhianna Gene's number into his cell phone when the flip side of the conspiracy began to drift into focus. Calling doctors' offices pissed off legitimate customers who felt they were being treated as if felons. It also pissed off doctors' offices who had to stop what they were doing, find the chart, and read through illegible notes to confirm the prescription. It also got back to management—it always did—and, inevitably, there would be a call from the district manager to remind that a pharmacist's job was to sell medications, not play DEA agent.

He sat in his mother's chair playing and replaying what he'd do with the money, and then wondering if Irena's softening would go one more step, and at least allow his relationship with Aaron to grow. It surely would not if Irena got word through the medical grapevine that he was honoring opioid scripts he knew had been written by pill-pusher M.D.s. He also took stock of his personal track record, and how often plots that seemed so foolproof went south overnight. Though he had tried to keep himself on the periphery, or so he tried to convince himself, the outcome of those forays had always been the same—a chunk out of his butt.

His thoughts returned to Aaron. There were not that many years before the boy would be in college, out of his life forever.

He made his decision to let the scheme die of neglect. When his cell phone rang with nightly calls from Rhianna Gene, he ignored them. Over the next month, her number showed up less and less frequently then stopped altogether. Elliott breathed thankfully each morning when he woke, his chest no longer squeezing uncomfortably as he opened his eyes. At work, while there was no change in the chronically inflated flow of Oxy prescriptions, he was calm, knowing it had nothing to do with him. Elliott put the offer of big money out of his head. He was at peace for the first time in his life.

CHAPTER FIFTY-TWO

On an indifferent, cold, Tuesday afternoon, a woman staggered in, a crushed paper prescription held tight in a bony hand. Elliott's eyes played over her cachectic frame for less than half a second before glancing, by reflex, toward the shelved bottles of OxyContin. A half second later, he turned back to the woman, unclear if her trampled mien was a function of having been beaten figuratively, by life, or literally, by a metal cudgel. He could not tell if her rubicund face and eyes were a function of her drug habit, or if she had been crying incessantly for days. Unsympathetically, he took the prescription and turned to fill the order, calculating under his breath the bottom line of his savings account had he enrolled in the pills-for-profit collusion he'd foresworn. It brought an acerbic smile and a low mumble that, with the money already rebuffed, he would have been able to take a cab after work to the BMW dealership on 57th Street.

The script's doctor line bore the name of Wahida Abadi, M.D., an internist, and one of the local mavens of tarnished medicine. As he walked numbly to the medication shelves, he rationalized that even she would not be underwriting this star-crossed woman's demise. He pulled the supply bottle of OxyContin off the shelf and started to twist the top free. His chest squeezed unpleasantly with the same apprehension he'd felt when considering the most recent pill scheme. He peered between stock bottles of oxy and hydrocodone to stare at the woman. Though twenty-five feet away, he could not ignore the worsening rattle of her hands and the building line of perspiration on her upper lip. He placed the bottle back on the shelf.

As he returned to the counter, the woman's eyes fixed on his empty hands. Beads of sweat now jetted abruptly from her upper lip to stream along the corners of her mouth, finally dropping like bombs to splash on the filthy counter. It was all Elliott needed to confirm his diagnosis. He whispered almost audibly, "Now they're forging signatures, not even bothering to see the pusher doctor. Wonder how Abadi'll feel about that." He spoke less than kindly to the woman, "Ma'am, are you positive the person who signed this prescription is really Dr. Abadi?"

"How should I know? His office gave it to me."

"Okay. I need to give *her* a call. It'll just be a minute." He walked to the back of the pharmacy and dialed. As he began to speak, the woman heeled about and darted from the store.

An hour later, another disheveled soul presented a rumpled script for sixty OxyContin. Elliott called Abadi's office again and demanded to speak directly to the doctor. A woman with a heavy accent eventually took the phone, "What *is it*?"

"Doctor, did you sign a prescription of sixty, eighty milligram OxyContins for a seventeen-year-old girl, let's see, Patty Houston?"

The roared answer was short. "Yes, and who da fuck make you doctor?" The voice disappeared. Elliott filled the order.

The quandary was that his professional mandate did not include second-guessing medical doctors. Unless he had reasonable suspicion that a prescription had been forged, the most he could do was advise the physician. It was out of his hands after that. And if the doctor had really written for so much dope, how could he confront her? It was not only futile, it was poking a bear that would someday bite his ass—probably sooner than later. He thought about raising the alarm the patient was getting opioids from more than one source. He could, but only with solid proof. If that patient had no other recent scripts for opioids in that store, he had no responsibility to practice medicine over the head of a licensed prescriber. If he called around to see if there were scripts at other pharmacies, that would be a clear HIPPA violation, for which he would lose his license.

Yet there were occasions when pharmacists were expected to inform the medical board in Albany if convinced a law in the criminal code had been breached. "Convinced," though, was fraught with snares; it did not mean gut feelings. If you presented more than your suspicions, the question always was, were you playing DEA agent on the side? All of a sudden you had made yourself part of the equation. Was this a personal vendetta? Had one of the parties rebuffed your sexual advances? In this case, he had far less than sufficient evidence to make the poison call to Albany. Not willing to create another unhappy patient or fuming doctor that day, he filled the teenager's script with a smile.

It was several hours before the next juvenile addict stepped to the counter. Elliott noticed she was accompanied by a stone-faced, soiled man, who waited until she was called forward then mechanically about-faced and disappeared into the supermarket portion of the store. Reaching the medication shelf, Elliott was able to see the derelict scrutinizing the pharmacy from behind boxes of Cheerios. He felt a squirt of adrenaline as he reached up instinctively and grasped the supply bottle of Oxycontin. It was lighter than it had been when he'd filled the last Oxy order from Dr. Abadi. Having become hypervigilant in his felonious world, his shoulders tightened, and his eyes peered about the dispensary searching for culprits. The place was a madhouse, and perhaps another pharmacist had come to work early and covered while Elliott was on break; perhaps it was a tech, possibly a maintenance person sent to change a light. While Elliott was the only person in the store authorized to open a Schedule II magnum, authority no longer trumped behavior. His adrenals involuntarily shot another dose of adrenalin through him, for if he knew there had been a diversion of OxyContin, he was required by federal law to report it immediately to the DEA's twenty-four-hour line. That action would trigger an accounting of everyone's dispensing files, and probably for the past two years. Cell phone records would be examined, alibis checked, savings and credit card accounts perused. He promised himself he'd look into the matter after hours.

He filled the prescription for the teen. The vagrant joined her as she left the store.

Elliott hardly had time to think about all the personal consequences of a simple phone call before his presence was requested at the counter. A burly man, tattoos extending north of his T-shirt collar, stood glaring at the tech. His artwork terminated in swastikas at his jaw line. It was not, however, the Nazi motif that gripped Elliott's attention. What concerned him were the tiny, inked teardrops, one beneath each eye. They evoked the prison tats in the visiting room at Sing Sing. Filled in teardrops implied, his father had whispered, the bearer had committed murder. Elliott imagined two meant a second homicide, not an attempt to balance the customer's physiognomy. What confused Elliott was that if the man had committed two murders, why was he already out of prison?

He stared for a bit then snapped back to full consciousness when the man shoved a folded piece of notebook paper in his face. Elliott took it clumsily. A crinkled prescription fell out to the floor. Before he bent down to retrieve the script, he noticed printing on the cover sheet. "Better to stay in lane." Elliott retrieved the prescription and filled it quickly. Not a squeak had escaped the client's lips, nor did his frigid countenance warm a single degree before he marched out, heftier by the eighty OxyContins Dr. Abadi had prescribed.

Elliott announced he was going on break. In the men's room, he dug into his pants to withdraw a full Xanax matted with cotton threads and pocket grit. He barely pulled free the detritus before the pill was in his dry mouth. It lodged in his gullet, so he ran to a sink and washed it down with a palmful of lukewarm sink water.

It went to work quickly, his stomach growling, the gastric muscles called suddenly to duty. His gut was otherwise empty, its last challenge, a cold McRib sandwich from the McDonalds around the corner. He sat in the break room for a few minutes until a tech popped her head in and groused, "Elliott, you need to move your ass. They're pilin' up."

The tens and tens of thousands of scripts he had filled over the years had armed his brain and hands with the facility to bypass the miserable handwriting of the local, harried doctors. He could presage what was written just by the eyes of the patient. Yes, he would sometimes confirm it with a glance at the paper, but he fashioned himself a seer with little need to actually read the gibberish. But even the great soothsayer Edgar Cayce had uttered prophecies that had been remotely correct only four out of ten times, and a medical batting percentage of less than ninety-nine point nine-plus percent sent a practitioner out of even the worst of clinics on his ear, next stop, dishing up McRibs for pharmacists.

Though the line of patrons was suddenly elongating, the Xanax had slowed his thinking to the point that he had to invest a second or two in actually deciphering the scrawl. He filled the scripts one after another robotically, and even in his decelerated state, his hand moved faster than the eye could follow, more a short order cook than a psychic.

With the queue finally under control, one of his frequent fliers, a sylph-like woman who suffered from bipolar depression, stepped up to the counter. Elliott's eyes rolled. When she was off her meds, she often presented in the manic phase, sidling up to Elliott, cowboy shirt unbuttoned halfway down, braless, leaning far forward to whisper the same enticement, "I wouldn't kick you out of *my* driveway." Today, though, she was quite subdued, so much so that she made him feel more depressed and anxious than before he had taken the Xanax.

Lithium for her madness was but one of six prescriptions she placed silently on the counter. As Elliott was filling them, he muttered that he liked her better when she was in the manic phase, and in the miasma of the Xanax and his sexual fantasy, his attention wandered. His mind blurred the dosage appropriate for her size and present symptoms, numbers that happened to be written, this time, clearly on her script. Nonetheless, he muddled the three hundred milligram tablets three times a day for thirty days into nine hundred milligrams three times a day for thirteen days, a slug of lithium that would have quelled Andre the Giant.

While that dose quickly assuaged her lunacy, it was only several blocks after she mounted her city bus as a driver that evening that she crashed into the crowded McDonalds around the corner from the pharmacy. Quarter Pounders and McRibs bounced off walls and the bus windshield. Elliott heard the sirens right before leaving work. He wondered if that meant Irena was about to receive a fresh hit in the ER. In fact, she was to attend several passengers and Micky Dee diners that night.

On his way home, he thought about calling Irena at work but decided to wait on her next move. That call came in the morning. She told him about the accident, and that the woman bus driver had become so disoriented, several passengers had bailed at the stop before the McDonalds.

Elliott sneered, "Probably drugs. Where will it end?"

She laughed, and he asked if he could see Aaron. She hesitated, his hopes rising when she spoke gently, "Passover's coming. Let's see."

It was only hours before the bottle of lithium found in the woman's pants pocket was turned over to detectives. It was a long-ago dated prescription but was filled to the brim with pills. The cops obtained the ER records and with it, the woman's stat lithium level. It was higher than the machine's top value.

This opened a Pandoras Box of worms. First, the Metropolitan Transit Authority did not permit active bipolar patients, or inactive ones for that matter, from driving trains or busses. The woman was fired on the spot, even before she got to the hospital. The union turned around and filed suit against the City, demanding the woman be reinstated, a clear case of violation of the Americans with Disabilities Act. They insisted she be fully compensated with back pay, and this was before she'd lost a dollar in wages. In fact, the legal form-filling had been completed and submitted to the corporation before the bus was extracted from the restaurant.

And that was not the extent of the Sturm und Drang. Not only had she failed to report her disease on her yearly physical, an oversight that could easily rise to the level of a felony; she had also been cited for reckless driving in her private car twice in the past year, once again, a manifestation of her bipolar disease. Both times, she claimed to have been speeding to get to a sale at Penny's. The woman's shrink testified on her behalf that the poor soul suffered a cruel disease that made all processes in the mind accelerate. As far as the patient was concerned, he argued, she was not speeding at all. From *her* perspective, she was a law-abiding citizen moving smartly on a crucial errand. She was fined eighteen dollars the first time and thirty-six the second. Only a sleight of hand by a computer geek in the union's head office, with whom the driver had a carnal relationship, kept the charges out of her personnel file. With a supposedly clean record and threats of an immediate strike, MTA forgave her the incident, though reassigned her to the barn as a dispatcher. It appeared the matter had been buried.

But that was not the end of it, not by a long shot. One of the passengers had suffered a broken wrist. When an MTA adjuster tried to argue the old lady had awful osteoporosis, and the fracture was hardly their fault, the woman's daughter stepped in. She happened to be the very clerk Elliott had spoken to at the offices of the New York State Pharmacy Board years before. She was now an investigator for the Board. Insisting she be informed if scheduled drugs had been involved in the incident, she was rebuffed by the union—personal medical records involved. She brought the matter to her boss, and up it went through the health department's chain of command and down the transportation department's. The woman was finally assured that no scheduled medications were found in the driver's blood, and therefore no offense that could reasonably come under the jurisdiction of the pharmacy board had been committed. The daughter was told to mind her own business.

She did not. By citing the investigative powers of the board and forging signatures, she secretly gathered the bus driver's medical records and compared them to the ER notes. How, in God's name she asked herself, could the bus driver's lithium level have jumped from her usual, normal 1.2 milli-Equivalents per liter noted in the chart her M.D. kept, to 2.3 mEq/L, a toxic level, on the first blood draw at the ER? She could find no change in the dose prescribed by anyone over the past years, including the prescription written on the day of the accident.

She called the patient, who denied having taken additional tablets. The investigator asked the woman if she still had the bottle of pills. She explained that she had tossed the most recent bottle; she always did, preferring to put the new tabs in an old bottle, one without a child-proof cap.

The next step was to talk to the prescribing physician. That turned out to be Dr. Abadi, who chaffed at the thought of a cretin from the pharmacy board questioning her medical judgement. Dr. Abadi hung up on the investigator but not before issuing a string of expletives.

The only way forward was to review the pharmacy records. That meant sticking her nose in the business of one of the largest retail drug dispensaries on Earth. *Any* request for records drove the national office's legal team into a defensive posture more forbidding than a herd of yaks. They hid behind a whirl of time-squandering algorithms: delay of service, motions to dismiss, motions to change the forum from New York City to Toledo, and threats of appeals of every decision made by the assigned local judge.

Fooling the MTA's administration, and local hospitals and doctors, into releasing confidential medical information was child's play. She was dealing with real money now. So, she went to a young member of the medical board in the next office down the hall, wound up in bed with him that afternoon, and begged for help.

She made sure the pharmacy board, toothless in state politics, turned the matter over to the powerful state medical board. Her new friend forced an investigation, and they were eventually granted a few of the pharmacy's records. When the medical board investigator compared the prescription from Abadi to what Elliott had dispensed, the pharmacy board was finally in a position to act. The medication error was brought before the board, which subpoenaed every eighth script filled by Elliott. Shocked that every fifth was for OxyContin, they suddenly demanded every third. Here, they discovered many a script for testosterone replacement gel, a scheduled, controlled medication used for Low-T in men, but also abused by bodybuilders. Elliott had dispensed gobs of the stuff, a majority of the scripts having been written by a long-deceased local general practitioner. The pharmacy's attorneys argued Elliott wasn't a keeper of local death records. The board was forced to shelve that portion of their investigation.

When questioned about the OxyContin, though, Elliott argued he was simply doing his job, and that they might look more closely into Dr. Abadi. And off they went to her office. It was an unfortunate coincidence that just that week, yet another Hollywood luminary died of an OxyContin overdose, and that endowed the examiners sanction to tramp into Abadi's office, chests puffed, as if they owned the place. She screamed at them to leave, citing patient confidentiality. But the investigators, culling the opioid crisis, held their ground, warning the staff haughtily they might easily be considered complicit if they did not cooperate. As they dropped pharmacy board business cards on each desk, one of the investigators threatened, "There isn't one of you who can't easily be led out of here in handcuffs. Just try me."

That was too much for Abadi, who howled another string of guttural expletives and launched handfuls of charts and pens and blood pressure machines at the examiners. They sprang for the door, but she followed into the street, still swearing, still throwing, chasing them past the platoons of supplicants milling outside awaiting their fifty dollar Oxy scripts.

It took only days for the investigation to bear fruit. Elliott was approached by Twuck and the regional pharmacy manager. He was placed on unpaid leave until further notice. "For what?" he asked. They were unsure—the board had not told them.

Weeks passed and he heard nothing. Then came a Special Delivery letter from the New York State Board of Pharmacy. His license had been summarily suspended pending a full investigation of his medication error. *And now*, his opioid and anabolic steroid dispensing practices would be included in the analysis.

Having watched other pharmacists run afoul of the board, he knew this meant a year before he would hear from them again, one during which he would be without income. He thought of giving his cheese-averse former girlfriend a call.

Most of all, he was petrified of confessing to Irena, fearful she'd remember the incident of the bus parking itself in the front window of the McDonalds. As it turned out, he needn't have lost sleep over that part of his wrongdoing.

Most of what ER physicians see is ludicrous, a bus accident no more unusual than a Coke bottle ensnared in some guy's rectum. As with most ER patients, once they were disposed of into or out of the system, the staff simply did not have time to follow up on the hundred and some souls a night who had crossed their threshold, no matter how outrageous the case. This was especially so if no one was maimed for life or died. It was simply another facet of the ER beast. Irena had, indeed, forgotten about the incident by the time she called Elliott and asked him to come for Passover dinner.

CHAPTER FIFTY-THREE

A day later, Jimmy called to tell Elliott the Feds had been to the pharmacy with a warrant. They had demanded copies of all the opioid prescriptions Elliott had filled for female patients over the age of sixty. Jimmy did not understand the connection. Elliott claimed he did not, either. He ended the call straightaway, explaining he was late for court as an expert witness.

Actually, he spent the morning ridding his place of meds and questionably begotten cash, cleaning as if he was removing the last crumb of leavened bread before Passover. He thought again of uncovering filth-shrouded nooks and crannies in the prehistoric basement that had not been accessed since Grover Cleveland's second term. He placed his money in several Ziplocs, doubling up until he ran out of bags. Then he poured Tabasco between the first and second bags to deter rodents and insects but ran out of hot sauce on the last one, and so sprinkled ages-old hot pepper flakes on the singles. Wrapping the marijuana and his leftover meds, even the Tylenol, in old Sarge's Deli take-home bags, he descended to the basement, his treasure buried at the bottom of a clothes basket beneath dirty T-shirts and underwear. He placed the bags in a series of fissures in the crumbling walls, jotting coded directions to each. It took over an hour, and he emerged covered in late 19th Century soot. To get back upstairs, Elliott had to pass the super's basement apartment. He approached it cautiously and, seeing the door shut, lifted his hand to press the elevator button. Before his finger touched it, though, the super's door flew open. Old Man Holtz took a step into the hallway, looked Elliott up and down, and grunted, "I heard somethin', grindin', chippin'. That you?"

Without the slightest hesitation, "Oh, that. That was me, yeah. I was chasin' a cat."

"What cat? You don't got no cat in your unit, do you?"

"No way. I came down to do laundry. Walk out of the elevator and a cat ran by. I don't want cats down here. They piss on the laundry." He straightened his shoulders and raised his voice. "Little fuckers get into the machines—shit inside."

The super listened silently, looked into the basket of clothes, and snarled, "Machine broken?"

"No, why?"

"Clothes ain't clean." He stared at Elliott for a moment and added, "You just leave cats and dogs and whatever to me."

Elliott withdrew silently into the elevator.

Elliott's subterranean labors had come none too soon. A few days before Passover, there was a harsh knock on his door at six A.M. Though he choked on his heart, he forced himself to calm, remembering a fellow pharm student from Puerto Rico, Diego's, admonition, "Dress me slowly, Mother, I'm in a hurry." He methodically pulled on his pants, slipped into a clean T-shirt, brushed his hair, and opened the door. He fell backwards at the sight of the ugly DEA sergeant, Grady Uveges. Nonetheless, Elliott steadied himself and smiled a very warm, very plastic greeting, bending forward to retrieve the search warrant the sergeant had dropped at his feet. The same dog who'd menaced Elliott on the previous visit waited until Elliott leaned over then bared his teeth and snapped at Elliott's face. The sergeant smiled more broadly than had Elliott, the hair-filled, acne potholes deepening with the distortion of his skin.

The sergeant taunted, "Can't stay out of trouble, huh? Second time's a charm!"

Elliott stared directly into the man's hard eyes. "Fuck you," Elliott hissed under his breath. The sergeant, sensing Elliott's rage, hardened his expression and coldly ordered one of his underlings to the bedroom floorboards, and one each to the kitchen and bathroom. The dog was commanded to sit but refused, tugging on his leash and sniffing wildly toward the recliner. Elliott smirked, but the handler bobbed his head knowingly and allowed the dog to assault the chair. He pawed the crease at the side of the cushion until it shredded then whined and took a posture of rigid attention in the Lazy Boy, as if guarding the President of the United States. The sergeant stood over the handler's shoulder as the man took over ripping into the upholstery with a knife. He dug and dug until coming to a tiny dot of what appeared to be the nearly microscopic remnant of a rolled joint. The dog tried to remain still but was overcome with passion and bolted toward the speck, snuffling so zealously, the evidence was sucked into its nose. The creature shook its head wildly, the speckle promptly blown out of the left nostril, enveloped by mucus. Uveges picked the glob from the floor with bare fingers and jammed the amalgam into an evidence test tube. He held the glass up to the light but couldn't see the speck for the dust bunnies, carpet fibers, and phlegm. The whole sample could not have weighed a milligram, grime and all.

Nonetheless, the excitement could be cut with a knife. High fives cracked the air as the agents huddled. When they broke, the sergeant gloated, "There's a motherload in here; and we're gonna find it, dickbird. You confess, save us time, we won't destroy the place, *and* we'll go easy on ya." Elliott stared wordlessly into the corner.

It took an hour, but not a trace of drugs, prescription or otherwise; paraphernalia; scales; or cash was uncovered. Even the hunt for computer evidence was an abject failure, but only because Elliott had placed his laptop into a carrying case the night before, planning to go out looking for a job. He had left the bag on a chair at the kitchen table, the case's black, knotty material blending in with the frayed, now black-with-stain, forty-year-old, seat cushion. It took the agents another half hour to disconnect and follow the web of cables Elliott had woven into the back and top of his PC, wires that linked everything from an extra monitor to a computerized telescope he'd installed on the roof to look for supernovas.

This time, though, they put him into cuffs. "On what grounds?" Elliott challenged.

"We just got this thing about drug pushers stealing from hurtin', little old ladies. Don't know why that bothers us so much." Two of the cops laughed, but the sergeant howled, "It ain't fuckin' funny." The squad quieted, and Elliott was led downstairs into an unmarked, illegally parked, grey Chevy. They drove for an hour to the Metropolitan Correction Center in Manhattan.

"This is a federal lockup, for Christ's sake," the desk officer carped. "Take 'em to goddamn County. You shittin' me? All of a sudden grass is a fuckin' federal felony?"

Uvegas taunted the desk officer, "Yeah, well watch me now." Elliott was shoved aboard an open, caged elevator then into a leaky, freezing cell where he met his two cellmates. The skinny white teens spent much of the evening throwing moronic gang signs and talking shit, as if they'd come up in Bed-Sty. They directed not a single word toward Elliott, and when the five-minutes-until-lights-out warning came, the boys swaggered arrogantly to the single set of bunkbeds. One of them purposely brushed past Elliott, making the slightest sleeve to sleeve contact.

Elliott sat quietly until the boys were in bed then began snarling, louder and louder, finally letting loose a maddened-dog howl. With the racket from Elliott's cell, the tier dropped into an expectant silence. The boys' eyes had dilated some during the early growling then expanded far beyond normal limits as Elliott ripped the putz off the bottom bunk. The kid from the upper cot jumped to the floor and pushed himself into Elliott's face, hissing and spitting. Both boys now faced him, mouths foaming, but Elliott lifted his palms in peace and spoke calmly, "Hey, gents, I don't want no trouble, but I got a bad back. Can't sleep on no floor."

One kid sputtered, his hands still flashing inane twisted-finger contortions, until Elliott lifted his palms again slowly, his left continuing up until the teen raised his head warily to follow it. Elliott surreptitiously locked his right hand in a flat fist and shot it into the kid's exposed neck. The boy collapsed like a bag of greasy garbage, gasping and moaning until he was able to take a half breath. Elliott cocked his leg to kick at the boy's head, but the teen rolled into a fetal position and broke into a pitiful blubber.

Elliott started toward the other teen. The boy put both hands up in surrender. Elliott smiled and started to turn away but spun around like an ice skater, grabbed the kid's legs, and hurled him to the floor. The bang was louder than Elliott had expected, for Number Two had landed mostly on his pal, except his head, which smacked the chipped concrete floor. The thump drew a corrections officer, who thundered, "What the fuck are you two doing on the floor? Fighting? Get up. One more problem, and you'll spend the next thirty days hidden in Seg."

As the guard bristled away, Elliott smiled warmly. "Now, gentlemen, I hope you have learned some respect for your elders. Good. Both of you on the top rack. And, if I hear one of you start to get down from your bunk during the night, I will remove both your dicks, if I can find them." The tenor of his voice hardened exponentially into a near shriek. "Pull the mother fuckers right fucken off and shove 'em down your throat." While Elliott knew in his brain this was supposed to be merely an act, his heart was exploding with such fury, his voice rose into a very real shriek, his madness now driven by the screaming, and then by an excruciating pressure in his chest. Tears of rage building in eyes, he jabbed his finger in Number One's face. "That means, his dick in your stomach and vice versa. You'll be shittin' out each other's pricks by fuckin' mornin'." The boys stared at the floor as if a gym teacher had chewed their seventh-grade asses.

Aside from the mind-numbing screaming and sobbing of the tier's limbic-ignited guests, the night passed drearily for Elliott. In the morning, he asked when he was to be granted his one telephone call. At first, he thought of contacting Twuck, but that fantasy passed quickly, for Twuck would likely be the state's primary witness against him. So, also, did the thought about calling Jimmy; but it would not be long before his partner in crime was tossed into the adjacent cell.

He thought of the paralegal he'd dumped. He bet she knew a good defense attorney; of course she would help; they had had such fun together. Well, that was right up until the end, when, even during the middle of her cycle, she insisted he wear a condom. He did at first, but in his uncontrollable heat ripped it off. She tried to make him pay for the abortion. He didn't answer her text messages or voice mails.

That left Irena. And that was a non-starter, at least that's what he told himself as the guards led him to the blue pay phones in the hall. He knew she would not take his call, but the number flashing on her cell was nothing like Elliott's, and she answered. Before he could utter a single word to set the mood, a recorded voice on his side warned that the call was being made from the Manhattan Detention Complex. With the end of the alert, he began pleasantly enough, and it took a moment for Irena's voice to toughen as she processed it was Elliott.

"*Now* what is it?"

"Look, Irena, I'm in a spot. I need ten thousand dollars." Elliott could not tell if he heard the gasp over the phone or directly from her apartment twenty blocks away.

"Is that all?"

"Get me out, and I'll explain; and I'll go to the bank this morning and pay you back. I swear."

At her place, all he could talk about was a shower and a pastrami sandwich. She refused to let him sit down until he came clean. He was unsure where to begin; he was not certain for which crime he had been arrested. She snapped, "You mean there's more than one?"

"I think they said I was dispensing too much testosterone replacement gel."

"Elliott Sass, that is another puddle of your *govno*. DEA does not break down doors for testosterone."

"It's a controlled substance."

"I want you to leave. Even you being here involves me in felony."

"Who said it was a felony, for God's sake?"

"Tombs! You do not go for jaywalking. Elliott Sass, I cannot afford investigation. It is already bad I am Russian; worse, I know your name. Any problem, I am sent away."

"Okay, they found a tiny bit of…" Irena gasped. "No, just a tiny piece of rolling paper. Couple of micrograms, if that."

"More *govno*. Get out. Even cops in America do not file federal charge for undetectable, sub-atomic fumes of marijuana. Out!"

"No. I'll tell you what I know. There have been a lot of scripts coming in for OxyContin recently."

"Ah, so now it comes. I do not want to know."

"Look, it's not my job to decide which one is real, which is forged. I even called one of the doctors, lady named Abadi; you know her?"

"Yes, she is pusher. You are involve with her?"

"Yeah, we're getting' married. No, I am not. Just called her the other day to see if a script she wrote for a teen was legit. She told me, 'Who made you a fuckin' doctor?' and hung up. What was I supposed to do?"

"How many scripts you fill for her?"

"How do I know?"

"How many, Elliott Sass?"

"A lot, I guess."

"What else?"

"What do you mean?"

"I know you. You have not changed in more than decade. There is more. Tell me or go. You make money on scripts?"

"All I know is that my license has been flagged."

"Flag? That means…? No, stop." She opened her laptop and went to the pharmacy board's website "Your name is Elliott Sass?" He began to respond, but she cut him off. "Your license *suspended*, not flag—no such thing, flag. You must answer my question about making money to fill scripts."

"Look, all I did was no different than what everybody is doing at every pharmacy in the city, state, the whole goddamn country. Tell me your doctor friends aren't involved."

"No one *I* know."

"That's what you think. The scripts I fill, the narcotics, all of them come from a *doctor*. You think your high and mighty physicians are seeing thirty teens a day with chronic pain? No, I'm no different than any other health professional around here. I do my job and keep my mouth shut."

"Yeah, health professionals. I do not doubt is going on. But why is license suspended before proving one thing? More. Tell me!"

"Okay, okay. Do you remember the lady who drove the bus into the McDonalds?"

She thought for a moment. "Which one?"

"The one with lithium intoxication."

"Oh, yes." She paused and looked up. "I don't know. I guess so. What about her?"

"I misfilled the prescription. Gave her three times the dose she was supposed to have."

"They tell us at ER was doctor screw up."

"Yep, it was written by Abadi, but they are saying I just transposed a number."

"Just transpose? You mean you read wrong. You are not paying attention? You are high? Drunk? I know you. First little problem, out comes chemical to make poor little darling whole again. What is it you *Amerikanskiy* say, 'snowflake'?"

"I just read it wrong. Yes, it was during a period of great stress. Not my fault. These things happen."

"Elliott Sass. You have learned nothing." She leaned back and was silent for a while. "So, what will you do, beside pay me back? You have to defend yourself."

"Well, I have malpractice coverage through the pharmacy. I guess they have to represent me."

"No chance. Read policy. It is like doctor insurance, only good when you are sued. I do not think is good for…" she stopped and looked at the ceiling seeking the word, "behavior misconduct."

"Well, I'll get a lawyer and pay for it myself."

"Very brave. I know you. Not much left of diamond money. How are you to pay for lawyer? No big payday for guy; you just give him five hundred for one hour. You think he is going to work quick?"

"They wouldn't do something like that!"

"You did with insurance company, and you are not even lawyer. Maybe you go to government legal service. Get law student—only two-fifty for hour, I hear."

Elliott asked if he could spend the rest of the day with her. The answer was a clipped, “Cashier’s check.”

CHAPTER FIFTY-FOUR

The first order of business with Elliott's attorney was the forking over of a retainer—ten thousand dollars. That ten was on top of his cash bond to get out of the Tombs. Elliott talked the man into accepting twenty-five hundred that day, the rest to be produced in a week. The lawyer agreed with a grumble then instructed Elliott to sit in the waiting room while his secretary ran to the bank to cash the check.

With the money in hand, he listened to Elliott's tale and sent him home with the promise to call the federal prosecutor. He was able to glean only that Elliott was being charged, amongst other things, with theft of a controlled substance, specifically oxycodone. This was connected to one of the old ladies from whom he had allegedly pilfered opioids. The story the lawyer had obtained from the DA's office was that the woman had come to Elliott to fill a prescription of pain pills for her back. Elliott had purportedly convinced the woman she should be able to control that pain with Tylenol, then talked her into letting him break the tablets into tiny splinters so that he could skim full tablets off the top. Somehow, she had slipped in the street fifty meters after leaving the pharmacy and fractured her wrist, for which she was transported the two blocks by ambulance to Irena's ER. The nurse tending to her found the pill bottle in her pocket, saw it was impossible to count the fragments, and sent the bottle to the hospital pharmacy, where they weighed the contents and came up with the weight of fifty tabs, despite the number sixty printed on the label. The nurse accused the woman of having taken the equivalent of ten full pills. "Honey, that's why you fell and broke your arm. We need to pump your stomach!"

The woman, though in great pain, absolutely swore she had not removed a single nubbin from the bottle. The nurse then assumed she was a chronic user of opioids, loaded before she left home. She posed that scenario. Now the woman was sufficiently miffed to struggle mightily trying to lift herself off the gurney and demand blood be drawn. There was not a trace of narcotics.

A call made to the pharmacy was fielded by Jimmy, who essentially told the nurse to kiss his ass with her accusations. The matter was turned over to the Pharmacy Board, then to the DEA, where all recent opioid scripts for patients over sixty years of age were subpoenaed from the pharmacy. Investigators visited their homes for med counts. Though it was patently clear in case after case that the number of pill fragments did not jibe with the patients' spoken report of use, there was no firm evidence to make connections that would survive cross-examination. That was based on the old medical rub that if a patient tells you he smokes five cigarettes a day, triple it for a start. Admission of a single drink of wine with dinner is consistently three cocktails a night; and two slivers of pain pills once or twice a day was really eight or nine full tabs during waking hours. It was a well-known rule, and a patient's sworn claims simply would not hold up in court.

When Elliott's attorney finally spoke with the DA, Dan Laird, he suggested that the old lady had probably been guilty of the under-reporting rule. Perhaps she had not replaced the cap properly after she looked into the bottle as she left the pharmacy, then fell and spilled a spoonful of the fragments. "Do we have any testimony that the nurse looked into the bottom of her pockets?"

DA Laird croaked, "I don't give a shit. Your client is guilty," and forthwith charged Elliott with diversion of narcotics. "And I'm askin' for the max."

Next came the marijuana charges. Laird snarled that had been placed on the back burner, but only because the sample was so small, it had to be sent to the FBI lab in Quantico. Though the DA had demanded expedited results, the speediest that could be promised was measured in months.

Elliott's attorney also determined that the State of New York Board of Pharmacy had suspended his license for the medication error regarding the woman to whom he had dealt the lithium dose sufficient to calm a maddened rhino. They knew nothing of the pending diversion charges—yet.

Finally, Elliott's lawyer got wind of a civil suit being prepared against Elliott for false testimony regarding Ampfloban. Several more suits against Marlancor had been filed, and new evidence uncovered. The Cromartie family complained that Elliott had provided the court with bogus statements about the drug, calling it benign, when he was in possession of all the damning data published in myriad medical journals weeks before his testimony. And if he wasn't aware of that data, he had no right to pass himself off as an expert.

He had also lied about how Ampfloban had been chemically fabricated, claiming under oath that it was his professional opinion Marlancor had spent untold millions finding a way to join two harmless molecules and, astonishingly, turn them into a benign wonder drug. The coming complaint against Elliott even included the sentence, "The so-called expert introduced statements into evidence that, at best, could be labeled misinformed, but were far more likely unprofessional, unprincipled, and amoral."

While Marlancor wasn't about to make public the chemical gymnastics they'd employed to create Ampfloban, and could not be compelled to do so, they were able to prove to the court's satisfaction in preliminary hearings that Elliott could not have had any idea how the drug was produced; that he had made up the entire narrative for no other reason than to bilk them of thousands in expert fees. When the judge asked why Marlancor's legal council had not corrected the witness in court, they pled, "We do not know the secret recipe, and even if we did, we do not script the testimony of our expert witnesses." The CEO even convened a press conference, mostly huffing that he was horrified by Elliott's testimony—it was not the way Marlancor did business.

Elliott's attorney shook his head. "Got a lot on your plate. You know, you may do a couple of years on the drug charges. Just do your time, keep your mouth shut, and plan what you're going to do with the rest of your life. On the other hand, this malpractice thing…what they usually do, at a minimum, is award the legal fees spent to bring the case to trial. And I studied your malpractice insurance. Everything's out of your pocket, lawyer's time, too.

"My best legal advice is to take the hit and come up with a payment plan, plans, for every soul that's got a piece of you. Get it over with. I can do the paperwork in say ten, maybe fifteen, hours. Give you a ten percent discount on that part. Probably no way they can turn the false testimony thing into a criminal case. If they did, it could easily be a felony, I mean perjury, in open court. But if you want me to, I'll get together with the lawyers and the judges. We'll work something out. 'Least keep it in civil court.

"Now, on the criminal charges, you know, the diversion and the marijuana, maybe it's better to do the same thing. Take a plea. Throw yourself on the mercy of the courts. Sometimes you can get them to put all the trouble together. Now, that would cost a lot of my legal time. Then again, if I can get it before a single prosecutor, they might roll the fine and incarceration into a single lump. Much neater all the way around. Judges like that. You demand a trial, goes to different prosecutors, they fight amongst themselves to look like the tougher guy. Good for the next election cycle. All up to you, though. I'm happy to play it any way you want."

"But I'm innocent. I never did any of that stuff, except screw up the prescription for the lady bus driver. Good, fine me. Make me write a paper on paying attention at work."

"Not so easy as that. DEA says they counted the pill fragments from the lady who broke her arm after leaving your pharmacy…"

Elliott exploded, "That's bullshit. She broke her arm before she came into the pharmacy. She went to the hospital when she fell and hurt her back after leaving."

"Whatever, the point is, as you know, they came up with enough pieces to make fifty. Bottle label has your number on it, and the label reads a count of sixty. Where did the other ten go?"

"I never took a single fuckin' pill from her, not one! Lady was a squirrel; I remember her. She opened the bottle, just like everyone does to peek at the pills as they leave the counter. Don't know what the hell they're lookin' at. Probably dropped a few. Not my fault. I'm innocent."

"Yeah, as the freshly fallen snow." Elliott's face burned. The man raised his palm. "Okay, okay, I'll see what I can do."

By the end of that week there had been several calls from the attorney, not one with a breath of good news. Most were increasingly strident demands for the balance of the ten thousand. There was no choice but to raid his money cache in the basement. He absolutely refused to allow himself to take a penny more than he needed to pay for his defense.

By the time he got them upstairs under clothes in the laundry basket, he discovered rats had gotten to the bills, gnawing them to near shreds. He had to split the money into chunks and visit several banks to have the damaged bills replaced. At each, the cashier sent him to the manager, who asked endless questions and made Elliott fill out reams of government forms, present his driver's license and one other piece of identification, and finally fingerprints. It would be weeks before the remnants were examined by a federal official and a final total calculated. Elliott explained this to his attorney. Work on his case ground to a halt.

When he could not endure another endless day of soaps, bologna sandwiches, and his own company, he bought flowers and walked downtown to Irena's apartment. She let him in hesitantly, sent Aaron to his room, and sat across from Elliott in a hard chair. He hashed and rehashed his legal troubles then begged for advice.

Irena did not hesitate. "To normal human being, I refrain from inflaming situation by speaking mind and saying out loud, 'You reap what you plants,' or 'And you have big surprise from your behavior?' *But*, Elliott Sass, for you I say out loud, you reap what you plants, and you have big surprise from your behavior?"

"That's your advice?"

"No. That is hors d'oeuvre. For you, I make entree suggestion. Follow advice of lawyer. Find least amount of energy. Take that highway. That is way of nature, and p-chem, if you had pay attention."

"You mean plead guilty and beg for leniency? No fight?"

"I don't know what is leniency but sounds like they can give lean sentence. That is best hope. Or, you can spend all your money, go into debt, pawn everything. Still you go to jail and owe more money than Mayor Bloomberg has in saving account. That is advice from Irena."

Elliott's face reddened. "And what about Abadi? You guys don't turn her in; you're as culpable as she is."

Irena put her feet up on the coffee table. "Mr. Elliott Sass, you should not talk if you do not know."

"What don't I know?"

"We report over and over. Medical Commission turned over to District Attorney. You see, Elliott Sass, DA is up for reelection. He must show cultural sensitivity in New York City. In this day, here, because Abadi goes to medical school very, very far away from America, he must pretend to listen to *govno* story she tells. She testifies that is how medicine practiced in her country. She says her country loves common people so much, doctor is not allowed to let patient suffer for even one second. Her lawyer asks DA to show single sentence in examination for foreign medical graduates that warn about use of pain medicine. She has professor from medical school write to DA. Professor says pain medication in treatment of suffering patient is prime responsibility of doctor. Letter written in Abadi's native language. DA had Abadi translate. End of it. Judge says Abadi is caring human being.

"In case of Elliott Sass, maybe you should get letter from Romania."

Elliott sat silently. "May I say a real quick hello to Aaron?"

"Okay, but he is in my doghouse. Paid kid to do book report. Sour genes! Oy. Everywhere I turn."

CHAPTER FIFTY-FIVE

After several weeks, Elliott received a check from the Treasury of the United States with a note that it had been able to account for around nine thousand dollars in damaged bills. He went back to the bank and railed that he had turned in twenty thousand in damaged bills. The teller snorted that he should file a claim with the government if he was dissatisfied. Her window slid shut with a crack. Elliott paid the attorney, who had added seven percent interest to the balance.

When the secretary returned to the office nodding that the check had gone through, the lawyer came out of his office and stood in front of Elliott. "I got you a sweetheart deal."

"You get me off?"

"Mr. Sass…are you sober?"

"Yeah, why?"

"I said I made a deal, as in plea deal. First, the charges concerning your perjury in civil court, you know, when that poor family got duped. You're lucky. The plaintiff wasn't worth all that much. Already taken out a lot of his teacher pension. Basic income was Social Security when he died of Ampfloban, that snake oil you lied about. Family has grounds to appeal the decision. So, you're not responsible for what they might have gotten in settlement. But you cost them a lot of anxiety. Daughter-in-law's claiming loss of consortium with her husband over the worry, and it goes on and on. I got them to settle for twenty-five thousand. Then there's the attorney's wasted time. He may or may not make a killing on the settlement if he wins the appeal and takes it back to court. I also got you a deal on that one. He's only going to claim twenty-five thousand in legal fees. Comes to fifty thousand you owe them. I talked them into accepting a payment plan, get it done in three years. They will forgo interest on the stipulation you swear not to declare bankruptcy. Do you agree?"

"I guess I have no choice, do I?"

"No, you don't. Now, regarding the criminal charges, the federal prosecutor has taken a less magnanimous tack. He's pissed. Told me, 'Here's an asshole who's profiting from the illegal sale of diverted, controlled substances, basically stolen medicine from dying elders. I'm going to make an example of him.'"

Elliott snapped, "I didn't sell a damn thing!"

"Well, *their* theory is that since you swore to them you don't touch opiates, and there were none in your drug screen at the Tombs, they gave you the benefit of the doubt and believed you. Now, since there is no question that you shorted her ten pills, and you certainly weren't watering your plants with dope, the conclusion is that you sold them. They believe this is part of an ongoing criminal enterprise.

"But lucky for you, I made them wonder about winning on the diversion charge. Told them she was a wacky old lady. Minute she testifies in court, I'd impeach every word she said, even that she said she was eighty. In fact, she's eighty-four. I think I convinced them."

"*You*? That's what *I* been sayin' for a month."

"Not sure they believed your story."

"Do *you* believe me?"

"Mr. Sass, I believe what my clients say. Problem is, they got you in their sites. I worked on them for hours. Finally got the bastard to combine the charges of opioid diversion, sale of the products of that diversion, and illegal provision of thousands of Schedule II substances to people with bogus prescriptions. Guy said he'd deal up a single count of possession of a small quantity with intent to sell. Bottom line, serve some time and parole for a few years."

"How much is some?"

"Said he was gonna think about it. Said it wouldn't be much. Said if you didn't take it, the next time you'd walk the streets would be so far into the mists of the future, people would be living into their two hundreds. They'd even have invented time travel, and he'd transport himself back and prosecute you all over again. He laughed that he'd be able to arrest and rearrest you for millennia. Sort of like *Ground Hog Day*. I don't think he can really do that, but I gotta tell ya, he's pissed.

After the papers were drawn up, the parties came together in the prosecutor's office. The prosecutor smirked, "I understand you are willing to take the plea deal. You're lucky I'm feelin' benevolent. Still remains, you're a piece of shit. Stealing pain meds from a ninety-year-old with a broken hip. And let's get this over with. I need to drive my kid to soccer practice."

He shoved the papers across the table so hard, they skidded into Elliott's lap and then onto the floor. Elliott began to bend forward to retrieve them but stopped and hissed at his lawyer, "You gonna let him talk to your client like that? Both of you, go fuck yourselves." He threw the papers back at the DA and marched out of the room hollering that he was going to demand a bench trial. "I'll tell my story to one person, a judge. No judge could be as stupid as either of you."

Even though Elliott was already well down the hallway, the prosecutor kept yelling, "And a thousand prescriptions for dope you filled without questioning their authenticity. I'll have the charges run consecutive. Don't think I can? Watch me now." Elliott, however, did not hear that; the elevator doors had already rolled shut.

He found a new attorney that afternoon, Andre Dalton, a kid just starting in practice. He warned Elliott that he had no experience in federal court but would work his fingers to the bone to defend him. Elliott was taken by the man's deep black eyes and because he had served as a medic in Afghanistan, two tours, and had worked as a New York City EMT while attending law school at night after he came back.

Elliott shook his head, "Looks like you've seen it all, huh?"

"And then some. I got a pretty good idea what's going on out there, sir."

The young man pushed for a quick bench trial, making several personal trips to the courthouse to speed the process. He showed up for the proceedings perfectly groomed, spit shined, Elliott thought, the bearing of a major general.

When the District Attorney focused on the defendant's profligate dispensing of controlled substances, Dalton called a witness. Before the man could be brought in, the DA grumbled that, yes, he had deposed the witness, but argued that as Elliott's boss for years, the man could not be objective. He also scoffed, "This is a waste of the court's time. You can't understand a word the man says."

The judge asked, "Where is he from? Name sounds Vietnamese."

"Your honor, China, Korea, Viet Nam. Doesn't matter. The accent is impossible."

Judge Paddy McCormack nodded. "I know what you mean. My wife's got an accent, too. Met her when I served in the army. Nearly fifty years later, I must admit, accent's still there, but so's her brain. Lot smarter than me. Anyway, since we don't have a jury we're trying to bamboozle, I'll bet I can use hand signals to communicate with the witness. Oh, and if all else fails, I'll use my Vietnamese. That's where my wife's from, you know. We'll get along fine. Let's have him."

Twuck was sworn. Direct examination barely mentioned Elliott. Instead, Dalton focused on the opioid crisis. Dalton asked if he believed pharmacists were the source of the problem.

Twuck shook his head and turned to the judge. "Your Honor, I tell you with great respect, real problem, Dr. Abadi and like her. She the one who DA should be prosecuting. She a *doctor*. Mr. Sass and me, just druggist. No power on Earth. But, no, DEA and justice system let her walk. No spine. She is criminal, Your Honor."

Dalton asked, "But still, sir, isn't it the legal responsibility of a pharmacist to notify the authorities when a doctor writes unlawful prescriptions?"

"Your Honor, there no such law in New York State. That what DEA want, to make pharmacist policeman. Save them work. Duty they have fail to do so far. Miserable fail. So, blame little man, guy work in trench. No, sir, Dr. Sass not have duty to come between patient and doctor. Pharmacist not have medical degree, not have patient medical history, not have option to do physical exam, not permit to see patient medical record, not even lab, not x-ray, CT, MRI result. How to make medical decision to see if patient need pain control? Not possible.

"And where, Your Honor, is law or even algorithm that tell pharmacist when proper or not proper to fill prescription? No such thing. Now you have DA lawyer second-guess pharmacist for not second-guess doctor.

"So now have, in some case I read, patient say pharmacy prevent from get important medicine. Sue for million. Win! This not tolerable. Dr. Sass easy target. Not just."

Dalton paused to let the judge absorb Twuck's testimony. He thought of going on with the interrogation but spoke softly. "No more questions for this witness, Your Honor."

The DA jumped to his feet, waiting for his turn to maul Twuck. The judge, though, made him stand there for a full minute before inviting him to begin.

Spittle flying, DA Laird demanded, "Mr. Twuck…"

"Objection. Your Honor, that's Dr. Twuck."

"Sustained."

The DA's face, befitting his federal station in life, went first red, then white, and, finally blue, as he held his breath and his tongue, fearful of blurting an epithetical declaration that would cost him twenty thousand in contempt of court fines *and* his legal license. Dalton turned surreptitiously to Elliott and nodded faintly.

The DA exhaled over a few seconds. "*Doctor* Twuck, do you manage a commercial enterprise in which your staff is ignorant of the scourge of fraudulent prescriptions and felonious dispensing of scheduled substances by errant physicians?"

Twuck paused, and it was clear he was translating the sentence into Vietnamese.

"Well, Dr. Twuck?"

Dalton was on his feet. Objection, Your Honor. Badgering."

"Sustained. Doctor, would you like the question asked in a different way?"

"No, sir. Twuck just want to make correct answer." He opened his computer bag and pulled a fistful of papers free. "Here. Dr. Sass make note on patient chart. He call many time, ask doctor why give so many pill. Ask doctor why give pill to teenage." He searched through the pile and held up a single sheet. "Here. He call Dr. Abadi, but all she say, 'Who made you f-word doctor?' Twuck not use real word. Every time call, doctor give same f-word answer. Why we have to be abuse? Too many year in school, study, fight for Pharm D. No listen to f-word anymore. DEA do job, not us. No more."

The judge had to look down to hide his smile. "It's okay, Dr. Twuck, you may read what is written on any piece of evidence in my court. We are all adults here." Elliott was not sure if the man's eyes had rolled faintly. The judge bade the DA proceed.

"And do you condone filling prescriptions from deceased physicians?"

"Dr. Sass not county coroner, election official, or priest. Their job to keep track of dead. You want pharmacist to study obit every day at work? I tell you, that stupid question."

"My last question for you. Are you aware of the senior citizen from whom Dr. Sass pilfered ten oxycodone pills?"

"Twuck aware of *charge*."

"How many pills did Dr. Sass provide for the patient?"

"Fifty."

"How many pills did the doctor write for?"

"Sixty."

"How many pills were noted on the bottle?"

"Sixty."

"So, Dr. Sass diverted ten—right into his pocket. *Isn't that true, sir*?"

Twuck again rummaged through the papers. "Here. When Twuck pharmacy hear of story, we go over oxycodone pill count for three day before and three day after problem. You see, we do witnessed controlled medication count at end and beginning of day, every day, every weekend, every day of year. Yes, Dr. Sass write sixty on bottle, but when we count, we find he make clerical error. He only give fifty. Ten extra pill in stock bottle that night. We make note at 2116 hour same day. Here."

He held up the document, waved it at the DA, and added, "You see, Dr. Sass cannot read prescription. Even call doctor. Doctor not give answer. Again, so rude. Dr. Sass guess number of pill. Take lower number so not to hurt patient!"

The judge called for all the papers Twuck had presented, went through the process of having them introduced into evidence, then read them carefully. He turned to the DA. "Do you have anything further for this witness?"

The DA did but mumbled, "No, Your honor."

"Do you have anything further for this case? I notice there was a marijuana charge."

His head dropped. "Your Honor, that charge should have been stricken from the case. Even though the defendant is guilty of the illegal possession of a controlled substance, we were informed an hour ago by the FBI lab that the material we submitted was apparently too small to be evaluated."

Both Elliott and Dalton gasped. The latter snapped, "Your Honor, *we* were not informed of the result of the FBI assessment!"

Judge McCormack pressed the DA. "Prior to ruling on this case, Mr. Laird, I want to know what you mean by 'apparently.' Either it was marijuana, or it was not. If you did not have evidence to conclude it was an illegal substance, you may not try to spin your questioning to bury exculpatory test results. The court does not deal in maybes. Which is it?"

"It may have been."

"May? What did the report say—verbatim? Please read it."

"Your Honor, in an effort to save the Court time, we will withdraw those charges."

"Read it!"

"'A tiny sample, two-hundred micrograms of…'"

The judge pushed up his glasses. "Two hundred micrograms, did you say?"

"Yes, Your Honor."

"How did the DEA agents even see it? That's no more than the weight of a single human hair." He shook his head and undertoned, "Trial of the century," then stiffly, "Go on."

"They are very dedicated to their work."

"Yeah, I'm sure. Continue, please."

"'A sample crafted from rag fibers;' may I add your honor, that is what joint rolling paper is made of…"

"So is a hand-rolled tobacco cigarette. Do you smoke, Dr. Sass?"

"Yes, Your Honor."

"Well, you shouldn't, sir. Anyway, continue reading."

"'A sample blah blah, crafted from rag fibers, is submitted for stat evaluation. We can say only that it is non-wood plant fibers. We were unable to determine if the material is flax, sisal, or esparto. There was a good deal of viscous fluid surrounding the specimen. It was determined to be non-human mucus, probably of canine origin.'

"'Because of the sparseness of the sample, the usual determination of the presence of suspected illicit material was deferred. We can say only that if the molecular presence of opiates, cannabis, or other chemicals is present, it would be sufficiently nominal to fall below the minimum sensitivity of our testing capacity.'"

"Is that the end? It looks like there's more."

"That's just a note, Your Honor."

"READ IT."

"'Note: Further, the cost and time required for this lab to fully examine the specimen was not commensurate with the charges as listed by The United States Attorney for the Southern District of New York. We also note the providing authority demanded, on several occasions, that the severity of the crime associated with the sample warranted full chemical analysis. Those studies would require an investment of twenty-five thousand dollars, for the specimen would have to be forwarded to MIT to be evaluated in their atomic research lab. We respectfully ask that in the future, the DA only request emergent/stat evaluation of evidence that has significant legal implications.'"

The judge's face hardened. "Anything else? Do either of you wish to deliver closing arguments?"

Dalton stood at attention. "Your Honor, I will abstain if prosecution agrees to do so."

DA Laird did. The judge said he was ready to deliver his verdict immediately. "Not guilty on all charges. Dr. Sass, I apologize to you for the overzealous prosecution you have had to suffer. I will be making a full report to the proper authorities. And, Mr. Dalton, please thank Dr. Twuck for testifying. Can you imagine how hard it would be if any of us had to stand before a court," he turned to the DA, "in Viet Nam, or China, or Korea? Does it matter? Court adjourned."

Elliott called Irena that night and asked if he could come over. She refused, but they talked on the phone for hours.

CHAPTER FIFTY-SIX

Elliott Sass's two-sentence request to the pharmacy board for reinstatement was summarily denied. He appealed. They countered that he had not shown any effort to beat his drug habit. He disputed that he'd ever had, or been accused of, suffering from an addictive disease. He reminded them that his certificate had been suspended for filling a prescription incorrectly. It was, he argued, an honest, though unfortunate, mistake, his only misstep in years of professional service.

They rejoined, "We are well aware of your conviction in federal court on drug charges. Cannabis was found on your person per court records. It is clear you have not come to terms with your opioid dependence. Until you accept and treat that illness, we will be unable to consider your request."

That night, it came to him in a dream. Since it was clear years would evaporate before the pharmacy board acknowledged their mistake, he would, instead, throw himself at their mercy, suck it up, admit his culpability, and pose the following: "If I successfully complete a licensed drug rehabilitation program, might it be possible to have my records sealed so that I may return to my important profession? I want to be a contributing, tax-paying member of society more than anything else in life."

Elliott found a two-month rehab situation in a comfortable hamlet on Long Island. The Board was so pleased, they offered to pay for the program and include a small stipend to relieve him of money worries while he was an inpatient.

He met a woman on the second night and off they snuck after curfew, both frantically hungry after the endless celibacy brought on by their legal troubles. They got only as far as the program's nine-hole golf course before the games began. Fueled by a bottle of smuggled champagne, divots were hacked out all over the 6th tee. The administration was livid, assuming patients had slipped out to play golf under the stars. While they could forgive these tortured souls for having ignored the rules, they would not tolerate criminals who failed to replace divots. Golf was suspended for the next two weeks.

Elliott finished the program without trouble, graduating at the head of his class. His lady friend was not far behind, and they celebrated in a proper hotel on the last night. Elliott paid. She had, unfortunately, run out of birth control pills and conceived that night. This time, it cost Elliott thousands for the remedial action, to say nothing of the psychiatric bills she accrued over the months and months of "recovery." She forced Elliott pay her directly. The funds would be dispersed strictly for medical purposes, she promised. Since the woman knew his entire story, especially about his shaky relationship with the pharmacy board, he pinched his nose and paid her ultimatum.

Elliott's license was restored but with an asterisk. He applied to over thirty New York City pharmacies yet landed not a single interview. He even tried a few in the suburbs, and while there were no offers, one HR woman told him he would need to work for three years without a complaint before they could consider him. He asked how he was supposed to do that if he couldn't get a job in the first place. "Maybe you shouldn't have used drugs. You must have heard that somewhere." She hung up before Elliott could formulate an answer.

Next, he turned to industry, particularly research, but admitted his only experience investigating new chemicals was back in high school and college. The interviewer was so cordial, they began to chat informally, the woman asking what sort of substances he'd produced. He snickered, "Oh, some stinky stuff sometimes, then again a test tube or two of really sweet distillations could come at the end of the afternoon. It all depended."

"Depended on what?"

He laughed, "When I was pissed at the teacher, whole damn place stunk for a week."

After that rejection notice, he applied for technical writing positions at drug manufacturing corporations. He was hired by a startup in Brooklyn. His first assignment was to write a few lines of the patient handout for a generic form of Viagra. The work he turned out was notable for his obvious paucity of training in the liberal arts. Though he spoke English with only the most subtle Eastern European inflection, one perpetuated by the extended stay with his parents, it would have taken a polyglot to discern it in everyday conversation. On the other hand, the lack of writing skills was hardly vague.

In the warnings section, he was to discuss possible vision changes associated with the drug.

> *If you suddenly register changes in sight, maybe everything you see is blue, don't become blue. Go to your doctor, better, an emergency doctor. Remember, rare problems of blindness from this medication are not found commonly.*

Before challenging Elliott and running afoul of federal guidelines that prescribed how a boss interacts with employees, the company faxed the paragraph to a university linguist. She was of the opinion the candidate was originally from behind the Iron Curtain. When Elliott's supervisor called him in, he asked, "So, Mr. Sass, are you from Russia?"

Elliott's face hardened. "Fuck no. I'm Romanian."

Another opportunity for Pharm Ds was in sales, particularly to high-ranking supervisors in hospital pharmacies. At this next gig, he was sent out to hawk a new intravenous antibiotic in Westchester County. His marching orders were to present himself to the staff at Mamaroneck General Hospital bearing gifts. This simply meant a truckload of delicacies from local restaurants, the tab and his travel expenses to be taken out of a per diem account, usually a flat five hundred dollars. Instead of ordering the platters from a caterer, he visited the local A&P and spent several hours the evening before making three dozen sandwiches, heavy on the lettuce, and a tub of potato salad. He had a million bags from his years of take out from Sarge's, the famous deli few suburbanites were able to visit more than once a decade. The staff would be delighted.

Since he had been eating strictly fast food for the past months, the bottle of imported Bulgarian mayonnaise in the corner of his fridge had not been opened in ages, nor had the Romanian spices left behind by his mother. The second scotch, and then the blunt he enjoyed while making the potato salad from scratch, slowed his mind, altering the fronds of green mold on the surface of the mayo from a toxin to fascinating examples of natural beauty. The notion of salmonella or staphylococcus never occurred to him, for it was not seen those days in Hellman's or Kraft's. The Bulgarian brand, however, was more than a drop short of preservatives.

He was able to produce the whole meal for less than thirty dollars, his calculated take at bit more than a hundred bucks an hour. He never did learn the cost of the doctor visits, the antibiotics, and Imodium racked up by the pharmacy staff at Mamaroneck General, because the bills kept coming long after he had parted ways with his employer. They did, however, demand the return of the five hundred before they let him go, threatening to inform the pharmacy board if he did not make good on that obligation.

CHAPTER FIFTY-SEVEN

As the months without work wore on, Elliott's savings dwindled. For a time, he absolutely refused to even bring to mind the rest of the money in the basement. He knew that when he was forced to dip into that cache, it would not be long before he was looking for work at the McDonalds near the old pharmacy, and two months later, he'd be homeless. If he lost the apartment, along with it went the rent control, and even a room in a boarding house would cost three times what he was now paying for shelter. After the monthly disbursement to the Cromarties for his false testimony, the rent, and utilities, there was nearly nothing left for food.

At the end of May, with what remained of his pocket change, he bought a cheap bottle of wine and knocked on the door of 5-H. Gladys gasped as she recognized him. When he asked if he might come in, the blood drained from her face. Without a word of explanation, he dropped onto the couch and opened the wine. She refused at first, but he moaned he didn't know what to do, that he was reaching the end, that he had not a single friend in the world, and that the two of them had shared something special. With misty eyes, she reached forward and took the small glass he'd poured for her. He started to explain all that'd happened, punctuating every third sentence with his fear that he was about to die friendless, completely alone. She was silent, almost breathless, staring at him. He waited until her eyes lowered before he let his hand rub casually over his crotch two times. That brought the color back to her face.

He spoke softly. "We had some good times, huh? I think of them over and over. Relived them." He paused. "Do you, I mean, do *you* ever think about it?"

For a moment, she said nothing then swigged the wine. Her eyes reddened. "Yes."

He put his hand back on his crotch. "Do you want to see me?"

"Oh, my God!"

They were in the shower for just seconds before he ran, she limped, to the bedroom.

She made lunch when they were done. As they sat finishing the wine, she asked what he was going to do, and if he needed help. He mumbled sadly, eyes fogging, that he did, and she disappeared into the kitchen, the next sounds, rattling pots and pans.

That was enough for food, for a while, but it did not help a bit with his rent or the payment to the Cromarties. He lay in bed twitching, fretting yet another late fee from the court, and an increasingly threatening demand for the rent. He jumped up, took a swallow from the bourbon bottle, and ran the stairs to the cellar. With the weak light from the laundry room, he was able to move into the nether parts of the basement, picking his way anxiously through the detritus, choosing first the passage to the most deeply buried stash. He was surprised that the path was nowhere as congested with cobwebs as on his last trip. He waited to turn on his flashlight until it could not be seen from the laundry room or the super's. As the beam filled the corridor, he flinched, noticing the thick dust of the cement floor had in it a fresh print, a huge boot, perhaps that of an urban Yeti. He looked more closely and saw that his own sneaker outline from last time had been trampled beneath it. The trail of both continued to the cleft in the crumbling wall that was his hideaway. He'd tied string to the Ziplocs, rammed them as far as he could with a piece of scrap pipe, then curled the twine and placed the loops an arm's length into the hole. It was foolproof.

As he reached in, his arm scraped the shards of decaying concrete, but he did not mind. He let his fingers begin to close on what he felt were fibers of his retrieval string. He was, though, grasping only a cable of spiderweb yarn. He pushed his arm beyond even where the insects trod. Nothing. No problem, he reassured himself. It had been months—just feel around. When that failed, he slid the flashlight into the hole—no string, no bundle. His heart leapt into his mouth. He dug at the wall, expanding the fissure.

Not caring if he was seen or heard, he charged out of that part of the basement and along the path to the next cache. He choked when he saw boot prints leading there as well. Empty. At the stash of marijuana and OxyContin, he found the Sarge's take-home bags open on the ground, weed and pills lying in the filth.

He sat in his mother's chair for the rest of the night, taking an occasional swill from the bottle of bourbon. It made him that much more maudlin. This really was the end, insult heaped upon insult, not one of which was within his power to undo. He felt so stupid for having believed his karma had veered a few degrees north. It was turning out to be the opposite; his life now in, he was certain, its final nosedive.

He had a son with whom he had spent a grand total of less than four hours, and to whose life he had contributed nothing. And now he was again a pauper without a cent to contribute, even if Irena had not forbidden Elliott to support Aaron in any way.

He admonished himself to stop drinking, but his arm raised to his mouth. When that swallow of venom reached his heart, his tears began. As hard as he scolded himself not to take the next step, with half the fifth of booze on board, his resolve vanished. He threw back the blanket and weaved to the dining room table where he had ditched the baggie of what was left of his dope. His alcoholic muddle was such, he wasn't able to calculate the lethal dose of OxyContin, the numbers simply would not stay in his head long enough to compute the sum of milligrams needed to arrest his breathing. He could focus only on the need to stop the pain, this time for good.

He took the bag and wobbled back to his mother's chair, crying an apology to her for not having been able to provide what she'd needed all those years, just a single ray of hope that her life had not been totally futile, irrelevant, squandered. He wished he could take it all back but knew well his failures were cast in stone.

He gathered himself and counted what was left—six, eighty milligram tabs. Again, he tried to do the arithmetic but was able only to work out that, if the dose was not sufficient, he would probably wake up in a couple of days with world-class constipation; on the other hand, because OxyContin did not contain liver-toxic generic Tylenol, at least he would not suffer acute hepatic failure and die a protracted death.

In the mists of history, he remembered a patient he'd seen in the hospital while still a pharm student. The young man had tried to end it all with Percocet, which did contain acetaminophen, and took enough to narcotize himself for two days, but not enough to cause death—yet. The end came four days later, but at the chemical hands of the acetaminophen, not the opioid. The poor man spent the last two days conscious and completely aware of his violent pain while waiting for his festering liver to fail completely. It was the worst death he had ever seen at the hospital.

He noticed the clock on the top of the TV. It was nearing 3:00 A.M. Sadly, he remembered his mother had always warned, "Nothing good ever happens after midnight, my shayna boy." He leaned the chair back as far as it would go and thought of her toward the end, how she sometimes wept that her only attachment to the universe, her son, had never enjoyed a single moment of peace. He had wanted to promise her he *would* make something of himself, that she could rest, that he *would* carry the baton of her spirit forward. But he hadn't spoken the words, for he knew it was nothing but a pipe dream, one at which she would nod gently but know it would never come to be.

A sudden mantle of stillness fell over him. His tears dried, and the sadness transmuted to determination, his decision finalized.

PART FOUR

CHAPTER FIFTY-EIGHT

As he tipped his head back to swallow all the pills at once, a harsh tone stabbed at his scrambled consciousness. The brief period of composure was gone that quickly. He thought he was already hearing the sirens of hell, but there was just enough smolder left in his brain to recognize the blare as his cell phone.

"What the fuck? HELLO?"

The voice on the other end was crying hysterically, the accent so thick, he was terrified he had begun the voyage downward, damned to hell, forced to make the trip on a Moscow city bus. He yelled brusquely for the creature to get ahold of itself. When the voice finally decelerated, Elliott realized it was a woman, and that maybe damnation held some promise. When he recognized it was Irena, his heart clenched. Aaron had died. Why else would she be calling?

But when she slowed, he absorbed a few of the gasped words. "I killed a patient, a child."

Elliott snapped, "You did not, Irena. That is not who you are," he slurred. "Now, please, my sweet friend, tell me what happened."

With those words, she related that a drug-addled mother, an OxyContin addict, had brought in a toddler whose breathing was shallow and labored. The baby was vomiting and conscious. Irena demanded from the mother if the child had gotten into her drugs.

"Yes, yes," the woman screamed. "He took my pills. Save him, goddamnit. Save him, or I'll sue you!"

Irena did not wait another moment before treating him with Narcan and positive pressure oxygen. When there was no response, Irena insisted the mother tell her again she was *sure* the kid had ingested opioids. She was, she shrieked, then jumped forward and slapped Irena for wasting time. There followed another dose of Narcan. The breathing, what there was of it, only deteriorated, the child slipping deeper into the coma.

Things were not adding up. Irena stopped and did a more thorough physical exam, planning to start on top and scrutinize all the way to the feet until she had the answer. She did not have to go far. There was an egg-sized swelling on the back of the boy's head and blood on her fingers as she withdrew her gloved hand from the never cut, matted hair. She asked the mother how the blood had gotten there. The woman dropped into a sob so profound, not a word was intelligible. Irena pried the toddler's eyes open. The pupils were dilated. No amount of light caused them to constrict. While it could have been other substances, antihistamines, decongestants, on and on, there was no time to cull the list from the interstices of her rare-disease memory. And, anyway, she knew. The child had an intracranial bleed, small blood vessels in the brain tearing from the trauma of the head being bashed with something very hard moving very fast. The skull was filling with blood that had no place to drain. The pressure was forcing the soft brain tissue to squeeze through the only outlet in the skull, the small hole at the bottom where the spinal cord began, where the head met the neck. As the compressed brain was jammed more tightly into the hole, less and less blood could flow into the crushed tissue, pinching shut a series of a million tiny hoses. With no blood to feed it, the few minutes of buffer before brain death had essentially passed. The clinical reality was that the precarious cushion had been squandered long before the mother called 911.

The emergency team needed to do a series of immediate maneuvers to slow the compression, get a stat CT scan, and have a neurosurgeon standing by to cut a hole in the scalp, then drill into the top of the skull to let the free blood out. But the child was gone before they got to step one. Irena cried that she had been stupid to listen to the mother for even the minute she had. She became silent again, but when her bawling resumed, Elliott began to cry.

When the emotion tapered, Elliott was able to speak, though with a tremor that made it hard for him to understand his own voice. "Irena, you listen to me. I am a medical professional, also. You did nothing wrong. That stupid excuse for a human did. She got what she deserved. I'm sorry to say it, but you are not God. There is no God. You did your job to the best of your ability. I know you. There is no chance on the face of this Earth that you did not put your heart and mind and empathy into this patient. You do it with everything you touch. Look at Aaron.

"No, Irena, that moron mother did it. She was probably so fucked up from drugs, she hit the kid or threw him on the ground and didn't even remember." He paused for a moment. "Look, when do you get off? I will sit with you and drink tea. Buy you breakfast. I want nothing from you. You've already given me more than I ever deserved."

Between sobs, she whispered, "I get off at seven. Maybe at Paula's Nook?"

CHAPTER FIFTY-NINE

Elliot could not sleep. There were still three hours before the end of Irena's shift. He sat in his chair and stared at the pills. Yes, he would take just one, a touch of OxyContin, the perfect solution. It would wear off in time for him to shower, shave, and dress nicely. He lifted a tab to his mouth but realized he had nothing with which to wash it down. He started to lift out of the chair but was swept back by a wave of sudden rage. It did not take long to realize he was the target of the fury, for his weakness, his selfishness, and once again, his weakness. He repeated the words Irena had used to describe him, though had been kind enough to aim at, "…you American snowflakes." He threw the pills across the room, wobbled back to bed, then tossed for the next few hours.

He met Irena at Paula's Nook. She was half an hour late, crying again, swearing, then apologizing that she had not purposely kept him waiting. She had been a captive of the coroner and three hospital administrators, all non-doctors, who had grilled her for hours. They had relieved her of her shift, one of the supervisors giving up the weekend with her grandkids to fill in for Irena. The woman did not mind, in fact, she took Irena into the lady's room and reassured her, explaining there wasn't an ER doctor on Earth who had not gone through the exact same scenario.

Elliott wanted to take Irena's hand, to touch her, but he knew better. He asked how she felt, "Okay now, thanks to you and medical director. Horses' ass from administration, they hit me with bat in head over and over, but I remember what you said last night. I do best I can do, always, Elliott. I work hard as any doctor." She nodded to herself in affirmation, but her head slumped, and she began to cry again.

With each sentence her English deteriorated, and when she tried to speak again, Elliott could not tell what she was saying. "Order me not to work. Investigation. Criminal."

This time he took her hand. It was soft and warm, and he was disgusted with himself for wanting to take her home and make love and *then* talk more about what had happened. She put her head in her hands on the table and did not move for several minutes. When her phone rang, they both jumped. The ringtone was a blast of bells and whistles, set as high as it could go so that she heard it even when she was fast asleep after a horrible night shift. She looked at him as if asking if she could, or should, answer. He put both hands out, urging her to take the call.

As she listened, her face calmed for a moment then took on the most relieved semi-smile. She spoke for a few more seconds and murmured, "Thank you so much. Yes, goodbye."

As she looked up into Elliott's eyes, she shook her head. "That was medical director. Every doctor saying to her that if administration stop me from work, even one shift, they march out—everybody!"

Elliott smiled knowingly. "What'd I tell ya?"

"So, Elliott, I am glad to have called you. The truth, but I call my surgeon friend. His first question is why I not order CT? He said sloppy work. Is who he is, perfect but no feelings. Maybe not so perfect. He did not tell me, but I found he sued two years ago. Patient came back for recheck one week after knee surgery. He never did physical exam. Patient had deep vein thrombosis in leg. Clot broke free, into lungs for pulmonary embolus. She get up next morning, I mean she got up next morning, pain in chest, but husband wait to take wife to ER. Too expensive. She dies in home, in bed. My friend get, got away with. Jury blames husband. Yes, he is not punished by judge, and he is happy. End of story.

"Today is last straw. He is gone. Never see again. I do not love him. He was safe harbor. Not one neuron of caring in whole heart." She leaned back and smiled. "No, Elliott, I am buy…ing breakfast. Big one."

They finished an hour later, and she asked him to walk her home. They held each other in bed, fully clothed, for hours, until she was so dead to the world, he was barely able to wake her to say he was leaving.

As he hiked back up to the Bronx, despite his awful hangover, there was a steadiness to his step. Gladdened they had not made love, his mind brightened, clearer than it had been for a decade, maybe two.

CHAPTER SIXTY

Elliot's chest was also as tranquil as he had ever remembered. But when he flung the door of his apartment open and took a step inside, he realized the only one there to greet him was Elliott Sass. He dropped into his mother's chair, eyed the pills scattered across the room, and brooded about how far his own hand might be lodged in the death of that child. Drugs had wounded him once again, but screw Elliott Sass he whispered heatedly to himself; they had killed a guiltless baby. And how about Irena? He shook his head, understanding that she would suffer fresh torment for the next week; and while the throbbing might fade to an ache, it would remain there for the rest of her life. The pills with which that awful woman had destroyed her life, and far worse, the toddler's, may very well have come from a script he, himself, had filled, and for which he had been paid and used the money to buy booze and marijuana. It drove his mood as dark as the night before.

Irena called late in the day. He confided that she had saved his life. She urged he think about seeing someone for his depression, but he explained that all the talk in the world was not going to pay down his crushing debt. Irena listened to his tale of having promised the judge not to declare bankruptcy. Before Elliott could take a breath to go on, she suggested that pledge was not worth his life, and that if he was the man she thought he might be becoming, he had time to pay his debts, even after he was not legally bound to do so. When he did, it would be with a level of interest that would make people ask, "Who does that?"

By the end of the next week, he'd made his decision and gathered papers to declare himself insolvent. Elliott told his legal aid law student about his sojourn in federal court and the promise he'd made not to file bankruptcy. The young man winced, cradled his jaw in his hand, then advised it was his legal opinion a judge could easily enforce the promise he'd made, and that Elliott could go to jail over the matter.

Elliott looked him in the eye and demanded, "Did you consult any of your law books about that?"

"Don't have to. I'm in law school."

Elliott fired him on the spot and spent a day in the law library at NYU, discovering that no court, at any level, could prevent him from filing bankruptcy. While there was no individual *constitutional* right to declare bankruptcy, all citizens enjoy statutory rights; that is, laws not in the constitution, but rules that have been enacted by a legislature or other governing body. They are laws, and cannot be superceded by a judge's desires, despite the belief of most judges that they have the power to do so, and often try. To be sure, he sidled up to an attorney in the library and asked for advice. The man laughed that there was no way on Earth the civil judge in Bronx County who had informally agreed to Elliott's promise not to file for bankruptcy could force him to do a damn thing. The bankruptcy judge before whom Elliott stood a few weeks later granted the relief and ordered that Elliott pay reparations at a drastically reduced level.

With Elliott's debt restructured, the ceaseless nagging in his solar plexus lifted, and he shook his head at how little trauma he'd suffered to make so considerable a difference in his life. With quantum levels less worry in his chest, he walked from the courthouse back home, stopping for the first time in many months at Sarge's for a pastrami sandwich and a beer. At home, he rolled a joint, stared at it for a while, then undid the paper, dropping the threads back into the Tupperware container. His life had changed radically in one day, and he decided to carry that transformation forward, accepting it was time to break with his troubled past. He leaned back and dialed Irena. She must have been in the hospital, for there was no answer. She never took a personal call at work.

In bed that night, despite the weariness from so many days and weeks and months of anxiety, he felt himself falling off to sleep quickly. He was, however, back up forty-five minutes later, his usual spiral of invasive thoughts pushing out any notion of rebirth. The bankruptcy ruling, he suddenly realized, removed but one spike of the truncheon still hanging over his head. His mind churned as the minutes and minutes dragged by on the clock radio.

How did a man undo blunders as appalling as those he'd left in his wake? He roared in his head that surely others had risen from such mistakes, many far worse. Or had they? The more he ruminated, the more he accepted his transgressions as exceptional, in a league with the most dreadful of people. A glass of scotch provided the reverse of the intended effect, leading him into a cage where his affronts to society were inescapable. His self-talk slowly spiraled into an endless loop of reproach, one in which he was convinced his wrongs had harmed so many, the rules of forgiveness that applied to common offenders, everybody else, were an amnesty to which he was not entitled.

At 1:30, he was wider awake than when he'd left for court in the morning. He wobbled into the bathroom to his Tylenol bottle. The six oxycodone had not been touched since the time he'd picked them off the living room floor the day after Irena's tragedy. Two pills were in his mouth before he took a step in the dark toward the kitchen. As he brought a glass of water to his lips, he regretted his weakness and thought about spitting them out, but it was too late, for they had already dissolved, or so he told himself. He cursed halfheartedly but also knew there would soon be release, hours of dreamless sleep.

While he waited the half hour for the oxycodone to muffle his consciousness, the notion of time captured his thoughts. As the minutes droned on, his tangled brain began to fashion an escape from his struggles by conceiving scenarios that culled the most bizarre elements of sub-atomic physics. Given these inexplicable notions, that a particle could be where it was going before it got there, might it be possible to reverse years of poor decisions, take them back by simply willing it to be so?

His first experiment was to crook his index finger and an instant later use his full consciousness to will the movement undone, to erase it from the record of man on Earth. As he failed that test, and the ones after it trying to remove even his thoughts from the chronicle of time, he laughed sadly at the absurdity, at the years of scientific knowledge he'd supposedly stuffed into his head, especially the greatest law of science that all educated souls on Earth had internalized: time flowed in but one direction. As that principle had prevented him from undoing the two pills twenty minutes earlier, he began to accept that if time marched only forward, all past acts were locked in an impenetrable tomb, never to be altered. Nothing could be erased. He was doomed; there was no escape.

As the oxycodone dragged him into a semi-stupor, a few more thoughts rattled about his head. His future, also sealed in a vault, was not accessible. But in the last wisps of awareness, it came to him that everything people thought they *knew*, every *certainty*, was simply a belief, nothing more than a few primitive electrical impulses in the brain, each a mere 0.07 volts, seventeen times weaker than what was left in a used-up battery for a transistor radio. How could this mere fleck of energy be the supreme power that had driven the human world for six million years?

Then again, he remembered how easy it had been to make people believe the rubbish he'd peddled over the years, so in a last burst of consciousness, he decreed that while he would never again make the same mistakes, he would use these principles to create words to spin the stumbles already part of the record. He fell off with a sense of hope.

The next morning, he arose early, a bit groggy, as it had been a long time since he'd used an opioid. He forced himself out of bed to shave and shower, for today he was going to find a job. He'd make whatever alterations to history were called for. The gullible would be made to believe that any sleight they could dig up on him was nothing more than zeros and ones converted to blips of light on a computer screen. The words, he would swear unbendingly, were no more trustworthy than the government data entry drones, souls like the rest of us, who mechanically input our work, rarely checking for mistakes, for to do so might delay going home.

Even the official seal on the bottom of the pages of his trial records, the documents that had so gravely affected his life, was nothing more than an illusion, a clump of pixels on a computer screen run together to appear to be the sacred emblem of the United States. Somehow, those computer dots suddenly endowed the records with authority and mandate. In fact, though, even the Great Seal glued to the president's podium had been created in some workshop by some worker bee who probably came home at night to one of the apartments of his decaying building. Like the president who hid behind the Seal, especially the president, there was nary a soul who wasn't dragging along the same skid marks in their drawers as the bums on Canal Street. Of all the letterheads, words, the seals, not one document, not one judicial decree, was imbued with a drop more God-given sanctity than a discarded newspaper. It all boiled down to the perceptions and deceptions we perpetuated in our minds.

He would swear as false any breath of history that stood in his way—the justification, his power not to make the same mistakes again. He had never once, ever, generated an intention with that much finality.

Deep in thought, he shuffled toward the door to leave. As he passed the landline, the decades-old bell clanged harshly. Unable not to reach for the receiver, he thought that there was still time to ignore the intrusion, but the provoked motor reflex was unstoppable.

A stuffy female voice spoke over his greeting. "Dr. Sass, I am Nona Cardinal from the New York State Pharmacy Board." She did not pause long enough to let Elliott jam his heart back into his chest. "I'm calling to let you know there was a request for your case to be reviewed. Apparently, we were given inaccurate information in regard to your legal status. It appears you have not been *convicted* of the charges we have on record. We're very sorry for any inconvenience…"

Elliott had by now regained his concentration. His jaw tightened as he spit, "Very sorry? Any inconvenience? You took my license *by mistake*?"

The woman interrupted, "Sir, there was an issue, we recognized it, and we are taking measures to adjust the outcome. I am simply calling to say that we are prepared to remove the asterisk by your name. The one condition is that you pass a drug test."

"Drug test? I didn't take any drugs in the first place!"

"It is our right as a government agency to request any non-invasive medical test we see fit to insure we are able to carry out our mandate to protect the public."

He took three slow breaths and forced a smile. "Okay, no problem. When would you like to schedule it?"

"As you are aware, drug tests are unannounced. It has to be immediate. There's a clinic a block from your residence that has been alerted to expect you within ten minutes."

Elliott's voice wavered, his mind sprinting through the time required to metabolize oxycodone in a person who had not used in a couple of months. He was a week away. "I'm sorry, I'm on a bus. I have a job interview—in mid-town."

"Well, you had this number listed as a landline."

"Nope, had that number transferred to my cell. Look, I'm at my bus stop. I'm not going to miss this interview to go back uptown. You know how long it took me to get a chance for a job because of *your* asterisk?" He let his voice break up as if he was losing the connection then waited until he thought he heard the woman end the call.

He dropped into the recliner. He had no idea if the board was authorized to order a drug test. It did not, though, matter an iota. He had now refused one, a clear admission of guilt. If he waited for them to renew the offer, he would be in his sixties before the phone rang again. It was not possible to call the board and speak to a representative. If he sent his request by email, the only way they accepted communications from licensed pharmacists, he would be on record as having delayed the test. No, he would proceed with the asterisk, find a drugstore desperate for a seasoned pharmacist.

He went to several pharmacies in the less polite areas of the Bronx. Turned away from those eyesores, he took the subway to lower Manhattan. The manager in one store spoke of the possibility of a trial working alone on weekends and nights, though there was a requirement that he obtain a New York Pistol License. Elliott grouched that obtaining a permit to carry a concealed gun in New York was next to impossible.

The man shrugged. "Without a pistol under your white coat, you won't last eight hours."

Elliott thanked him and promised to call back after he had looked into the permit.

CHAPTER SIXTY-ONE

There was a message on the landline when he got home. Irena asked him to call. She was crying that she'd been served late that afternoon with notice of a malpractice suit in which she had been blamed for the death of the little boy. She asked Elliott to go with her to see the defense lawyer assigned by her malpractice carrier. She was afraid her English wasn't strong enough.

They sat with the attorney two days later. The office was on the forty-second floor of the RCA Building. It overlooked much of lower Manhattan. They were served espresso and offered Danish pastries. When the lawyer stepped out for a moment, Irena whispered, "Malpractice insurance company is paying."

The attorney told them this was nothing more than a money grab, that Irena's actions were easily defensible, especially given the mother's lying about the little boy's ingestion of her OxyContin. "She was just trying to cover up, keep the cops from finding out about the head injury. They'll eventually charge her with child abuse, murder. You are going to have to testify against her." Irena blanched, but the attorney waved his hand. "Not to worry, what they'll do is offer to drop the charges against you if you agree not to testify against her."

Irena's face scrunched. "Can these people keep me from testifying if police call me?"

"Of course not. The stupidity never ends, extends from the defendant to her lawyer, Dan Laird..."

Elliott gasped, "Dan Laird! He's the DA!"

"Not anymore. Had some difficulties over there. Happened pretty fast. Had to find a new gig. Now he's a medical malpractice authority. What he's done is take any case, anything. Way these guys live is, the case may not have merit, but it does have potential—every legal action does. Works for a discounted settlement, quickies, and if that doesn't pan out, gives the case to a group of trial lawyers, and they cast the dice. Throw everything up against the wall, see what sticks. I'm sorry our profession has such people, but we do. I guess all the professions have their twenty percent. Betcha most of it is drug related."

Elliott's face drained of color. Both the lawyer and Irena noticed.

The attorney went on. "They don't have the autopsy report, so her lawyer took the case based on her story. Doctor, you are not to worry. But speak to no one except Dr. Sass here, who will not mention a word about it to any breathing, or dead, soul. That clear?" Both nodded.

They went to Sarge's for pastrami sandwiches. Elliott wanted to tell Irena of the call from the Pharmacy Board but knew she would see through his excuse to avoid leaving a specimen that day.

Three days later, it was his turn to seek legal advice. He went to an attorney who listed himself as a business lawyer. The dingy offices occupied a storefront in the seedy city of Yonkers. The man collected five hundred dollars, sat back, listened for a few seconds, and interrupted, "I'm not going to sugarcoat it. You should have taken the drug test. You would have passed, right?"

"Ah, of course," the infinitesimal delay in Elliott's reply answered the question more honestly.

"Well, you're going to have a hard time finding a job in retail. Asterisk automatically raises a pharmacy's malpractice insurance premium, not only to cover you, but everyone in the store. Their rates go up, big time. Sort of, your sins'll rub off on the rest of them."

Elliott snapped, "That's a bunch of bull!"

The lawyer chuckled, "Not really. And why would you want to go back to retail? You must love dealing with the public, where was it again?"

"Lower Manhattan."

“Woah. Anyway, welcome to the computer age. You know what I mean?”

“Ah, no.”

“Look, these retail pharmacies. Whata they pay you?” Before Elliott could answer, the man sneered, “Don’t tell me, I already know. You’re a measly worker ant. One dies, one gets caught with his hand in the cookie jar, one gets an asterisk next to his name, who cares, doesn’t affect business one dime. Just push the next chump onto the treadmill. Endless supply of saps who can’t butter their own toast. Look, almost anything you can sell in person, you can sell over the internet. I mean, maybe not haircuts or tattoos.” He stopped and looked pensively at the ceiling. “Thinking about it, you can even get those things. You pay enough, barber, tattoo artist, happy to come to you. No reason to ever leave your home, never again. Die there, have someone come and pick up the remains.

“What you need to do is look into getting a license to sell medications online. In my wildest dreams, I can’t imagine an asterisk would have a damn thing to do with it. You are buying from shell corporations, boxes within boxes. Most of them overseas, India, China, Indonesia. Can’t even spell asterisk. May think it means you’re a senior pharmacist, special award for thirty years of blemish-free service.

“All you need to care about is your due diligence to find out if the stuff they supply is real, works, at least some of the time. I mean, you could even come to some deal with them to have samples tested by a lab here in the U.S. Or they can prove to you they already have provenance and chemical analyses. Bet most of them do. Probably falsified, but such is the way of today’s world. If they have certificates, you’re probably covered legally. Why, you could sit at home and make a million.

“Now, there would be some paperwork, incorporation and the like, but we can set you up with that, no problem. Few other things you’ll need, like liability insurance, tax registration, business account at a reputable bank; and you’ll need a warehouse, and insurance on the stuff you store there, unless you can get them to ship direct. Gets a little complicated. Oh, and don't forget about advertising. Dog eat dog in the medical field anymore.

"But, like I said, we can get that all done for you, real estate, insurance; we have the connections. Now, we'll need a retainer." Elliott's face drooped. The man waved his palm again. "All attorneys work that way."

Elliott looked up. "Yeah, I know all about that. Lemme guess. Ten thousand."

The man tensed. "Well, we could do a bit less, of course. Eighty-five, if that would make you more comfortable."

Elliott stood. "I'm gonna go home and think about it. But thanks, you've been very helpful."

The man added quickly, "We could even go a bit less." But Elliott was already through the door.

He called Irena. They talked for an hour. She was proud he'd dodged yet another abyss. Elliott shrugged, "I mean, he seemed nice enough, but I don't have that kind of money."

CHAPTER SIXTY-TWO

Irena suggested he, once again, do a computer search of non-retail jobs open to licensed pharmacists. He started that evening. There were the usual offers: hospitals and pharmaceutical companies, a list so long, it depressed him thinking there were so many openings, that each one likely meant an unhappy soul had fled, or been tossed out of, the profession. With a new cup of coffee, he sat back down and refreshed the screen. There were several new emails. Other than spam, no one ever emailed him. He was shocked to see messages from CVS, Rite Aid, and one from Pharm Associates International.

The two from retail stores were auto returns from corporations that paid to have the email address of anyone who had opened a pharmacy hiring website. The salary ranges of the stores were far less than he'd been making at his old job. He deleted both then opened the one from Pharm Associates. It was a quasi-personal note and started out with an apology for not knowing the recipient's real name, and a second apology if the information offered was unwelcome. As he skimmed down toward the unsubscribe button, he passed a paragraph heading that caught his attention.

CONCIERGE PHARMACEUTICAL SERVICES

It touted Pharm Associates International as an established corporation a doctor could call from anywhere on the globe, anytime, day or night, seven days a week, and make arrangements for essentially any medication to be sent to a patient in essentially any country in the free world. The on-call Pharm Associates International pharmacist guaranteed to locate the medicine somewhere, most often the US, in less than twelve hours, and have it delivered no later than twelve hours after that. They freely admitted there were extreme cases in which the delivery time could be up to forty-eight hours.

Elliott read on. They boasted about delivering life-saving insulin to a climber on Mt. Everest who had lost his meds in an avalanche. The expedition leader knew of PAI's services, and he immediately emailed them via the Wi-Fi available in many places along the trail to the top of the world. The PAI pharmacist took control, contacting the patient's personal physician in Chicago to get a prescription approved immediately. There was a footnote at that point urging the reader to click on a link to learn of the heroics that had gone into the project.

Elliott was intrigued and went to that page. There were pictures of a helicopter adorned with the PAI logo picking up the medicine from the US Embassy roof in Beijing, and one of its transfer to a UPS jet for the flight to Kathmandu's Tribhuvan International Airport.

The rhetorical question emblazoned across the top of the page was why the client simply didn't order the medicine from a Kathmandu hospital. A note was made that much of the medicine produced in Asia was no more what it purported to be than if it came from North Korea. Far more than half of the pharmaceuticals available at neighborhood drugstores throughout the Eastern World, especially Nepal, were simply sugar pills—a fair percentage laced with poison from the manufacturing process. Pharm Associates International, though, was not subject to the vagaries of the Third World market. They had a relationship with the American government that allowed U.S.-produced medicines stored for use by the consulate staff to be dispensed in emergencies, but only for American citizens in dire need.

The website went on to describe how the insulin was flown from the Kathmandu airport by helicopter to the Everest Base Camp at 18,192 feet. Of course, the air was far too thin for the aircraft to hover and land at such an altitude, so the helicopter had to over-fly the base camp and drop the medication. But the air was also too thin to support a parachute. It was time to click on the video titled, "Extraordinary Delivery."

The footage began with the picture of an Augusta helicopter dropping what looked like a five-foot-wide popcorn ball onto a flat, open patch of snow. The ball landed with a soaring, slow motion bounce, a NASA probe landing on Mars. From there, the package rolled across the plains outside base camp, Sherpas, Elliott imagined, charging after it on stocky ponies. He noticed there were no mountains in the background and thought it strange, but only for a moment until he presumed the video was made facing the lower elevations, where hundreds of miles of plateau were devoid of towering peaks.

Pharm Associates International allowed that the cost to the client, who eventually summited, was forty-two hundred dollars for fifty buck's worth of medicine. But they reminded the viewer that the man had forked over sixty thousand for the trip, and if he had not received the insulin, at best, he would have been lugged on the back of a Sherpa to the lowest base camp, where a helicopter would have evacuated him to a local "hospital." At worst, he would have died in place, his body lugged on the back of a Sherpa to the lowest base camp, where a helicopter would have hearsed the remains to Kathmandu. In other words, in the end, it was money well spent, and probably only a few dollars over the alternatives.

Elliott immediately thought of the chance to travel, to practice his profession, and clearly be part of an exciting corporation that addressed human need across the world, the latter growing out of his craving to reverse history.

Though there was no home office address on the email or the website, there was a phone number and a signature, Edward F. McCracken, CEO. Elliott realized the man who had sent it was awake and perhaps awaiting a return communication.

He dialed the number, a 242 area code, accepting that wherever that was, it made no difference in the age of cell phones. And, in fact, the call was answered on the first ring by a woman who spoke briskly and professionally. "Pharm Associates

International. This is Colleen. Do you have an emergent need for medication?"

Elliott introduced himself and explained his interest in employment. The woman softened her tone. She explained that Mr. McCracken was not at that location, but she would contact him immediately. "Please standby, Dr. Sass."

Two minutes later, a chipper male voice took the line. "Good evening, Doctor. This is Eddie McCracken. Thank you for your interest." Elliott thought about the marvels of modern technology, that a call from halfway around the world, maybe in a desert or fourteen thousand feet above sea level, could be so crystal clear.

McCracken asked if Elliott was working at present. Elliott said he had left his old employer, "a mammoth retailer. Got so tired of the rote. I'd like to get out and see the world."

McCracken laughed. "I was there not all that long ago. So, tell me a little about yourself."

Elliott mentioned NYU, the Pharm D., and his years in retail.

"Your license up-to-date?"

Elliott felt himself hesitate for a millisecond but then smiled into the phone, "Good as gold. All caught up on continuing pharm education credits, too."

"Well, what can I tell you about us?"

Elliott dared not ask about compensation but did about office locations, travel, and expenses.

"Well, you would be hired as an independent contractor to get ahold of meds wherever you can find them and have them shipped to customers in need right away. You supply your own office, staff, insurance, and the like. The beauty in that is you are your own boss. You eat what you kill. Our agents love that. We provide customers, and let me tell you, that's taken developing an international reputation. Didn't come cheap or easy. Took years. We give you those customers, and it's all yours after that. Sky's the limit.

"And we don't start out our new team members in the international division. We have a six-month evaluation phase, sort of an internship. You work on your own. We coach you when requested or needed. We're always available, as you can see.

"We have two divisions at present. First is the delivery of emergency medications almost anywhere in the world, the one on our webpage. The other arm of PAI provides bulk medications to small retailers in foreign countries, generally not on an emergent basis, but within a couple of days. You would be involved in the latter. We do the former after the internship. Basically, what we're looking for is a hard-working, self-motivated entrepreneur.

"If you're interested, let me email you an application. Get it back to me as soon as possible."

Elliott was excited and thought about calling Irena but knew she would not answer at work. More than that, he fretted she would query the lawfulness of what he was about to do, and he had no idea how to convince her it was all legitimate.

He filled out the application at midnight but waited to fax it back until morning, hoping it would make him appear less needy. Aside from his state pharmacy license and DEA numbers, there were no questions about the currency of his certificate, or even requests for notarized copies of his diplomas, original license, or letters of recommendation. There was a place to enter his Social Security number. He left that blank.

At noon the next day, a woman called. She introduced herself as Kathy from PAI. She was bubbly, gushing that they were impressed with Elliott's credentials and would like to offer him a trial position. If he was interested, they would have Mr. McCracken call him that evening, that is, during the day where he was presently travelling.

Elliott asked where the woman was calling from. She was less effervescent. "We have offices all over the world. We look forward to working with you." And she was gone.

Eddie McCracken called at 8 P.M. He explained the job. "Now, Elliott, if I may call you that, what we do is list jobs on a restricted website. Like, for instance, if a private pharmacy in the Maldives wants a shipment of, say, lisinopril for high blood pressure, you call various wholesalers and Jew 'em down to the lowest price, then contract the cheapest reliable shipper. You pay for meds and shipment with your own credit card. That's for tax purposes. It's complicated, but it's what our legal staff requires, and it's *all* above board, I can assure you. You do the follow-up, inform us when the product has been shipped, which you do with a fax, and we contact the pharmacy or the customer. When you're done with that acquisition, you go to our order board and choose another project. Sounds complicated, but it isn't at all. Be doing dozens a day in no time. Don't worry, we compensate you with bit coin before your credit card balance is due. I'll get to that in a minute.

"Most of our Pharm Ds get good with one type of medication from two or three suppliers and two or three delivery services. Jobs get easier, almost rote; you set up your computer with the right software, it'll just be a matter of pushing a few keys and the drugs are heading for corners of the world you've never dreamed existed.

"Now, of course, you want to know how you get paid. This part *is* a little complicated. Sorry. We have a list of what a certain drug should cost and the usual shipment and delivery fee. You will have that information. If you go over, you get less of a percentage of the sale, and vice versa if you undercut them. If it's the usual price for both, you get twenty percent of the profit. Actually, it's a bit less while you're on probation. But that's only for six months. Time'll fly. You'll see.

"Now, like I said, we pay you in bit coin, which as you know, is going up in value as we speak. So, just like we do, you take a small risk on the bit coin market, but it hasn't disappointed yet, not one bit, no pun intended. Give us the monthly business credit card due date, and we will credit that card with whatever you've made in the past month. Questions?"

Elliott did not know where to start, so he didn't. A contract appeared by fax minutes later. He signed it and received a copy in return signed by a Richard Clary, CFO.

He did not hear from PAI until late in the afternoon two days later. It was an email that led to a downloadable program giving access to a list of available projects. He chose one so simple, Aaron could do it. He was to send HCTZ, hydrochlorothiazide, an extremely common blood pressure medicine, to an address in the Bahamas. The whole deal was worth about sixty dollars, including next day delivery, and that meant he'd clear about four dollars. He made calls to suppliers from numbers on the list, made no attempt to barter, allowed the suppliers to choose the shippers, and it was done. He took another task off the board, this one fancy aspirin to Bolivia. Another few dollars.

By now it was 8 PM in the Bronx, too late to make any more calls to suppliers. The next morning, he received faxes from the shippers confirming the goods were airborne. He faxed PAI with the information, and in the return fax, a note scribbled in the margin urged him to take on more challenging requisitions. He did, and by the end of the day, he had earned eighty dollars. He was, though, getting up there on his credit card limit, and in a call to PAI, they recommended he open a new account.

He did this as well, and a few days later, when payment was due on the first card, PAI sent him a few hundred dollars in bit coin certificates over what he had spent on purchases and delivery. It was far less than he'd counted on. His call to PAI was put on hold for several minutes until a gruff male voice came on the line to remind him, "You're in the probation period." Elliott waited for another sentence, but the line went dead.

CHAPTER SIXTY-THREE

As the depositions for Irena's malpractice suit neared, she spent more and more time with her attorney. When the practice questioning becoming increasingly intense, her English deteriorated, and she finally asked Elliott to come along again as an interpreter, for he was familiar with her style of speaking. The lawyer agreed.

A colleague stayed late to role-play the plaintiff's attorney. He pushed Irena until her answers became unintelligible. At that point, he'd throw his arms up in frustration, turn to the make-believe jury, and plead, "I wonder if Dr. Ledderova understood a word of what my poor client was trying to explain about her beautiful son." Irena's lawyer would, of course, shout an angry objection and explain to Irena that the comment would be immediately stricken from the record, and the lawyer threatened with a fine, but also that the bell had been rung.

Irena became so aggravated with the trickery, she blurted, "Your justice sick like in Soviet Union."

That begot a stern warning that if she lost control during the trial, the plaintiff's attorney would simply turn to the jury and ask if they wanted a doctor like her, a so-called cool-headed professional, operating on their kids. That rendered an even more contorted face, and she nearly raised from her chair to advocate her theory that drug use was a volitional act, as much of a real disease as scuffed shoes. If the mother had given a fig about her precious baby, she wouldn't have beat him in the head and fractured his skull. Any doctor, any rational person, would lose his temper thinking about so irresponsible a mother.

The room went silent until Elliott grunted. She turned indignantly to see him shrug and mumble the words, "Guy's right ya know." When he looked back down at his computer, she apologized to the attorneys, her voice slow and deliberate as the interrogation wore on.

It was good that Elliott had come along. He was placed at the far end of the mile-long conference table, where he buried his nose in a laptop plying his new trade, sending off orders around the globe. One of the lawyers finally asked, "None of my bee's wax, but you writing a book or something?"

Elliott gave him a thirty second explanation of his international pharmaceutical endeavors, leading the man to nod acceptingly then screw his face in skepticism, asking if Elliott had a big insurance policy covering liability for his risky work. Elliott shook his head, as if something of that insignificance had never crossed his mind. "Risky?"

The attorney sat up. "You bet. Again, none of my business, but you might want to look into protecting yourself." Elliott's head canted. The lawyer became utterly serious. "What if a patient in Algeria asks for something simple, say a blood pressure medicine, say plain old lisinopril. Just had a case about this. Safer than water, right? Especially in Algeria. You get the U.S. embassy to supply a few tabs to cover the patient, who turns out to be an American oil executive. They give him enough for a couple of days, until you FedEx him a full prescription. You are confident of the purity of the meds, and you're the hero—right up until the guy drops dead of an anaphylactic reaction.

"Now, you say, 'That's not my problem. Guy's been taking the stuff for twenty years. Never had trouble with it before. How should I be able to read the crystal ball?' Right?" Elliott nodded, but an instant later, his face lost its color. The attorney smiled. "I see you figured it out. All sorts of bizarre foods and insects in Algeria. Our executive gets bitten by a bee-like creature, would normally only have had a mildish reaction, but lisinopril can push the problem from an insignificant itch into life-threatening anaphylaxis in a matter of seconds. You think you're covered?"

"I assume my company is covered."

"Famous last words. Never assume when it comes to this great game of baseball. Dead, multi-six-figure executive? Like I say, none of my business, but I hate to see people screwed when they did nothing wrong except live in our litigious society. That's why we do defense. Hope we don't need to get to know each other better.

CHAPTER SIXTY-FOUR

That night, Elliott called McCracken and asked for a copy of the PAI liability insurance contract. "Elliott, we really like you, but you have to understand, you're an independent contractor, like every professional who works with us. I'm sure I explained that to you at the beginning that we don't provide health insurance, life insurance, or liability insurance. Just like we don't provide an office, supplies, computers, or internet. We couldn't pay you as much as we do if we had these other expenses.

"But let's not worry about that. Glad you called. I know you're chomping at the bit to become a full agent, get off probation. I'm going to take that step right now. Let's get you on the A team. You ready to join us?" He ended his question with a hard break of his voice.

Elliott allowed the positive strokes to warm him for a few seconds, though it was not long before a cold shiver wafted over him as he waited for the tally of what it was going to cost him. McCracken, though, said nothing, and to break the embarrassing quiet, Elliott finally grunted, "Yeah, yeah, of course."

"Good. I have to tell you about our new project. We're going to offer small overseas pharmacies the latest U.S. cancer medications, the check point inhibitors." Elliott pulled a breath through his teeth. McCracken laughed. "That make you uncomfortable?"

"Nah. Just a little surprised. I thought only the big boys dealt in that stuff. It's pretty spendy from what I've heard."

"Elliott, we are the big boys. And yes, it costs far, far more than an equivalent weight of gold. Probably milligram for milligram, the same as diamonds." Elliott gulped; McCracken heard that as well. "Not a big deal, Elliott. No different than shipping blood pressure meds in bulk. The only modification is form-filling because it is so expensive; there are customs regulations at both ends. You familiar with them?"

"Some. I had to do a little of that for the meds I sent overseas. Since it wasn't scheduled stuff, it wasn't that big a deal."

"That's right. But when you are shipping sensitive stuff like cancer drugs, it's not nice to lose a shipment. I mean, this isn't rubber dog doo. Your responsibility continues after the meds leave our transshipment point until they arrive at the correct port of entry, and at the correct time. Even though that's where your official responsibility ends, it's very important to find a reputable freight forwarder, and to make sure they have people at the foreign end to walk the shipment through their customs. Good for customer relations. More return business.

"Yeah, it's more time intensive, I won't lie, harder than what you've been doing, but the other side of the coin, the profit is dramatically higher—*if* you stay organized and get things done in the cheapest way. It'll be up to you. Million other people are doing it and getting stinkin' rich. Sky's the limit, Elliott."

"How about the finances? Do they have to pay in dollars? Do they have to report it to the IRS? Do they report my name or yours?"

"You don't need to worry about payment. We take care of the transfer of monies here in the home office. See, it works like this. When they find our website, they read our conditions. First rule: pay up front, so they know ahead of time, before you contact them, what's what. Since this stuff is so expensive, when we receive the funds you have negotiated with them, we divert some of that money to our field agents, i.e., you. Also, when a foreign pharmacy puts in an order, *they* have to attach the documents from their country guaranteeing they are eligible to receive the medications, *and* that their customs have agreed to let the product through. Sort of double protection for us."

"What if they forge the documents?"

"Not our problem. Most likely they'll be stopped when they go to pick up the shipment. Truth is, there's lots of bribes going on.

None of our business. And, again, who cares? Like I said, they pay up front, we have the money in hand before you make the first call to the wholesaler.

"You find an interested foreign pharmacy on our website, negotiate a price. Fax us like before. We inform you when their payment has been received and cleared into our account. You negotiate with the wholesaler and purchase product from them; we pay most of that charge directly to them. You arrange for delivery to our transshipment center. It's in Bayonne, New Jersey. Because we also use it for controlled substances, it's a federally approved facility. You send a fax to give them a heads up. They take *very* good care of these shipments. Then you notify the recipient and ship it out via however you want, but we have been using UPS exclusively. A bit more expensive, but they're the most reliable—in the world. They've got good people on the other end. Lotta little stuff to do, more bureaucracy, yeah, but much better money than shipping water pills."

Elliott hesitated. "I'm not sure where to start with the red tape."

"I'll send you the details in a fax, but the bottom line is, get on the internet and read the regulations. It's all there. You can even download the forms and get them prepared mostly beforehand. Look over the FDA and export regs. Bullshit paperwork, not graduate school in chemistry. Basically, filling in forms; your clerk can do ninety percent of it."

"And all of this is legal?"

"Yes, of course. Told you, federally approved, even for controlled substances. And this stuff you're dealing with is expensive as hell, but it's about as controlled as jock itch powder. Feds really not all that interested."

"Good. I don't want to end up in Sing Sing."

"Me neither. Like I said, when the packages are received at the transshipment facility in Jersey, they send the confirmation to you, and then another when it's shipped. You inform the consignee overseas by fax, and they fax back verification of receipt. You simply put copies of all the paperwork in an envelope and send it off snail mail to the records place in, ah, I think it's St. Louis. End of your responsibility."

"Okay, where do I find wholesalers? When I was in retail, for exotic meds like that, we ordered directly from the manufacturer."

"Of course. That's okay for the huge retailers you worked for. This is bits and pieces, carpet remnants, *but* you will be amazed at how much international business there is in it. Doctor in Namibia has a rich patient with lung cancer—prime minister's father. Only needs enough for that one person. Money, oh, my God. Right up there with Warren Buffet, willing to pay *anything* for the latest panacea. Probably be replaced with salt water and sold on the black market before it leaves the airport, but who cares.

"Lotta people want to send product overseas, and even more foreign pharmacies that need it. We'll get you started with some names."

"Ed, okay, sounds like it's on the up and up, a garden variety import-export venture. But let me ask you a simple question. Why can't you guys just go direct to these wholesalers and cut me, yet another middleman, out of the loop? I'm a profit drain."

"Elliott, that is a good question with a simple answer. You're a *pharmacist*, a health care professional. You have the public, and governmental, trust to purchase and dispense drugs responsibly. I'm just a businessman. Juggle numbers, scrape for customers. You did the work to get the degree. You think the FDA's gonna give me a license to buy cancer medicine because I ask nicely? You know, you may think it's nothing, what you've accomplished; but I'm here to tell you, it's a big deal.

"Also, guys like us, we don't understand the dosing or the chemistry. We can't communicate with foreign pharmacies like you can. You speak the language—you're fluent! So, what do we do? We hire those who do have the credentials *and* the professional expertise. United Airlines' s CEO doesn't fly the plane. Not trained, and too busy with other things like running a business. So, he hires pilots. That's what you are, a medication pilot.

"Now, I will send you wholesale contact numbers and the other stuff by fax. And you contact them and go over the details. Everything from them is encrypted, so there's no funny business with intercepted orders, no people changing addresses and the like. We run a tight ship. Hope that relaxes you. You're about to make a very nice commission.

"Look, I have to catch a plane. Gimme a call if you don't understand the material in the fax. Should be there in no time."

The line was silent before Elliott thought to say good-bye.

A fax came in the morning. The cover page was plastered with official-appearing verbiage allowing only the intended recipient to peruse the contents. Printed on the actual document was a fax number with an 849 area code and instructions to send a test fax. A reply came in minutes listing an internet site he could enter to find pharmacies overseas requesting pembrolizumab, Keytruda, the most widely used, non-traditional chemotherapeutic agent available. The fax provided a login name, "esass", and password, his birthday. Opening the site, he found requests from foreign pharmacies for Keytruda, the list as long as the menu at the Waldorf.

He thought over the job for many hours in bed that night, mostly about how unlikely it was that he'd ever again be granted DEA permission to fill a single narcotic prescription. Essentially, his retail pharmacy days were over. He wondered if the state pharm board's website still listed his license as corrupted. He opened the site—the star was there, hovering indifferently after the last letter of his name. Might that portend he was not going to obtain FDA clearance to purchase even non-controlled medications like Keytruda? Tainted at both state and federal levels, he accepted there might be little he could do to make a living as a pharmacist. The Keytruda wholesalers would check him out before consigning a single vial of so fantastically expensive and dangerous a medication.

He thought of getting up for a glass of bourbon, but his head suddenly cleared, and he asked himself how many times he had allowed catastrophizing to derail his life. No, there wasn't a single cogent reason to beg off the job yet, not on the basis of an unfounded supposition. Setting his jaw, he sneered into the darkness, mouthing a harangue to set the wholesalers straight, his voice rising, arguing as if in court, that nothing had ever been proven against him, that he had no criminal record, not even a parking ticket. If they refused to do business with him, they could be accused of restricting his right to make an honest living, thus denying his constitutional rights.

As weeks passed awaiting approval by the FDA, his checking account continued to drizzle toward zero. The forms were returned several times, more fees extracted. He paid them only because he had not yet been summarily turned away. At the FDA internet site, where he could watch the progress of his case, there had been no change in status: "Preliminary Evaluation." He made the firm decision to wait six weeks, until his birthday. If he hadn't been approved by then, he would withdraw the application, get back what he could of the fees he'd squandered, and take the job slinging McRibs McDonalds.

As the screen opened on his birthday, the same "Preliminary Evaluation" opened in big letters. He barked, "***Shit***," and smashed a fist against the desk. The screen went blank, so he screamed louder, "***Shit, shit, shit***," this time beating both fists against the table. Bursts of light danced across the screen, and the word, "Processing" suddenly appeared in the status box. The image was coming and going, but he was able to read a footnote suggesting that phase generally lasted between forty-five and sixty days. Down again came the fist, the crash followed with a "***Goddamnit***" that shook the walls. A bright flare played across the screen, the status box went blank, then "Preliminary Evaluation" reappeared for an instant. Before he could pull the monitor free of its wired harness and slam it against the wall, a puff of smoke curled from behind the screen. What might have been the letters, "A P P R O V" flickered, but it was less than the 50 milliseconds the human retina takes to register a visual impulse. The light was totally gone, and a vapor of burning electrical components wafted toward the ceiling. He spent the rest of the day at a big box store replacing the monitor.

CHAPTER SIXTY-FIVE

The approval for foreign sales of Keytruda stared back at him when he fired up the new monitor late that afternoon. Elliott opened PAI's protected website cataloging foreign pharmaceutical requests. The list ran from Angora to Zimbabwe. There was no way all these countries had been approved by the FDA to receive sensitive, U.S. anti-cancer drugs, and he took a step back, spending hours reviewing FDA regulations for international sales. By sunset, he was still unable to find a definitive list and decided to quit until after dinner. He got three paces from his desk before the phone rang.

Irena was quite subdued. It took a moment to pry out of her that one of the other ER doctors, who was to be deposed in her case, hated her.

"How do you know that? Who could hate you?"

"He is Bible Belt boy—Southern Illinois."

"And?"

"He hate all communists, most of all Russian. I never talk to him for years. One night I walked into doctors' lounge. Empty only for him. He said to me, 'You have found Christ?' I said, 'Thank you very much for wanting to know, but I am very well in my spiritual life.'

"He did not stop. 'Do you not want salvation? Go to heaven? You need to accept Christ in heart. Do you people not know this?'

"I left room. Now we pass in hall, he always looks at ceiling. Why is he to be in my case?"

"Irena, listen to me. Your malpractice case has nothing to do with the care you provided. I told you before. I know you.

There can be no situation in which you did not do your best, which is better than everybody else. This is about money and politics. The country is coming apart. Truth is not important. You need to act like a Russian, not an American snowflake, like me."

There was a giggle. "I know I should have call you first. You are only one to change mood."

"I thought you weren't supposed to talk to anyone about your case. Why, your surgeon pal let you down again?"

Elliott's heart clenched as Irena answered defensively, "Before, he has been sued. He knows ropes."

"I guess you're right." His pause was longer than intended. "Hey, I gotta get going. My new job's a hassle, and the kids got the flu."

"What are you, going nuts?"

"Nope. Gotta go." He ended the call. When she rang again, he let it go to voice mail.

The next morning, he awoke with a terrible headache from the bourbon surfeit. Barely able to focus on the computer screen, and completely unable to make smart tactical decisions, he simply clicked on a pharmacy in Bucharest. For fun, he typed part of it in Romanian. A reply fax came in less than an hour. There was no sending number. It was in English, and at the top, "All correspondence will be done in English."

Elliott faxed again. The pharmacy requested one hundred doses of Keytruda, offering seventeen thousand for the lot. He faxed McCracken. PAI released eight thousand in bit coin. A follow-up fax to McCracken was answered succinctly. "Suggest obtain additional credit cards."

Elliott faxed the first wholesaler on McCracken's list. They settled on a price of fourteen thousand, but only because Elliott was a new customer. They promised the consignment would leave their depot via UPS within eight hours. So many faxes were sent and received, he ran out of ink; and it was several hours before he returned from the big box store with a new printer, the salesman having convinced him it was cheaper than buying the two cartridges required for Elliott's antediluvian model.

He spent the afternoon applying for a dozen new credit cards. Three were approved, though the limit on the highest was ten thousand, and the interest rate on outstanding debt topped seventeen percent. He made two medication purchases the next day and three the day after that. The faxes zoomed back and forth between Elliott and PAI, Elliott and the wholesalers, Elliott and the warehouse, Elliott and UPS, and Elliott and the overseas customers. By the end of the week, the fax machine started thumping and eructing sheets folded like Chinese hand fans. He called the big box store. "Sorry 'bout that. Bring it in. We'll have it back to you in a week, maybe five days."

He decided to buy a new machine on the internet and have it delivered that day, but his checking account was bare, so he opened his Bitcoin tally only to find it had been inactive since the day PAI injected the eight thousand.

While it was already late, unable to fax PAI, he called McCracken to beg for enough to buy the new fax machine. The call went to voice mail, the greeting explaining that Edward McCracken was out of the country and that all correspondence was to be strictly by fax for the next week.

There was no choice. He called Irena. He was so surprised when she answered, he was tongue-tied for the first thirty seconds.

She asked stiffly, "Are you drunk again, Elliott Sass?"

Finally, "No. Just happy you took my call."

"Why, you think I am special like Vladimir Putin?"

"No, it's just that, you know..."

"You know what?"

"I was upset last time."

"Ahhhh, you are calling to say sorry?"

Elliott's hesitation was palpable. "Yes. I am very sorry. But I had a lot on my mind."

"You are the only one?"

"That's what I wanted to ask about. What's going on with the lawsuit?"

"If it matters to you, my lawyer deposed mother. She was, you Americans say, 'shipwreck.'"

"Does that mean it's over? That they have to give up?"

"No. Lawyer says may even work in mother's favor. May show jury how sad mother is. Cannot answer even simple question."

Elliott sighed. "Well, I am sorry to hear that. When is your deposition?"

"Next week."

"Do you want to have coffee and talk about it?"

"No…Maybe."

"How 'bout this afternoon? Starbucks around the corner from your place?"

A long pause. "What time?"

"Two."

When they sat down, Irena looked across the table at him. "You are in trouble again."

"No. What are you talking about?"

"Yes. I can see your eyes when you pay for coffee. Like last dollar. Elliott Sass cannot lie to Irena."

"Let's talk about your deposition."

"No. I do not care anymore. I absorbed so much Yankee outlook. Here, the bad one is always the victim. But no more. If mother wins case, I will not care. It is why I pay malpractice insurance. I do not talk to others about case, but others come to me and say they are sued, some say three times. The great lesson? They tell me if only know before how corrupt system is, how greed drives court, they would never cry one tear, not one argument with wife or husband or kids. Everybody tells me. So, now I put on big-boy pants. They go to hell." She paused, set her jaw, and stared at him. "Elliott Sass, what is problem?"

He filled her in on his promotion with PAI.

She twisted her lips. "So, Aaron's father is shipping drugs."

"Yes, madame, but not the kind you think. Cancer meds. Doing some good in the world."

"Finally."

"Was that nice?"

"No. I know you are working hard. I can see in your face. You are tired."

He rebuffed her pointed questions about the process, afraid she would see through what he was finally beginning to suspect was not a kosher operation. “Irena, pretty lady, this time it’s all aboveboard.”

She was kind enough to simply grunt, “Uh huh.”

She lent him the money, “Only because you were good for it last time.”

CHAPTER SIXTY-SIX

It did not take long for Elliott to generate a debt of thirty thousand dollars. Still, there was no word from PAI, including McCracken, who had not changed his voice mail message in two weeks. Elliott sat at the kitchen table with a pad of paper writing scenarios, including finding McCracken and threatening to shoot him if he didn't reimburse him in forty-eight hours. And so began the round-the-clock calls to McCracken's phone. Finally, a new message blared. "This voice mail box is full."

Maybe he could trace the calls, bribe a worker at the phone company to find the towers off which the sonofabitch's signal was bouncing. Maybe there was a needy cop who could fake a warrant for telephone records if the payoff met NYPD standards.

In the meantime, Elliott began his investigation on the internet, first looking up the area code 242. His gut clenched when he saw it was the Bahamas, and he nearly vomited when he paid twenty bucks for a two-week subscription to a people finder website and discovered there was no such person who even remotely resembled the man who owed him so much money.

The fax number also bore the 242 area code, but hours of internet research uncovered no Pharm Associates International. He tried variations: Pharmacy, Pharmacist, Pharmacists, Pharmacist's, Pharmacists'; Associated, Association; Internal, Interveners, Internist, Internists; McKracken, McCrackan, McKrackan, McCrackun, McKrackun, MacCracken, MacCrackan, MacKrackan, MacCrackun, MacKrackun… He opened another people finder, one that claimed to cover international sites. He first checked the Bahamas then the other Caribbean islands. He went to the U.S. business directory, pulling up the Secretary of State websites in all fifty states and territories to research every list of corporate licensees in the country. He thought of doing the same for Canada, Mexico, Great Britain, and the EU, even corporations in China, the ASEAN, and the sub-continent; but it was 2 A.M., and while he told himself to begin again in the morning, he knew it was just more wasted spirit. So, he faxed all the wholesalers provided by McCracken. That elicited not a single response. He tried the overseas pharmacies, asking where they had remitted funds for their purchases. Nary a reply.

He realized the only address he had anywhere in North America for PAI was the private box number of the transshipment center in Bayonne, New Jersey. It was on Hook Road, near the docks. He checked Google Street View. While the area was industrial, the actual building appeared to be more a convenience store than a warehouse. He looked up rental cars but realized his credit card limits had been buried. He checked bus schedules—it would take five hours to get there.

Maybe he could borrow Irena's car. She answered his call. "Have to meet with you. A challenge has floated to the surface."

"No more money!"

"No, no way. Not asking. But I gotta talk over what's going on. I need a cool head. A smart head, a beautiful head."

"*No money!*"

"Can we have coffee again?"

"No. *No money!*

They met at the same Starbucks. She sat closer and closer to the edge of her chair as he spun his story. It wasn't as though she was enthralled; it was because she was positioning herself to run when the other shoe dropped.

He asked if she would like to spend the day in elegant north Jersey. She asked why he didn't rent a car and go by himself. "And don't tell me you want my company."

She picked him up at 9:00 the next morning. It was the first time he had ridden in the Volvo. The air was laced with her scent. He spent the hour on the Henry Hudson Parkway remaining quiet, the lost years playing over in his mind. Like his father and his mother, he had wasted his life, one barren decade after another. He had nothing to show for all the tax dollars spent on his education. Now, he didn't even pay taxes, and hadn't on the myriad side gigs that had consumed so much of his creativity and sweat. All in all, he had not contributed to make the world a better place than when he arrived. He looked at Irena out of the corner of his eye. From nothing, from less than nothing, from the Russian tundra of which the world had not the slightest knowledge or interest, born a demon, left to die, and here she was saving lives in a hospital in Manhattan, doing God's work on Earth, and he was sitting next to her. He did not have the right.

As they slowed in the thick traffic waiting to enter the tunnel, his continued silence surprised her, and she turned toward him. His eyes were glassy and red. She said nothing at first, but as they coasted slowly to the nadir of the tunnel, she reached over and brushed his arm. He startled but just as quickly a wave of emotion seized him, and his chest blazed with release, as if he had been acquitted of a terrible crime. He sighed then caressed her hand as gently as he had ever touched a woman. He reached slowly toward her face but stopped as he was overcome by a gush of tears that alarmed her. She slowed and pulled into the right lane. "We stop in Saint Aedens for breakfast. I know nice greasy spoon. Borsht, but American sour cream." When he did not answer, she laughed, "Not to worry, Elliott. I am paying today."

He let his seat recline and rested for a bit before confessing he knew very well that he had made a bollix of the years, that she had been right in rejecting him for so long, that he had no business sitting next to her—and never had.

She was also quiet for a minute. "Elliott, there have been spotty times. But you cannot look back, as you *Amerikanskiy* say, and 'trip on past.' Like rest of us, many mistakes. I thought all night. You have done no big deal bad thing. Not one time. You are not alone in having past; there is no one without skeleton in closet."

She went on softly. "I have been cruel to you. Always negative comment. It is not way to help person you love." She took her eyes off the road quickly and shot a fleeting glance at him as his face blanched. "I am sorry, but it is because you always scare me, that you could do such harm to my heart. One single day, one single minute, one word, one look from you, my life changed forever." She began to cry quietly but quickly gathered herself. "Not rational you could do that, not after lifetime of people say and do much, much worse to me. But you did." She paused again. "Elliott, maybe not so tragic. Your few words turn around my life. So, you see, I owe you very much."

They spoke little at breakfast, and after a few bites, she reached across the table and took Elliott's hand. They sat there like that, staring at each other for so long, their eggs were cold when they finally looked down. They pushed the plates aside and spoke about the trip to Russia, soon laughing so hard the other patrons shot them looks.

As they entered Bayonne, Irena looked around and grunted, "Nice place. Maybe I can get job here—heroin clinic."

"And I can work at the CVS over there on the corner and fill prescriptions to keep you busy around the clock."

"You already do."

They came upon a postman and asked him directions to Hook Road. When Elliott showed him the address, the elderly black man winced. "I'll tell ya, but y'all be careful down there, hear?"

They found Hook Road in a vast area of fuel oil storage silos, railroad tracks, and warehouses, some mammoth, many larger. Interspersed were dilapidated, long-abandoned, brick factories. As they drove deeper, they passed no cars, no signs of life. Irena mumbled to herself, "Nice neighborhood. Location, location, location." As they rounded a curve, now less than half-a-mile from their destination, Elliott caught a glimpse of a few parked black SUVs hugging the far side of a gargantuan fuel silo. For a split second, he saw what appeared to be the silhouettes of several men in jumpsuits, but Irena was driving so fast, he could not really be sure what he had seen.

The address Elliott had written down was a ramshackle, single story, clapboard affair, certainly less than two thousand square feet. The roof was covered in missing and peeling shingles encrusted in clumps of repulsive, pea green moss. It had the appearance of a World War II basic training barracks that had been abandoned half a century before. A nearly toppled, three-foot-high, chain link fence enclosed a muddy yard. Two abandoned beaters, a Chevy and a Ford, sat in the enclosure, their tires flat, windows long since smashed out. Completely out of place, though, was a new Beemer parked on the crumbled cement driveway. Even more unexpected was the glow of lights inside the building.

It was a dreary, cold day, and the car windows became opaque in a patch of low-lying harbor fog. As they rolled slowly closer, unable to see the structure clearly, Irena warned, "Elliott, I think we must drive by first. Not welcoming. What do you think?"

"All of it's out of place, isn't it? You're right, let's keep going."

As they trundled past, while Elliott was on the wrong side of the car to see inside clearly, he was convinced a face in the window stared at them until they had passed the next building.

That structure, feet farther on, was a public storage facility, not much more charming than the barracks. A pole rose out of the roof, four cameras atop, two pointed toward the barracks.

Irena drove a quarter mile farther on Hook Road. They looked at each other, went back and forth nodding uncertainly, then firmly shook their heads no. But Elliott stiffened and blurted, "No! I'm goin' in there. Fuck 'em. They owe me a lotta money."

She touched his arm. "My brave soldier. Please remember, *I* am one who is owed money. And I do not think this is good idea."

"Irena, I'm just going to ask if they know where PAI is headquartered. If it looks dangerous, I will turn around and run out. You stay in the car, be the getaway driver. Okay?"

She bobbed her head weakly. As they reapproached the barracks, Elliott noticed flashing red lights on the cameras. "Irena, were those things blinking when we drove by a minute ago?"

"What things? I barely can see road."

They stopped in front of the failing fence. He patted her hand. "Don't leave town." She smiled wearily and turned the radio off.

The gate was half open, hanging at an obtuse angle and held by a single bolt. He slinked through, careful not to touch it. He semi-knocked on the warped door and opened it at the same time, the grinding of its corroded hinge loud enough to be heard inside Irena's car. Sitting on a high stool behind a counter was a scruffy, semi-bearded, morbidly obese man. A cigar smoldered in an ashtray next to a pile of cigarette butts. A stained coffee mug sat by his right hand. The place stunk of stale tobacco, stale beer, and, strangely, cardboard.

The man was already staring at the door when Elliott pushed it open. It stopped Elliott in his tracks, though he drew a breath and took a sheepish step forward. Smiling foolishly, he stopped feet from the stools on his side of the counter. The man's eyes opened wider. He said nothing. Finally, Elliott spoke brightly, "Hello, sir," though that was greeted only with a thickening of the man's glower. "I'm trying to find PAI, you know, Pharm Associates International."

"And who wants to know?"

"Oh, yeah. I'm Elliott Sass. I work for them." There was not the slightest flicker of an expression change. Elliott danced faster. "Yeah, see I'm tryin' to track down some cargo I sent to this address," and he took a step forward, pushing a bill of lading toward the countertop.

The man did not glance at it. "I don't know no Farmer Association. You got any other business here?" Before Elliott could answer, the man put his weight on his fists and pretended to start lifting himself off his stool. At the same time, his enormous head bobbed toward the door.

Elliott protested. "But sir, I send all my stuff here."

The pressure on the man's fists built until his tobacco-stained knuckles blanched. As Elliott took a step back, he stopped reflexively at the harsh sounds suddenly coming from behind the cinder block wall to the rear of the service counter. Seconds later, two greasy men emerged. The counterman had not taken his glare off Elliott, who was now backing quickly toward the door.

In an instant, Elliott's attention was whipped away from the men as the front door banged open. A body dashed into the building and collided with Elliott from behind. Both men fell to the floor. Elliott turned his head to focus on a UPS deliveryman who stared back at him heatedly. Elliott babbled an apology, came to his feet first, and put out a hand to help the man.

He also picked up the driver's clipboard. As he started to hand it back, he noticed the letters PAI in the address box. The UPS man's hand closed impatiently around the clipboard, but Elliott yanked it back to focus on the document. It was one of his own shipments, a consignment for Burundi.

Elliott asked the UPS man, "Hey, are you the driver that delivers PAI stuff here?"

"Why do you want to know?"

"Because these are my shipments. Just trying to find out a little bit more about where they came from."

The delivery man pulled hard and reclaimed his clipboard. "Talk to my supervisor if you got questions."

"What's his number?"

The driver screwed up his face. "Look it up."

Elliott was essentially surrounded by people not terribly thrilled with his presence. Despite that, a pleasant feeling swept over him as he realized Irena was waiting in the car. He stopped to think about her words. In that instant, he felt as though he had a future, and if he wanted to experience it, he had better turn and run.

Abruptly, though, a hunk of black filled the doorway. It took less than a breath for him to realize it was the silhouette of a large man dressed in a black jumpsuit. Elliott did not have the opportunity to look at the face, for his attention locked on the 9-millimeter Glock aimed between his eyes. An instant later, the barrel swept to the left, toward the counterman's head. Gasps came from the corners of the room. The two men spun about and retreated behind the wall. A moment later, he heard the back door fling open and then screeching. Elliott made out only the words, "DEA…arrest…shoot you." The UPS driver dove frantically into a corner, curling into a fetal ball, arms rigidly crossed about his chest.

The intruder shoved Elliott toward the man at the counter so he could hold both with one pistol. As Elliott's back hit the tall stools, he lost his balance. His flailing arm launched one of the stools away from the counter to bang into the invader's legs. The man tripped on it but maintained his balance and kicked it behind him toward the door.

He screamed, "DEA, warrant, get your goddamn hands up where I can see them!"

The counterman let his shoulders relax, his lips curling up subtly. "Officer, no problem. You don't get no trouble from me. It's this guy," he nodded toward Elliott, "who's been shakin' down all the storage places."

The agent swung his weapon back and forth between Elliott and counterman before the latter grimaced, "Officer, please don't put that thing in my face. I'm already a heart attack lookin' for a place to happen. You don't need that, sir." His left hand came up from behind the counter. He pointed. "He's the one you want. I guarantee it. Thank God you're here."

With the pistol now trained at Elliott's forehead, the agent screamed, "On your fuckin' knees, ass…" The bellowing, however, stopped short as the man's eyes rolled into the back of his head. "Are you shittin' me? You're that asshole from the Bronx. You little fucker, you beat that rap, convinced that fuckin' homo judge that we set you up. It won't fucken happen this time, cocksucker."

It was at that instant that Elliott recognized the agent, Uveges, with the supremely repulsive mug who had twice raided his apartment. While the man's face was frozen in anger, Elliott detected movement in his lower field of vision. His eyes dropped to see one of the cop's fists tightening around the pistol butt, the other winding up to deliver a punch. When the blow didn't come, he wondered if the agent was waiting for the attack dog to arrive.

"Get on the fuckin' ground."

Elliott did, but the instant his nose touched the filth on the rotting linoleum, there was shouting from the back of the building. Two shots followed. The agent turned his gun toward the partition and took steps in that direction. With the agent positioning to take a furtive look behind the concrete divider, the fat man's right hand pulled a .38 from under the counter and set about the procedures required to rotate his four-hundred-plus pound mass. When his belly caught on the edge of the counter part way around, he panicked and pulled the trigger. The round hit the cop in the back, the entry wound much closer to the shoulder than the agent's midline. It looked to be a superficial wound, but it had entered at an angle, and there was no way to know what internal path it had taken. Regardless of where it had gone, the man went down with a thud, and the 9-millimeter flew out of his hand, caromed off the wall, and slid to rest in the middle of the room. The fat man turned his head forward, starting to pivot to shoot down at Elliott.

At that moment, Irena flew through the door. She stood absolutely still for two seconds, assessing, then suddenly came into violent motion, lifting the toppled stool to launch it at the fat man. It hit the counter with a bang that shook the room. The man, though, had ducked to the side and become wedged between the chair and counter. The UPS driver took the sudden silence to spring toward the door, fast-crawling on his belly toward the delivery truck. Before he was fully seated in the van, the vehicle screeched off down Hook Road.

Irena tugged at Elliott, and they bolted for the door and straight to the Volvo. As they were about to jump in and drive off, Elliott stopped. "Irena, that guy's gonna get executed." He turned and sprinted back in to see the fat man lifting off the stool, one hand on the counter, the other still gripping the pistol, the barrel of which was swinging toward the DEA agent.

Elliott immediately dove for the agent's pistol, which was still sitting in the middle of the floor. While on the ground, he rolled to his side, aimed toward the counter, and pulled the trigger so hard he thought he had broken his finger. Nothing happened, but the business end of the barrel staring at the fat man sent the thug down onto the floor, flailing like a beached whale, thrashing toward the partition.

It gave Elliott time to grab the agent's shoulders and pull with a fury he did not know he had within him. As he dragged the cop through the door, a shot rang out. He felt a burning slap in his right lower leg. He ignored it and dragged the agent two more steps from the building before collapsing backward into the mud, his consciousness battered by booming explosions, flashes of light, shrieks, and more explosions. Elliott looked up into Irena's reddened eyes. It was the last thing he remembered.

CHAPTER SIXTY-SEVEN

He woke in the hospital three days later, his right leg throbbing. He tried to flex it to relieve the pressure, but it did not move, and the ache only worsened. The nurse put a few milligrams of analgesics into his IV when he moaned, "Pain," then sat with him and explained that he should expect to hurt, a lot, and that it was normal as his wounds healed. He heard only the first words of her counsel before nodding off, oblivious to what she meant by wounds. In fact, he spent most of the next two days asleep, unaware that Irena, Aaron, and several DEA agents sat by his side, hoping to be there when he roused.

Nearing a week in the hospital, he finally became sufficiently alert to recognize Irena. She began to weep when he held out his arm to take her hand. He pulled her toward him and kissed her fingers. He reached for Aaron but quickly mumbled, "Don't worry, I ain't kissing you, Sonny."

He looked around the room and saw three, dark-suited men. That jarred a flurry of memories. The trip to Bayonne began to seep into his mind, and then the image of the DEA agent who had threatened him with what sounded to be life in prison. He spoke slowly to the men. "Are you here to arrest me, take me back to prison like the last time?"

They shook their heads, and one of the men spoke kindly. "No, Dr. Sass. We're here to make sure you're safe, and to make sure you get better. DEA owes you a lot. Country owes you a lot. If we're going to be taking you anywhere, it's to the White House to get your award, and Dr. Ledderova's, for heroism."

Irena pulled her chair closer to the bed. "You were something, Elliott." She turned to the men and Aaron, nodding for them to leave the room.

"What's going on, Irena? How is that agent that got shot? Are you about to tell me he didn't make it?"

"Not at all. Because of you, he is alive. He's asked about you."

"Yeah, I'll bet he did."

"Really. He knows whole story now. They all do. We have even heard from pharm board. All apologies and smiles. Shitheads. They have nerve to ask please not to go to newspapers. But that is way down list of things." She took his hand. "Listen, my brave soldier, there is something I must tell you…" The pause drained what little blood was in Elliott's brain. "You were shot in lower leg. It was special bullet made to explode inside. It hit bone, artery, vein, mostly took away any chance to keep leg. They talked with me for very long time. You had lost so much blood so fast…I tried so hard to stop it…" She began to sob. He kissed her hand again then squeezed it harder and harder, her touch all that he cared to sense.

She slowly gathered herself. "Elliott, your leg could not be saved. It was clear it must be taken off because you could not go through long, long surgery to try to fix it. I will tell you truth. It is my decision in end. I lied and told them we are husband and wife." She stopped and let him think.

He rolled toward her and asked, "Is that what you want?"

"With all my heart."

CHAPTER SIXTY-EIGHT

Irena forced Elliott to stay in her condo until he graduated from physical therapy, became facile with his prosthesis, and was deemed safe to live on his own. She finally let him go home, but it wasn't thirty-six hours before he was back, both crying on the phone that they missed each other too much.

At the end of the third month after Bayonne came a call from the DEA. They asked if they could come to him and talk about the case. He agreed, though his heart squeezed in dread.

When they showed up at noon the next day, they brought Chinese food, enough to feed the Peoples' Liberation Army. Agent Uveges led the delegation of three. When he saw Elliott standing behind Irena, his eyes clouded. "Dr. Sass, of course, I don't have the words to thank you for your bravery. And I don't have the words to ask your forgiveness for my behavior that day…and the other times. I hope you will understand it is rare that we deal with good people. Our bedfellows are the most contemptible creatures in the country. We have to assume the worst of behavior from every person we are ordered to investigate. And since this is the great melting pot, what we deal with are the lowest forms of life on the planet. It is not a justification, I promise. It's how jaded we've become. Again, no excuse for my behavior."

They shook hands and bumped shoulders. Uveges stopped suddenly. "Oh, and I almost forgot. Let's get Fluffy in here." Still sitting in the hall was the German Shepard. The agent motioned for him to sit two feet from Elliott. His ears were relaxed and his tail thumped the floor.

The handler commanded. "Flufster, give the nice doctor a kiss." He stood, wagged his tail, and Elliott scratched his head. The dog took a step closer and sat again.

As they ate and talked, the agent explained what they had uncovered about PAI. "We found a lot of pharmacists like you, you know, guys with that asterisk stuck next to their names. When someone with a pharmacy license was looking for a job, they paid Google to get notified. Then they looked up the person, and if there was a problem with the license, or there had been legal issues, they knew that guy was desperate and would be putty in their hands.

"They had this cockamamie payment scheme, which I'm afraid you fell for. I know, you needed work. Not judging. So, they ripped people off for a couple of months, had them send pills all over the place. That part was close to being legal, but it was still practicing medicine in states and countries where the pharmacist did not have a license. As long as the meds weren't scheduled, the FDA ignored it. They weren't going to spend the money prosecuting single prescriptions for a week of water pills.

"But after a few months of that, they had you. Next came cancer drugs and big hitter cardiac stuff. They were all funneled through the warehouse in Bayonne. They had people there switching the good stuff for diluted injectables which they got from China. It was in a lab near the warehouse. Then they shipped overseas. Profit was obscene.

"When you did that for a while, they chose the ones they could trust, you know, good little boys and girls who didn't ask questions. Called them up to the big leagues—opioids. Same scheme, except here, they sold the pills back to American drug runners. There were no actual overseas shipments, but the pharmacists didn't have a clue.

"They submitted the paperwork to us and whoever, and it looked like the goods were transported to foreign pharmacies, but PAI had agents in those countries forging records to confirm deliveries that never took place. The phony documents then got stamped by government officials over there on the take and sent back here for submission to the DEA. Looked kosher to all the world. We didn't have a clue about the opioids, and the FDA had no idea about the cancer drugs. Embarrassing.

"Oh, and don't let me forget your pal McCracken. Are you sitting down?" There was subdued laughter. "Ain't no such dude. Doesn't exist. The voice is actually one Ayman Bashir Shihab. He did all his work through burner phones and burner fax lines all over the Caribbean. Cell phone records down there can be manipulated to meet the needs of the highest bidder. No trace of *their* faxes to anyone, but there are of yours. Nothin' dishonest at all there on your part. No sweat.

"Anyway, the website's protected by more VPNs than Carter's got little liver pills."

"Liver pills. FDA?"

Uveges quipped. "You don't know what that means, wrong generation. Just a shitload of VPNs. No way to untangle it, least not on our budget.

"We had no idea about any of this until an opioid wholesaler who got screwed by PAI came to us. It took us a year to work that lead. Then one came from a Bitcoin employee we arrested. When she realized she'd gotten herself into a pile of manure, we gave her immunity, and things started to come together. Sorry it took so long. Sorry you got sucked in.

"And that's what we were doing down in Bayonne that day. We waited until the UPS delivery. Figured we'd get a load of narcotics and maybe boxes of diluted meds, start making arrests. You know, give our brothers at the FDA a little boost. Hit these bastards from two directions.

"Well, that was our plan. Supposed to be just the fat clerk and the UPS driver. Where those other two came from…our bad. And then, of course, there you were. Cost us the agent who was covering the back door. But I don't wanna talk about that."

Elliott shook his head. "Shit, I didn't know about that." He paused. "I hope you got the two grease balls."

"Yeah. Sad to say they didn't make it either."

"And how about the fat man?"

"He's no longer with us, gone to his final reward at the big pizza shop in hell. I mean, he didn't get shot or anything, but we had a hard time transporting him. Poor man had a heart attack right there in the transport van on the way to the federal lockup in Jersey City. Lived for a few days, enough time to give us what we wanted from him."

"He didn't seem like the kind to talk."

"Well, we know the nurses up there in Jersey City. They get a lot of our customers. Heart attack is painful. Traded two milligrams of IV morphine per sentence of information. See, usually takes three or four milligrams to stop the pain. This elephant took seven or eight. Got reams of stuff outta him before he was called home. Saved the government millions."

"The UPS driver?"

"Oh yeah, that prince. Corporation gave him a certificate of bravery or some such bullshit. We had questions about that, so we took a deep dive into his part of the operation. Seems he accepted a few bucks to deliver the cancer and heart meds directly to the lab in Bayonne where they did the watering down, instead of delivering them to the drop point with the fat man. Saved the driver a lot of time, which he spent with a gal in town. As far as we could tell, he wasn't aware of the scam, so officially, he did nothing illegal, but UPS dropped his ass like a hot potato and so did his wife. Maybe there is a God."

"Agent Uveges, what's goin' on with McCracken or whatever his name is?"

"Shihab. Well, he's on the run. Has several passports and, we think, millions stuffed away in a trust in the Cook Islands."

"Cook Islands? Does that mean I'll never see any of the money they owe me?"

"Let me be honest. Probably not. The Cook Islands are more secure than Fort Knox. Ten percent of their yearly income comes from keeping funds hidden for rich foreigners. A pain in our ass. When we got snippy with them some years ago, their government passed legislation to insure the anonymity of all the accounts. Can't touch 'em.

"Now, we think Shihab is in the Middle East. His father was a muckety-muck in the Maronite Church in Seattle. It's a sect of the Catholic Church that's centered in Lebanon. Shihab grew up in Seattle from the time he was six. His family's clean, but they have untold relatives in Lebanon. I think forty percent of the country is Maronite. We don't have an extradition treaty with Lebanon, and even if we did, there'd be no cooperation in finding him. But I will say his family here in the States is so embarrassed, better to say, ashamed, they agreed to cooperate with us. Good people. I believe they will.

"But Dr. Sass, like I said, we came for two reasons. The second is your future." Elliott's face drained of all color. "Not what you're thinking. I'll let Special Agent D'Amico here discuss that."

An older man shoved forward on the couch. He opened his briefcase. "Dr. Sass, I want you to know that the Agency owes you big time. Thank you, but let me get right down to it. We want to offer you a position, Forensic Chemist, starts as a GS-11. It's government pay. You're not gonna get rich, but work's steady, and the bennies are great. See, we could use your chemistry experience; your pharmacy expertise; and, to be honest, we did some digging, and your computer skills are impressive. We know you're not formally trained in computer science, but we need someone with imagination. Pretty obvious you think outside the box. Oh, and you got guts."

Elliott was speechless until he looked at Irena, who nodded briskly several times. He finally opened his mouth. "Agent D'amico, I'm flattered, but let me be honest, I have used drugs in the past. Not for a long time, and never any heavy stuff, but still, I don't think I qualify. And my leg. Wouldn't be too good at chasing down perps."

D'Amico shook his head. "Not as a sworn agent, as a civilian employee. Look, we are very aware that there would be a total of about fifteen people in the DEA, FDA, and FBI combined, if every candidate that had ever used a drug was exempt from service. What we are looking for is recent, ongoing substance abuse. And what we demand is *absolute honesty*. You will have to complete the Drug Enforcement Administration Contractor Drug Use Statement. I will admit it's a bear, goes on forever; but if you decide to let it all hang out, you will not be subject to prosecution by the DEA, and we will not provide the information to any other agency. That will be given to you as a written guarantee.

"Our human resources panel evaluates each case separately. Now, if you've committed other crimes, I'm not talking about shoplifting bubblegum when you were fourteen, or a few speeding tickets, we would ask you to state you aren't interested in the offer. There would be no further investigation. That, I, we, promise. Save everybody a lot of time.

"What do you think?" He opened the briefcase, pulled free the Drug Use Statement, and handed it to Elliott. "You can look this over right now and decide. Again, we make no judgment. We know who you are."

Elliott turned to Irena then back to the agent. "Sir, do you mind if we look this over together?"

"Not at all. We can be in touch later in the week."

Elliott brought his gaze back to Irena. "Is that okay with you?" She nodded. He leaned forward and started browsing through it, shrugged nonchalantly a couple of times, and asked Irena, "Could we talk for a minute in the bedroom?" He turned to the agents and smiled. "Promise, just a minute."

They emerged less than thirty seconds later. "I will be happy to provide answers to every question. Thank you."

They sat drinking wine that night. Elliott asked Irena if she thought he could swing a bank loan for fifty thousand based on his new employment. She asked why.

"I intend to pay back the Cromarties, the family that got screwed when I testified. I need to make that right."

She stared at him for a minute, rose, and walked to the kitchen. He heard a cupboard open and a few seconds later, close. She came back to the living room, a cupped palm extended. He reached out to touch her hand, but she shook her head. "Oh, Mr. Doctor Elliott Sass, what is to be done with you?"

He looked more closely. It took a minute to get over his astonishment, and when he did, he lifted one of the two quite sizable diamonds and held it to the light. "Oh, I believe they are of Russian origin. Very nice cut, color, carat, clarity, and care." She rolled her eyes, and he countered arrogantly, “I know about these things, if you don’t mind.”

CHAPTER SIXTY-NINE

Twuck gave away the bride. Jimmy wore a suit for the first time in his life as he carried out his duties as best man. Agent Uveges; Abraham Baker, Arron's chess partner; newly retired Dr. Arthur Julian; and Attorney Andre Dalton sat in the front row of the small side room at a local Synagogue. The rabbi wouldn't let them use the main hall for neither Irena nor Elliott were members of the congregation. Three dozen of Irena's friends from the hospital stuffed in behind them. Irena had asked her friend, Antoinette Chugunkin, to be one the bridesmaids but her breast cancer had worsened unexpectedly, and she'd passed four days before the wedding. Her son, Gregor, though, was there.

The wedding party walked to the Russian Tea Room for a banquet after the ceremony. Agent Uvegas had a couple of beers and bellowed, "Bring on the borsht!"

While Irena had promised not a drop of beet soup would sully the feast, Elliott laughed and waved his hands. "I'll have a bowl!" He took a teaspoon but skimmed only from the dollop of sour cream. Still, he gagged.

A lawsuit was brought against the owners of the warehouse that had been doing the illegal business that cost Elliott his leg and the other agent his life. It settled for nearly a million dollars, a portion of which Irena and Elliott set aside for a scholarship fund at Isadore Goldstein. It was in Irena's father's and Elliott's mother's names.

Aaron continued to play chess with Mr. Baker on afternoons he wasn't working at the McDonalds near the old pharmacy. Irena could not understand where the money from Aaron's wages went each week, and at first, she worried drugs might be involved. The last day they played chess, Aaron asked his mom and dad to watch. At the end of the afternoon, the chess pieces put away, Aaron dug around in his backpack and pulled free a gift-wrapped box, chess pieces ornamenting the paper.

"Mr. Baker. I want you to have this, sir."

It was a brand-new Staunton Grand Master set.

Aaron left the next morning for the University of Geneva. He had been accepted to study medicine.

OTHER TITLES BY WILLIAM S. GOULD, MD

AT YONAH MOUNTAIN

Brand new Second Lieutenant J.W. Weathersby is on orders to depart for a combat tour in Viet Nam. At a West Point wedding, though, he commits a very public faux pas and is thrust as punishment into a class of 160 select young officers who sweat and freeze through months of brutal training at the United States Army Ranger School.

J.W. joins an African American PhD candidate and a Rose Bud Sioux Harvard graduate, the three pushed together to trudge the mountains, forests, and deserts as Ranger buddies. As half the class is weeded out, they share their disparate lives and dreams. J.W. struggles to be cut from the program, and at the same time fights desperately to remain.

At Yonah Mountain is a coming-of-age adventure, an examination of race relations in the military, and an authentic tale of Army Ranger training.

CAPTAIN IRON MUSTACHE

Captain Iron Mustache takes place in 1968 and 1969. United States Army lieutenant, J.W. Weathersby, just out of Ranger School, volunteers for duty in Viet Nam. It is not long before he changes from naïve youngster to hardened soldier.

Something about rural Viet Nam, though, captivates him, and he convinces his commanding officer to allow him to live as the sole American in a remote rice-farming hamlet. His mission is to win the hearts and the minds of the peasants. J.W. forms a deep friendship with the village chief, and falls in love with the schoolteacher, Miss Lin.

During a mid-night battle, Miss Lin is arrested and tortured as a communist agent. At the same time, the chief is critically wounded, and disappears after being flown out of the village by an American medevac helicopter.

J.W. and the chief's wife spend the last month of his tour driving the deadly roads of Viet Nam searching hospital after hospital for the man.

Nearly half a century later, J.W. and his wife return to Viet Nam in a surreal effort to find the chief. He also wants to see Miss Lin, but the Vietnamese government is suspicious of his motives, and the days of his sojourn are fraught with struggle and frustration until a simple act of kindness changes his life.

IN BLACK GRANITE

In Black Granite is set in the decade after J.W. Weathersby returns from the war in Viet Nam. He eventually accepts the assessment of family, friends, and medical school deans that he will never become a doctor. He drifts without focus until the miracle of his first child's birth rekindles the craving to study medicine.

This is a narrative of his dogged struggle to beat the overwhelming odds against a man in his mid-thirties gaining admission to an American college of medicine. In Black Granite scrutinizes the ruthless battle for places in medical school, and how the psyches of the chosen are sieved as they are herded through the decade as students and residents. The strain of endless days and nights away from family, of sleepless months, and of pervasive arrogance, distort the souls of even the strongest. Some find the path more treacherous than surviving a war.

C.O.L.A.

The day his father died, Dr. Solomon Forte promised his mother he would honor the man's memory by dedicating his years as a doctor to the treatment of injured workers. It seemed so clear a decision—his patients would be like his dad, stoic, honest, working-class stiffs who sought nothing more from a doctor than an arm around the shoulder, a word of reassurance, and an ally in dealing with the state industrial insurance system.

His life at the Whitaker Hospital and Medical Center is, though, the antithesis of his dream. He can't tell which of the roadblocks is most daunting: that posed by his medical colleagues, the threats of S.M.A.C., the State Medical Abuse Commission, the bureaucracy at C.O.L.A., the state's Commission on Labor Affairs, or the duplicitous patients, some of whom spend every waking moment trying to dupe him out of drugs and government benefits.

Occasionally, a case is obvious—the worker really was devastated by an industrial accident. It seems to Sol, though, that those are the very patients C.O.L.A. torments. On the other hand, claimants skilled at ripping off the Commission run free for decades. C.O.L.A. also examines the specter of serious medical errors, and how they are so much easier to make on patients whose care is mired in the aggravation of government-sponsored insurance plans.

Questions are also raised about the state-appointed morality commissions that determine which doctors relinquish their licenses for treating pain.

Finally, it is a disturbing look behind the scenes of a modern, multi-specialty medical clinic.

A HEART WIND FROM THE DESERT

Dr. Solomon Forte has lost everything. There is little left but to offer himself to the wretched in war-torn Sudan. Arriving in the desert, heart brimming with hope, it does not take long to recognize that the social and political beliefs that have spawned the war and famine are the very forces that prevent him from carrying out his dream of caring for the dispossessed.

At first, despite the warnings of the tiny European medical team left at the refugee camp in Darfur Province, he fights back with typical, strident, American resolve to save the entire population of refugees. The obstacles of life in Central African, however, soon draw the spirit from him, and he turns his efforts to preserving the lives of his Western companions.

He falls deeply for a gorgeous, but outwardly hardened, British nurse. When she disappears from camp, he spends what strength is left searching for her.

A Heart Wind from the Desert examines the need in all of us to accomplish something meaningful in the tiny fragment of time we are allotted, and the impossible hurdles faced when trying to change the way people have thought and behaved for the millennia.

It is a tale of beautiful, warm children, but also of the stark life in the sub-Saharan Sahel.

RAPHAEL'S BLANKET

Raphael Blumenkopf is born clandestinely at the Bergen Belsen Nazi death camp on the 14th of April, 1945. His birth is an unprecedented miracle, as is the liberation of the camp by British forces that very afternoon. He has only his mother and a few surviving villagers from their home in Checzonovska, Poland. While the majority of the refugees leave Central Europe for Israel and the West, his band travels across Russia to China. A relative has promised jobs in Shang Hai's old Jewish settlement.

The journey is fraught with threats from starving Russians, barbaric border guards, and destitute Chinese peasants. Just as the lives of the immigrants begin to normalize in China, the victory of Mao Zedong's communist army forces them to flee, this time to Hanoi.

Five years later, the communist movement in North Viet Nam topples the French government, and the Jews run again. They settle in Saigon until the unrest there compels them to emigrate to America. Raphael's years in the U.S. are colored indelibly by the poison that follows him from the Holocaust, and he formulates a plan to extract revenge from a federal judge with ties to the Nazis.

Who could have envisaged the price he'd pay?

LINCOLN FRIDAY

Lincoln Friday is born into nothing, an obscure, dirt farmer's son, destined to live dominated by the jagged edges of two wars. His early years are an endless series of losses, yet he struggles back after each blow, and slowly, a strongbox of dreams emerges from the fog of his hopelessness.

The harshest test of Lincoln's life, though, comes when the effects of his exposure to Agent Orange devastate both his and his daughter's lives. While the Fridays fight back passionately, the courts, Congress, and the VA turn their backs on them.

In the end, his deeds were neither profound nor dazzling, but he left his mark on disparate people in disparate lands. The world he touched chafed less for his quiet dignity.

SABRINA'S SUIT

Sabrina Friday, a gorgeous, young Doctor of Psychology, was born with a spinal defect as a result of her father, Lincoln Friday's exposure to Agent Orange in Viet Nam. Nonetheless, she leads a perfectly normal life until she becomes pregnant, and her care is botched. The complications change her life forever.

She and her husband finally bring suit against the doctor and hospital responsible for her tragedy. This is the narrative of that medical practice lawsuit, an anatomy of a case that lays forth the ends to which doctors and hospitals go to sidestep responsibility for shoddy care.

Made in the USA
Monee, IL
04 November 2026

67379930R00233